4th edition

immunology

The National Medical Series for Independent Study

4th edition
immunology

Richard M. Hyde, PhD

Department of Microbiology and Immunology
University of Oklahoma Health Sciences Center
Oklahoma City, Oklahoma

LIPPINCOTT WILLIAMS & WILKINS
A **Wolters Kluwer** Company
Philadelphia • Baltimore • New York • London
Buenos Aires • Hong Kong • Sydney • Tokyo

Editor: Elizabeth A. Nieginski
Editorial Director: Julie P. Martinez
Development Editors: Emilie Linkins, Donna Siegfried, and Lisa Bolger
Marketing Manager: Aimee Sirmon
Managing Editor: Marette Magargle-Smith

Copyright © 2000 Lippincott Williams & Wilkins

351 West Camden Street
Baltimore, Maryland 21201-2436 USA

530 Walnut Street
Philadelphia, Pennsylvania 19106 USA

The publisher is not responsible (as a matter of product liability, negligence, or otherwise) for any injury resulting from any material contained herein. This publication contains information relating to general principles of medical care which should not be construed as specific instructions for individual patients. Manufacturers' product information and package inserts should be reviewed for current information, including contraindications, dosages, and precautions.

Printed in the United States of America

Library of Congress Cataloging-in-Publication Data

Immunology / editor, Richard M. Hyde.-- 4th ed.
     p. ; cm. -- (The national medical series for independent study)
    Rev. ed. of: Immunology / Richard M. Hyde. 3rd. ed. c1995.
    Includes bibliographical references and index.
    ISBN 0-683-30662-6
    1. Immunology—Outlines, syllabi, etc.   2. Immunology—Examinations, questions, etc.
  I. Hyde, Richard M.   II. Series.
    [DNLM: 1. Immunity—Case Report.   2. Immunity—Examination Questions.   3. Immunity—
  Outlines.   4. Immune System—Case Report.   5. Immune System—Examination Questions.
  6. Immune System—Outlines.   7. Immunologic Deseases—Case Report.   8. Immunologic
  Diseases—Examination Questions.   9. Immunologic Diseases—Outlines. QW 18.2 I33 2000]
  QR182.55 .H94 2000
  616.07'9'076—dc21

                                                                          00-040554

The publishers have made every effort to trace the copyright holders for borrowed material. If they have inadvertently overlooked any, they will be pleased to make the necessary arrangements at the first opportunity.

To purchase additional copies of this book call our customer service department at **(800) 638-3030** or fax orders to **(301) 824-7390.** International customers should call **(301) 714-2324.**

                                                                00 01 02
                                                    1 2 3 4 5 6 7 8 9 10

Contents

Preface

This text, since its first edition nearly 15 years ago, has served as a useful syllabus to accompany Immunology courses and as a review for USMLE Step 1 preparation. This fourth edition has been modified considerably, both in light of new developments in this rapidly moving field and with valued feedback from students and colleagues. Several chapters have been combined to achieve greater integration and coordination. The chapters on transplantation and on the immune response and regulation have been revised to update information on the cytokines and membrane receptors that are pivotal in these events.

To help students apply what they have learned to clinical situations, case studies have been added as a separate section at the end of the book. Many new clinical study questions have been added and all questions, answers, and explanations have been carefully updated and provided in both print and electronic format to be used in preparation for the USMLE Step 1.

The text first presents a review of native immunity, immunogenicity, the mechanisms and products of immune responses, and practical considerations of immunization and the laboratory procedures employed in the diagnosis of disease. The remaining chapters are concerned with defects in native and acquired immunities, with diseases in which the immune system has been inappropriately activated or is autoreactive, and with transplantation and tumor immunology.

This book provides concise coverage of the fundamentals of immunology in a readily understandable manner. The material is presented in outline format, with key points emphasized in boldface. Complex material is presented in figures and tables to give the student useful summaries. Clinical relevance is stressed, both in the text and in the study questions and explanations. Because the vignettes and clinical cases may contain data that students have not yet encountered in their education, a table of laboratory values has been added as an appendix to assist interpretation of these data.

Acknowledgments

I would like to express my appreciation to Elizabeth Nieginski, Acquisitions Editor; Julie Martinez, Editorial Director of Review Books; to Emilie Linkins, Development Editor, for her guidance and support during the preparation of this text, and to Darrin Kiessling, Managing Editor. Appreciation is also extended to Donna Siegfried and Lisa Bolger for manuscript editing.

Many colleagues have contributed to the preparation of this book. Dr. D. Rex Billington served as the catalyst for the preparation of the original manuscript; he contributed innumerable ideas on organization and format and was invaluable in our efforts to evaluate the teaching effectiveness of the text. Valuable assistance in content revision was obtained from my dear friend and colleague, Dr. James T. Barrett. Dr. Kiley Prilliman was instrumental in the revision of the transplantation section. My sons Roderick and Scott helped in the editing of the clinical cases and vignettes.

The contributions of my wife Ruth are also acknowledged. Her patience and support were the foundations upon which I was able to complete this text. This book is dedicated to the many students, both past and present, who contributed to its preparation through their penetrating questions, thoughtful comments, and constructive criticisms.

To The Reader

Since 1984, the National Medical Series for Independent Study has been helping medical students meet the challenge of education and clinical training. In today's climate of burgeoning information and complex clinical issues, a medical career is more demanding than ever. Increasingly, medical training must prepare physicians to seek and synthesize necessary information and to apply that information successfully.

The National Medical Series is designed to provide a logical framework for organizing, learning, reviewing, and applying the conceptual and factual information covered in basic and clinical sciences. Each book includes a comprehensive outline of the essential content of a discipline, with up to 500 study questions. The combination of an outlined text and tools for self-evaluation allows easy retrieval of salient information.

All study questions are accompanied by the correct answer, a paragraph-length explanation, and specific reference to the text where the topic is discussed. Study questions that follow each chapter use the current United States Licensing Examination (USMLE) format to reinforce the chapter content. Study questions appearing at the end of the text in the Comprehensive Exam vary in format depending on the book. Wherever possible, Comprehensive Exam questions are presented as clinical cases or scenarios intended to simulate real-life application of medical knowledge. The goal of this exam is to challenge the student to draw from information presented throughout the book.

Books in the National Medical Series are constantly being updated and revised. The authors and editors devote considerable time and effort to ensure that the information required by all medical school curricula is included. Strict editorial attention is given to accuracy, organization, and consistency. Each book is actively reviewed by students currently attending medical school and having recently taken the USMLE, and medical student advisors drawn from schools throughout the United States. These reviews are carefully considered in the editorial development of each title. In this regard, the staff at Lippincott Williams & Wilkins welcomes all comments and suggestions.

Chapter 1

Introduction to Immunity and the Nonspecific Immune System

> ### *Vignette*
>
> A fussy, 18-month-old boy presents with labored breathing, a cough producing rusty sputum, and a fever of 38.4°C. He appears small for his age. His right tympanic membrane is inflamed, and he has rales in his left lower lobe. His mother reports that the child was normal until approximately 6 months of age, at which time he began to experience respiratory problems and repeated sinopulmonary infections.
>
> 1. Is there any clinical significance to the size of the patient?
> 2. Does the history of recurrent infections suggest anything of importance?
> 3. Why did the child begin to have infections at 6 months of age?

I. **IMMUNITY (RESISTANCE) is the sum of all naturally occurring defense mechanisms that protect humans from infectious disease.** There are 2 types of resistance mechanisms: nonspecific (innate) and specific (acquired). Examples of each are presented in Table 1-1. Impairment of these mechanisms increases an individual's susceptibility to recurrent infections often caused by "opportunistic" organisms (i.e., organisms not ordinarily considered pathogenic which take the "opportunity" to cause disease when host defenses are diminished).

A. Nonspecific immunity is innate.

1. The **physiologic mechanisms** of nonspecific immunity exist throughout the animal kingdom as inherent, or innate, qualities of the species. They are **present as normal body components** and are **not induced** by exposure to infectious agents, although their numbers may increase in response to infection (e.g., increased white blood cell numbers during the acute phase of many diseases). These mechanisms do not exhibit specificity— that is, they do not depend on specific recognition of a foreign material. Instead, a **single defense barrier affords protection against many different potential pathogens.** The components of the nonspecific immune system are discussed in sections II–V of this chapter.

2. The **complement system** is a series of serum proteins that interact sequentially with one another to augment resistance. Once activated, the components of the complement system work to rid the body of invading microbes by enhancing inflammation and phagocytosis. The protective function of this system of normally occurring plasma proteins is discussed in detail in Chapter 4.

B. Specific immunity is developed as a result of exposure to a variety of agents capable of inducing an immune response (immunogens), such as vaccines, microbes that colonize the body, and macromolecules in the diet.

1. **The specific immunologic response has two components and three essential characteristics.**
   a. **Components**
      (1) **Primary immune response.** Initial exposure to a particular infectious agent, or im-

TABLE 1-1. Resistance Mechanisms

Types of Resistance	Examples
Nonspecific (innate)	Skin and mucous membranes Phagocytic cells Enzymes in secretions Interferon
Specific (acquired)	
Naturally acquired	Placental transfer of antibody (passive) Recovery from disease (active)
Artificially acquired	Administration of antitoxin (passive) Vaccination (active)

munogen, is followed by an **induction phase,** during which precommitted **lymphocytes** proliferate and mature into antibody-secreting **plasma cells** (in the case of humoral immune responses; see I B 3 a) or specifically reactive **T cells** that secrete various mediators (lymphokines) on subsequent contact with that agent (in the case of cell-mediated immune responses; see I B 3 b).

    (2) Secondary (anamnestic) immune response. On further contact with that same immunogen, increased resistance develops through the abundant production of specific antibodies or sensitized lymphocytes.

  b. Characteristics
    (1) The ability to **distinguish self from foreignness** marks the specific immune response.
    (2) Specificity. This characteristic is the selectivity shown by antibodies and lymphocytes of the specific immune system in reacting only with matching **(homologous)** immunogens.
    (3) Immunologic memory. This characteristic allows the immune system to remember homologous immunogens and respond rapidly to them on subsequent exposure.

2. Specific immunity may be acquired by natural or artificial processes (see Table 1-1).

3. Specific immune responses are mediated by two interrelated and interdependent mechanisms. As immunologic barriers to infection, humoral and cell-mediated responses usually work together to destroy pathogenic microorganisms or neutralize their toxic products.

  a. Humoral immunity primarily involves bone marrow-derived (B) lymphocytes, or **B cells. Immunoglobulins,** as proteins in the plasma fraction of the blood, comprise the humoral (i.e., soluble) component of the specific immune system.
    (1) The B cell expresses specific immunoglobulin on its surface. When this surface immunoglobulin (sIgM) interacts with its homologous antigen, the B cell is triggered to proliferate and differentiate into **plasma cells.**
    (2) The plasma cells excrete vast quantities of immunoglobulin that is specific for the same antigen that originally triggered the B cell.

  b. Cell-mediated (cellular) immunity primarily involves thymus-derived (T) lymphocytes, or **T cells.** The T cell expresses on its surface a receptor molecule that is structurally similar to an immunoglobulin and is similarly specific for its particular homologous immunogen, but is not secreted from the cell.
    (1) When the T-cell receptor contacts its homologous immunogen, proliferation and differentiation of the T cell is stimulated. The end product of this developmental process is a variety of **T-cell subsets** with different functions (see Chapter 5 III B 3).
    (2) These T cells, which reside in the peripheral blood and lymphoid tissues, com-

prise the cellular (i.e., T-cell-mediated) component of the specific immune system. Interaction of these specifically sensitized lymphocytes with their homologous ligand (antigen) triggers the release of a variety of lymphokines.

C. **Acquired immunities are not always protective.** The immune response may be inappropriate, resulting in allergies (e.g., hay fever), or it may be directed against one of the body's own constituents, resulting in an autoimmune disease (e.g., thyroiditis). Thus, humans exist in an immunologic thunderstorm; some of the lightning bolts are beneficial, while others are not (Figure 1-1).

II. **MECHANICAL, CHEMICAL, AND PHYSIOLOGIC FACTORS** contribute to nonspecific immunity.

A. **Mechanical barriers to infection** contribute to innate immunity by inhibiting the attachment and penetration of infectious agents (Table 1-2).

1. **Intact skin** and mucus membranes are the first line of defense against infection. Consisting of the keratinized outer layer of dead cells and the successive layers of epidermis, undamaged skin is virtually impenetrable to all but a few organisms. A contiguous mucosal epithelium is also virtually impenetrable to microbes.

2. **Mucus** coats the epithelial cells of the mucosa. Bacteria and other particles are trapped in the viscous mucus and are removed by other mechanisms. For example:
    a. **Beating of cilia of epithelial cells in the respiratory tract** removes contaminating microorganisms that become trapped in the mucus. This mechanism can be damaged by air pollutants, smoking, and alcoholism, all of which may predispose an individual to opportunistic respiratory tract infections.
    b. **Coughing and sneezing** dislodge and help to expel the mucous blanket.

3. **Shedding of cells that carry microbes** provides a mechanical cleansing action.

4. **The flushing action of saliva, tears, perspiration, urine,** and **other body fluids** assist in washing microbes from the body.

5. **Vomiting, peristalsis, diarrhea,** and **other processes** also eliminate pathogenic organisms. These functions, however, also may act as vehicles for spreading disease.

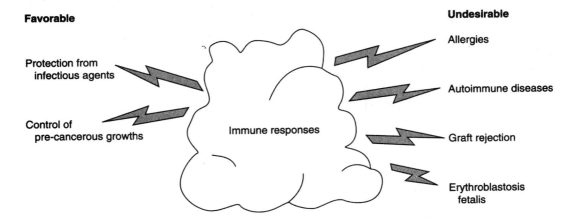

FIGURE 1-1. The acquired immune response (i.e., specific immunity) has both good and bad consequences, some of which are shown here. Natural, nonspecific resistance (i.e., innate immunity) is the foundation on which the adaptive responses have an effect.

TABLE 1-2. Examples of Nonspecific Defense Mechanisms

Site*	Protective Products
Skin	Fatty acid secretions
Oral cavity	Enzymes and antibodies in saliva
Respiratory system	Turbinations and hairs in nasal passage, which help trap microbes
	Enzymes and antibodies
Gastrointestinal system	Low pH of stomach
	Enzymes and antibodies in secretions
Eyes	Lysozyme
Genitourinary system	Low pH

*All of these body sites are also protected by their normal flora, which compete with pathogens for adhesion sites and nutrients.

B. **Chemical barriers to infection.** Numerous substances found in body secretions provide a natural defense against microorganisms that invade the body (Table 1-3). Secreted antibodies and the acid pH in most physiologic secretions prevents colonization by microorganisms.

C. **Physiologic factors contribute to innate immunity.**

    1. The inflammatory process is very important in protecting the body from foreign invaders. As a result of inflammation, body fluids and phagocytic cells are brought into a site of injury. This subject is covered in more detail in Chapter 4.

    2. Body temperature. Some organisms do not infect humans because the organisms grow poorly at 37°C.

    3. Oxygen tension, which is high in the upper lobes of the lungs, favors the growth of obligate aerobes such as the tuberculosis organisms.

    4. Hormonal balance. An increase in corticosteroids decreases the inflammatory response and lowers resistance to infection. Thus, people receiving corticosteroids to control autoimmune disease or graft rejection have a heightened susceptibility to infectious agents.

    5. Age. People who are very young (age 3 years or younger) or very old (age 75 years or older) are much more susceptible to infection because their immune responsiveness is suboptimal.

III. **PHAGOCYTOSIS** contributes to nonspecific immunity.

A. **Definition.** Phagocytosis is the process by which particulate substances, such as bacteria, are ingested by a cell and destroyed. Phagocytosis is one form of endocytosis (the uptake by a cell of material from the environment by invagination of its plasma membrane). The other form, pinocytosis, is the internalization of fluids and solutes. Phagocytosis requires:

    1. Energy generated through glucose metabolism

    2. Synthesis of additional cell membrane

    3. An active cytoplasmic contractile protein system

B. **Types of phagocytic cells.** Although neutrophils, monocytes, and macrophages are not the only cells that phagocytize, they are the most important.

    1. Neutrophils (polymorphonuclear leukocytes, PMNs) are granulocytes that circulate in the blood and migrate quickly in response to local invasion by microorganisms.

TABLE 1-3. Biologic Activities of Secretory Products Important in Nonspecific Immunity

Product	Mechanism of Action
Fatty acids	Denatures proteins* of the cell membrane
Saliva	Contains enzymes that damage the microbial cell wall and membrane and cause leakage of cytoplasm; also contains antibodies and complement proteins that opsonize microbes, and lyse cells
Tears	Contain lysozyme, which lyses bacteria by destroying the peptidoglycan layer of the bacterial cell wall
Lactoferrin and transferrin	Bind iron, interfering with microbial acquisition of this essential metabolite
HCl	Denatures proteins
Bile acids	Interfere with vital functions of the cell membrane
Trypsin	Hydrolyzes proteins of cell membrane and wall
Spermine	A pH-dependent polyamine found in sperm, seminal fluid and other tissues; inhibits growth of gram-positive bacteria

*Bacterial cell membranes contain essential transport proteins plus oxidative and biosynthetic enzymes.

    2. Monocytes also circulate in the blood, but in much lower numbers than neutrophils. They migrate to the tissues, where they differentiate into **macrophages,** which reside in all body tissues. For example:
      a. Kupffer cells are macrophages in the liver.
      b. Histiocytes are macrophages in connective tissue.

C. Movements of phagocytic cells

    1. Ameboid movement. Phagocytic cells migrate in and out of blood vessels and throughout the tissues. The process of cellular emigration from capillaries is called **diapedesis.**

    2. Chemotaxis. Phagocytes move toward other cells or organisms by cytoplasmic streaming in response to chemical agents called **chemotaxins** (Table 1-4). Two bacterial constituents are of particular importance.
      a. The **lipopolysaccharide endotoxin found in the outer membrane of gram-negative bacteria** activates the complement cascade (by the alternative pathway), which produces the potent chemotaxin **C5a.**
      b. Bacteria initiate messenger RNA (mRNA) translation with **N-formylmethionine** (eukaryotic cells do not). Phagocytic cells have a receptor that reacts with peptides blocked at the N-terminus with this amino acid, causing the cell to move toward the source of the signal.

D. Ingestion and vacuole formation (Figure 1-2)

    1. When a phagocyte makes contact with a particle, it engulfs the particle, surrounding it with part of its cell membrane.

    2. Opsonins in plasma and tissue fluids enhance this process (see III H).

    3. Once the phagocyte engulfs the particle, the membrane enclosing the particle compresses and moves into the cytoplasm of the cell, forming a phagocytic vacuole, or **phagosome.**

    4. Lysosomes, which are membrane-bound bags of enzymes, fuse with the phagosome to form a **phagolysosome.**

TABLE 1-4. Factors Chemotactic for Neutrophils

Chemotaxin	Source	Comment
fMet-Leu-Phe	Bacteria	Also chemotactic for eosinophils and macrophages
Endotoxin	Bacteria	Activates the alternative complement pathway to produce C5a
C5a, Ba	Complement	Causes degranulation of neutrophils; also attracts eosinophils and macrophages
Leukotriene B_4	Arachidonic acid	Products of the lipoxygenase pathway; also attracts macrophages and eosinophils
Fibrinopeptides	Fibrinogen	Generated via fibrinolytic pathways
Histamine	Mast cells	Chemokinetics; also increases capillary permeability
Platelet-activating factor	Mast cells, neutrophils	Aggregates platelets and causes release of serotonin and histamine
Eosinophil chemotactic factor	Mast cells	Peptide released on degranulation
Interleukin-8	Macrophage	Microphage derived cytokine that induces cell immigration into an area of inflammation

Ba = an activated split product of factor B; *C5a* = activated fifth component of complement; *fMet* = formyl-methionine; *Leu* = leucine; *Phe* = phenylalanine.

E. **Intracellular destruction.** Inside the phagolysosome, the engulfed material is digested by enzymes contained in lysosomal granules. The contents of the lysosomal granules are important in breaking down ingested material and in killing microorganisms.

1. **Oxygen-independent killing mechanisms are the result of granule contents. Two types of lysosomal granules exist in neutrophils.**
    a. **Primary granules** contain many hydrolytic enzymes, myeloperoxidase, lysozyme, and arginine-rich basic (i.e., cationic) proteins.
    b. **Secondary (specific) granules** contain alkaline phosphatase, lactoferrin, and lysozyme.
    c. The lysosomal granules of macrophages are not subdivided in this way, although they contain a similar array of enzymes and antimicrobial products.

2. **The granule contents destroy foreign particles primarily by enzymatic means.**
    a. **Hydrolytic enzymes** include cathepsin, glycosidase, phosphatase, phospholipase, and lysozyme (Table 1-5). These enzymes are able to digest cell wall components of some bacteria. Some enzymes also may act on viral protein coats or envelope membranes.
    b. **Defensins** are cationic proteins—not enzymes but basic peptides containing large amounts of arginine in polypeptide form—that kill microbes by interacting with the microbial cell membrane to form channels through which essential metabolites escape.
    c. **Nitric oxide synthase** activity is stimulated in phagocytic cells by the synergistic action of interferon-γ (IFN-γ) and tumor necrosis factor (TNF). The enzyme combines oxygen with the guanidino nitrogen of L-arginine to yield nitric oxide, which is toxic for parasites, fungi, tumor cells, and some bacteria.

3. **Oxygen-dependent intracellular killing** is a by-product of the respiratory burst that accompanies phagocytosis and produces several other microbicidal oxygen metabolites.
    a. **Events in the respiratory burst are as follows.**
        (1) **Oxygen consumption** increases.

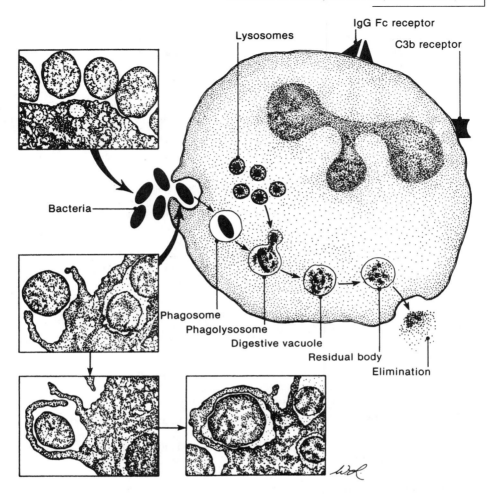

FIGURE 1-2. The process of phagocytosis. The electron microscopic views (*insets*) demonstrate the phagocytosis of a mycoplasma cell by a neutrophil. *IgG Fc receptor* = receptor for the Fc segment of immunoglobulin G; *C3b receptor* = receptor for complement component C3b.

TABLE 1-5. Lysosomal Enzymes

Enzyme	Substrate
Aryl sulfatase	Sulfate esters [e.g., the leukotriene slow-reacting substances of anaphylaxis (SRS-A)]
Cathepsin	Proteoglycans (e.g., collagen)
Cholesteryl esterase	Lipoproteins
Glycosidase	Carbohydrates
Lysozyme	Peptidoglycan
Phosphatase	Phosphate esters
Phospholipase	Lipoproteins, phospholipids

    (2) **Hexose monophosphate shunt (HMPS) activity** is stimulated.

    (3) **Hydrogen peroxide (H_2O_2) production** increases. H_2O_2 is a potent oxidizing agent that kills microbes by denaturing essential enzymes and transport protein in the cytoplasmic membrane.

    (4) **Superoxide anion is produced.** Superoxide anion is molecular oxygen that has picked up an extra electron.

      (a) Superoxide anion is extremely toxic to bacteria and tissue, but it is very unstable. It is quickly converted to H_2O_2 by superoxide dismutase. The H_2O_2 is broken down by catalase.

      (b) A defect in the cytochrome b system exists in the neutrophils of people suffering from chronic granulomatous disease (CGD) leading to reduced formation of superoxide anion and eventually of H_2O_2.

    (5) **Singlet oxygen is produced.** In singlet oxygen one of the electrons has moved to an orbit of higher energy.

    (6) **Hydroxyl radicals are produced.** Hydroxyl radicals are highly unstable oxidizing agents that react with most organic molecules they encounter.

    (7) **Myeloperoxidase,** in the presence of toxic oxygen metabolites (e.g., H_2O_2), catalyzes toxic peroxidation of a variety of surface molecules on microorganisms.

    (8) **Hypochlorite,** the product of the myeloperoxidase enzyme, is more antimicrobial than each of its three components [i.e., myeloperoxidase, H_2O_2, and halide (e.g., chloride ion)] alone.

4. Exocytosis. Secondary granules release their contents into the phagosome first, usually before the vacuole has completely pinched off. The contents of the secondary granules are partially expelled into the interstitial space; this reverse endocytosis is called exocytosis, or regurgitation.

5. Inflammation and tissue destruction. When exocytosis is accelerated and primary granule contents are also released into the extracellular space, inflammation and tissue destruction can occur, as is the case in immune complex diseases such as serum sickness.

6. Other mechanisms of phagocyte degranulation that can lead to tissue damage include:
  a. Neutrophil cell death
  b. Perforation of the cell membrane by ingested crystalline substances, such as monosodium urate in patients with gout

F. **Secreted products.** In addition to destroying foreign particles intracellularly, phagocytic cells secrete a wide variety of biologically active compounds (Table 1-6). The macrophage is the most active cell in this process and releases the following major secretory products:

1. Cell differentiation stimulants

2. Cytotoxic factors

3. Hydrolytic enzymes

4. Endogenous pyrogen

5. Complement components

6. IFN-α

7. Various plasma proteins and coagulation factors

8. Oxygen metabolites

9. Arachidonic acid metabolites

G. **Tests for measuring phagocytic function** are described in Chapter 6 IV A.

H. **Receptor molecules on phagocytic cells** (Table 1-7). Several biologically important receptor molecules exist on phagocytes. Some interact with lymphokines and cause activation of the cell to enhanced phagocytic activity; others increase the adherence of the cell to surfaces of other cells in the body.

TABLE 1-6. Secreted Products of Macrophages

Products	Examples
Enzymes	
Proteinases	Collagenase
Hydrolases	Lysozyme
Plasma proteins	Fibronectin
Coagulation factors	Tissue thromboplastin
Complement components	C1, C2, C3, C4, C5
Oxygen metabolites	Hydrogen peroxide
	Superoxide anion
	Nitric oxide
Arachidonic acid metabolites	Prostaglandin E_2
	Leukotrienes
Nucleotide metabolites	Cyclic adenosine monophosphate (cAMP)
Cell function regulators*	Interleukin-1
	Interferon

*Promoters of cell proliferation for T cells, B cells, and endothelial cells; inhibitors of cell proliferation of tumor cells and certain microbes (e.g., *Listeria*).

TABLE 1-7. Intercellular Adhesion Molecules in Phagocytic Cell Membranes

Receptor	Ligand	Function
Integrins*		
CR1	C4b, C3b	Aids target cell ingestion; allows factor I to cleave C3b to C3dg; important in clearing immune complexes from the body
CR3	C3b, ICAM-1	Aids target cell ingestion; important in cell adherence to endothelial surfaces
CR4	C3b, C3dg	Same as CR3
LFA-1	ICAM-1	Important in cell–cell interactions
Fc Receptors		
FcγRI	IgG	High-affinity opsonin
FcγRII	IgG	Moderate affinity
FcγRIII	IgG	Low affinity
FcαR	sIgA	Opsonization

*Integrins are cell-membrane glycoproteins that act as receptors for extracellular matrix proteins such as fibronectin, complement proteins, and some cell-surface glycoproteins. In addition, phagocytic cells have membrane-bound receptors for the crystallizable fragment (Fc) portion of immunoglobulins.

CR = complement receptor; *LFA* = leukocyte function antigen; *ICAM* = intercellular adhesion molecule; *FcR* = receptor for the Fc portion of an immunoglobulin molecule.

1. **Integrins** are surface proteins found on many different cells of the body that play a role in inflammation and in the immune response by promoting cell-to-cell interaction.

2. **Opsonins** are substances that bind to particles and make them more susceptible to phagocytosis. Opsonins found in serum include the following:
   a. **Split products of the complement cascade**
      (1) Complement component **C3b** is the most important complement-derived opsonin; components **iC3b, C4b,** and **C5b** also are active in this process.
      (2) Phagocytic cells possess membrane receptors for these molecules (see Table 1-7 and Figure 1-2). Thus, bacteria and other foreign particles with one of these molecules on their surface will have an enhanced interaction with the phagocyte.
   b. **Antibodies**
      (1) Phagocytic cells have a receptor (see Figure 1-2) for **Fc portion of certain immunoglobulin molecules,** thus enhancing the strength of interaction between the cell and the antibody-coated (i.e., antibody-opsonized) particle that is being engulfed (see Table 1-7).
      (2) The **IgG isotypes** IgG1 and IgG3 are the most active in this process; IgG2, IgG4, and IgA also may be opsonins for phagocytosis, but are less efficient.
   c. **Other factors enhance phagocytosis.**
      (1) **Fibronectin** is a glycoprotein that opsonizes and acts like glue to cause neutrophils and their targets to stick together.
      (2) **Leukotrienes** are derivatives of arachidonic acid; some of the leukotrienes are opsonins. Leukotriene B_4 (LTB_4) is chemotactic as well. Most leukotrienes increase vascular permeability.

IV. HUMORAL FACTORS contribute to nonspecific immunity.

A. **Antibody and complement.** Normal serum can kill and lyse some gram-negative bacteria. This property probably is the result of the combined action of antibody and complement, both of which are present in normal serum. The activity is destroyed by heating at 56°C for 30 minutes, owing to the inactivation of some complement components. The antibody is induced by subclinical infections (caused by normal flora) and by immunogenic dietary components.

1. **Bacteriolysis** begins with the lytic action of antibody-activated complement on the lipopolysaccharide outer layer of the cell wall.
   a. **A gram-negative bacterial cell wall contains two layers:** an outer membrane layer of lipoproteins and lipopolysaccharide and an inner layer of mucopeptide (peptidoglycan).
   b. **The antibody and complement disrupt the lipopolysaccharide layer of the cell wall.** Some complement proteins assume esterase activity, which may be involved in disrupting the integrity of the cell wall.

2. Once the lipopolysaccharide layer is weakened, **lysozyme,** a mucopeptidase present in serum, can enter and destroy the mucopeptide layer.

3. The **membrane attack complex (MAC)** of the complement system also may produce pores in the bacterial cell membrane that cause vital cytoplasmic constituents to be lost, resulting in the death of the microbe.

B. **Nonantibody humoral factors** (Table 1-8)

1. **Chemotactic factors** attract phagocytes; the chemotaxin **C5a** is an extremely important split product of C5 that is generated during complement activation.

2. **Properdin** is involved in complement activation by the alternative pathway, and it is believed to work to stabilize a critical complex on this complement cascade (C3bBb, a C3 convertase).

3. **IFNs** are proteins that are not antiviral themselves but induce an antiviral state in other cells in the area. Production is induced by viral infection or by injections of synthetic polynucleotides.

TABLE 1-8. Nonantibody Antimicrobial Factors of Plasma

Factor	Biologic Activity*
Complement components	
C3a	Anaphylotoxin that releases histamine from mast cells and causes smooth muscle contraction
C4a	Same as C3a, but 100-fold less active
C5a	Same as C3a, but also very active in inducing chemotaxis and degranulation of neutrophils; it also increases production of superoxide by neutrophils
C3b	Opsonization
Fibronectin	Glycoprotein that promotes the adhesion of cells to surfaces; it functions as an opsonin
Interferons	Group of proteins that induce the production of antiviral proteins in susceptible cells
Transferrin	Iron-binding protein which competes with microbes for the particular ion essential for bacterial growth
Lysozyme	Mucopeptidase that hydrolyzes the peptidoglycan cell wall of bacteria; loss of this structure makes the cell susceptible to osmotic lysis
C-reactive protein	Acts as an opsonin by binding to cell wall components of bacteria, especially phosphorylcholine as found in *Streptococcus pneumoniae*; it also can activate complement when thus bound

*Many of these factors are referred to as "acute phase proteins," which increase rapidly in concentration (perhaps as much as 100-fold) during infections. This increase is the result of active synthesis and not of release of preformed molecules. The acute phase reaction is induced by interleukins 1 and 6 as well as tumor necrosis factor.

   a. Type I
     (1) IFN-α is secreted by macrophages and other leukocytes
     (2) IFN-β is secreted by fibroblasts.
   b. Type II—also called immune IFN or IFN-γ—is secreted by T cells after stimulation with the specific antigen to which the lymphocyte has been sensitized.
   c. Protective effects of IFNs
     (1) IFNs react with receptors in the cytoplasmic membrane and activate cellular genes, inducing the cells to produce **antiviral proteins** that interfere with the translation of viral mRNA.
     (2) IFNs block viral translation by two enzyme-mediated processes.
       (a) Protein kinase transfers a phosphate group from adenosine triphosphate (ATP) to an initiation factor required for protein synthesis. This phosphorylation inactivates the initiation factor, and viral protein synthesis is inhibited.
       (b) Oligonucleotide polymerase synthesizes adenine trinucleotide, which activates an endonuclease that specifically cleaves viral mRNA and thus prevents viral protein synthesis.
     (3) Other protective actions of IFNs include:
       (a) Enhancing T-cell activity
       (b) Activating macrophages
       (c) Enhancing the expression of major histocompatibility complex (MHC) molecules on cell membranes
       (d) Increasing the cytotoxic action of natural killer (NK) cells
  4. Lactoperoxidase is found in saliva and milk. Its mechanism of action is similar to that of myeloperoxidase.

V. **LYMPHOCYTIC CELLS contribute to nonspecific immunity.** Certain lymphocytic cells are cytotoxic against a variety of targets in the absence of any previous exposure to the foreign antigen.

A. **Natural killer (NK) cells** are granular lymphocytes that appear to function in immune surveillance, the process that purges the body of precancerous cells.

1. **Source and location**
   a. NK cells are naturally occurring cytotoxic lymphocytes that exist in the body at birth. They are not induced by immunologic insult, although their numbers and activity can be increased by various lymphokines [e.g., interleukin-2 (IL-2)].
   b. NK cells arise from bone marrow precursors but are of a lineage distinct from that of either T or B cells.

2. **Functions**
   a. NK cells are **cytotoxic for tumor cells and virally infected autologous cells.**
   b. They also have been reported to play a role in **resistance to some bacterial, fungal,** and **parasitic infections** and to participate in regulation of the immune response through the secretion of lymphokines such as IL-2.
   c. NK cells are the major lymphocytic cells responsible for **antibody-dependent cellular cytotoxicity (ADCC).** These cells have membrane receptors for the crystallizable fragment (Fc) portion of IgG, and therefore can interact effectively with antibody-coated targets.
   d. NK cells do not possess antigenic specificity and do not acquire immunologic memory after exposure to virus-infected cells or tumor cells.

3. **Mode of action**
   a. NK cells kill their targets by perforating the cell membrane, causing pores to form. The molecules responsible for the pore formation are called **perforins.**
      (1) After intimate cellular contact, perforins are released from granules within the cell. The killer cell then disengages from the target and leaves to find other potential targets.
      (2) The perforins insert into the target cell membrane and polymerize (in the presence of calcium ions), forming polyperforin channels within the cytoplasmic membrane of the target cell.
      (3) Depolarization, abnormal ion flux, and essential metabolite leakage from the cytoplasm are the result.
      (4) The membrane of NK cells contains a protein (called protectin) that binds to perforins and prevents their insertion and polymerization in the NK membrane. Thus, the NK cells are spared.
      (5) Granular enzymes and toxic proteins are also released when the NK cell degranulates. A similar type of cytotoxicity is expressed by cytotoxic T (Table 1-9).
   b. NK cells have a broad target range, and they are **not subject to MHC restriction.** That is, cytotoxicity by NK cells does not require that the NK cell recognize MHC molecules on the target cells.
   c. The cytotoxic activity of NK cells can be significantly enhanced by exposure to IL-2 and the IFNs.

B. **Antibody-dependent cytotoxic cells** can kill target cells without the participation of complement if the target cells are coated with specific antibody. The cells that participate in antibody-dependent cellular toxicity (ADCC) have membrane receptors of the Fc portion of IgG molecules; this serves as an anchor between the cytotoxic cell and its target.

1. **Functions.** ADCC is thought to play a role in **antiviral, antitumor,** and **antigraft immunity.**

2. **Types of cells**
   a. ADCC has been attributed to a unique subset of large granular lymphocytes called **natural killer (NK) cells.**
   b. In addition to NK cells, **macrophages and neutrophils** also participate in ADCC.

TABLE 1-9. Major Cytotoxic Products of Activated Natural Killer Cells (NK)

Product	Effect of Target Cell
Perforins	Polymerize in the cell membrane to form polyperforin channels that allow cytosol out of and toxic molecules into the cell
Serine proteases	Degrade proteins in cell membrane
Nucleases	Degrade NA in cell
TNF	Depresses protein synthesis and causes production of toxic free radicals
FAS ligand (CD95)	Intitiates apoptosis by reacting with Fas protein in target cell membrane; nucleases are activated in cell cytosol and they kill the cell.

NA = nucleic acids; *TNF* = tumor necrosis factor

Vignette Revisited

Much of the information about the immunology of the 18-month-old boy has been presented in the chapter. However, some terms or concepts that go beyond the scope of the chapter or book are discussed briefly here.

1. Patients, particularly children, are often anxious and **"fussy"** when they are ill.
2. The child in this simulation is having difficulty breathing and is spitting up a mucoid, blood-tinged **("rusty")** material.
3. The child is **small for his age** because he has spent a great deal of his young life fighting infections instead of putting on weight and body mass.
4. He has an inflamed eardrum because he has **otitis media,** which often precedes bacterial pneumonia.
5. **Recurrent infections** are a very important clinical clue to immunodeficiency. **Cystic fibrosis** might also be considered in the differential diagnosis for this patient.
6. Finally, the **antibody-mediated immunity conferred from mother to fetus** should be waning by the sixth month of life, making the child more susceptible to infectious agents.

1. A 7-year-old child has hay fever. Each spring he has a great deal of respiratory discomfort; rhinitis is his chief complaint. Examination of his nasal secretions reveals a significant eosinophilia. The eosinophil granular enzyme that degrades slow-reacting substances of anaphylaxis (SRS-A) is

(A) aryl sulfatase
(B) cathepsin
(C) lysozyme
(D) myeloperoxidase
(E) acid phosphatase

2. A characteristic of viral meningoencephalitis is lymphocytic infiltration of the spinal fluid. Which of the following plasma proteins is secreted by these lymphocytes?

(A) Third component of complement (C3)
(B) α_1-antitrypsin
(C) Antibodies
(D) Fibronectin
(E) Coagulation factor IX

3. A major feature of acute bacterial infections is leukocytosis. Neutrophils usually predominate at sites of inflammation. Which of the following chemotaxins is a product of microbial metabolism?

(A) N-formylmethionine
(B) Histamine
(C) Leukotriene B_4
(D) Fibrinopeptide
(E) C5a

4. Natural killer cells are the cells of immune surveillance (i.e., they are the cells that rid the body of pre-cancerous tissues). Which of the following substances is found in the intracytoplasmic granules of these cells?

(A) Myeloperoxidase
(B) Interferon gamma
(C) Lysozyme
(D) C5a
(E) Perforin

5. Bruton's disease is a serious form of immunodeficiency in which the individual is unable to synthesize gamma globulins of all classes. These patients have an increased incidence of infections caused by opportunistic bacteria, and they lack normal opsonizing antibodies to help cleanse the organisms from the body. Non-antibody factors in plasma that act to opsonize microbes and compensate for the lack of specific opsonins include which of the following molecules?

(A) Aryl sulfatase
(B) Fibrinogen
(C) C3b
(D) Lysozyme
(E) Superoxide anion

6. Antimicrobial factors that are products of secretory glands include which of the following molecules?

(A) Aryl sulfatase
(B) Lysosomes
(C) Arachadonic acid
(D) Lactoperoxidase
(E) Interferon (IFN)-γ

7. Some cells that function in innate resistance contain granules, which play a major role in cytotoxicity and the ability of the cell to destroy tumors. Examples of such cells include which of the following?

(A) Basophils
(B) Natural killer (NK) cells
(C) Eosinophils
(D) Mucosal epithelial cells
(E) Plasma cells

8. The immune response is bimodal; B cells secrete antibodies and T cells secrete various cytokines. Which of the following is secreted by T cells from a patient with tuberculosis after the cells have been stimulated with PPD, the purified protein derivative of the tubercle bacillus?

(A) Complement
(B) Properdin
(C) Lysozyme
(D) Interferon (IFN)-α
(E) Interferon (IFN)-γ
(F) Lactoferrin
(G) Lactoperoxidase
(H) Lysozyme

9. Inflammation is one of the major responses of the body to injury. Which of the following is a derivative of arachidonic acid that is involved in the increased diapedesis of neutrophils from the blood into acute inflammatory lesions?

(A) IgG1
(B) Fibronectin
(C) C3a
(D) Lysozyme
(E) Leukotriene B$_4$

ANSWERS AND EXPLANATIONS

1. The answer is A [Table 1-5]. Aryl sulfatase hydrolyzes the leukotrienes C_4, D_4, and E_4—the arachidonic acid metabolites thought to be responsible for many of the symptoms of anaphylaxis. Slow-reacting substance of anaphylaxis (SRS A) contracts smooth muscle but at a slower rate than histamine. In addition, it is not inhibited by antihistamines. The remaining enzymes (lysozyme, myeloperoxidase, and acid phosphatase) are found in the granules of polymorphonuclear neutrophils and are involved in the destruction of phagocytized microbes.

2. The answer is C [I B 1 a (1); Table 1-7]. Antibodies (immunoglobulins) are secreted by B cells and plasma cells. Macrophages are the source of the other plasma proteins listed (C3, α_1 antitrypsin, fibronectin, coagulation factor IX).

3. The answer is A [III C 2 b; Table 1-4]. N-formylmethionine and lipopolysaccharide endotoxin are two bacterial products that are chemotaxins. N-formylmethionine binds to the cell membrane and induces calcium ion flux and activation of the microfilaments, thus facilitating migration. The lipopolysaccharide endotoxin of the outer membrane of gram negative bacteria activates complement by the alternative pathway, thus generating the chemotactic molecules C3a and C5a. Histamine is also chemotactic but is a product of mast cells; C5a is the major chemotaxin of the complement cascade. Peptide split products of fibrin also are chemotactic. Leukotrienes B_4 is a chemotactic product of lipoxygenase breakdown of arachidonic acid which has importance in atopic allergies (e.g., asthma).

4. The answer is E [V A 3 a; Table 1-9]. Perforin is the protein that is released from the granules and polymerizes in the target cell membrane forming polyperforin channels. Cytosolic contents of the cell leak out and toxic molecules such as nucleases and tumor necrosis factor enter the target cell. Myeloperoxidase and lysozyme are not contained in the granules of natural killer (NK) cells, but are found in body secretions and in lysosomal granules of phagocytic cells. Lysozyme is a mucopeptidase that hydrolyzes the bacterial cell wall, rendering the cell susceptible to os-

motic lysis. Interferon gamma, also known as immune interferon, is produced by T cells and induces an antiviral state in neighboring cells by inducing the production of enzymes that block the transcription of viral mRNA. C5a is the chemotactic split product of the fifth component of the complement cascade.

5. The answer is C [III H 2; Table 1-7; Table 1-8.]. C3b is the major opsonizing protein of the complement cascade; phagocytic cells have a membrane receptor for this molecule, as they do for the crystallizable fragment (Fc) portion of immunoglobulin heavy chains. Lysozyme hydrolyzes the cell wall of bacteria; it does not enhance phagocytosis. Superoxide anion is an antibacterial molecule that is generated during glucose metabolism in phagocytic cells. Aryl sulfatase is an enzyme found in the granules of eosinophils that degrades the slow reacting substances of anaphylaxis. Fibrinogen is important in blood clotting; fibronectin is opsonic.

6. The answer is D [IV B 4]. Lactoperoxidase is secreted by the salivary and mammary glands. Aryl sulfatase is an enzyme found in the granules of eosinophils that degrades the leukotriene slow-reacting substance of anaphylaxis (SRS A). Lysosomes contain many microbicidal substances, including lysozyme, which hydrolyzes the sugar backbone of peptidoglycan, an essential component of bacterial cell walls. Arachidonic acid is a product of phospholipase action on the phospholipids in mammalian cell membranes. It is broken down further into vasoactive compounds such as leukotriene C4 by lipoxygenase enzymes activated during anaphylaxis. Interferon gamma, also known as immune interferon, is produced by T cells and induces and anti-viral state in neighboring cells by inducing the production of enzymes that block the transcription of viral mRNA.

7. The answer is B [V A–B; Table 1-9]. The granules in cytotoxic lymphocytes such as natural killer (NK) cells contain perforins, tumor necrosis factor, and hydrolytic enzymes that are cytotoxic to target cells. Plasma cells, which produce antibodies, are a major component of adaptive immunity. They do not contain granules however, and their cytoplasm is loaded with rough endoplasmic reticulum. The granules of eosinophils contain basic proteins that are toxic to helminths. Basophilic granules contain heparin and histamine, the latter being very important in allergies such as asthma. Mucosal epithelium functions as a physical barrier to protect the body. It also contains goblet cells that secrete mucus and other materials that coat the lining of the respiratory tract and protect it from microbes.

8. The answer is E [IV B 3], Interferon (IFN) γ, also known as immune interferon, is secreted by specifically sensitized T lymphocytes when they come into contact with their homologous antigen. Macrophages secrete interferon (INF) α during an inflammatory response. The interferon induces an antiviral state in other nearby cells by inducing the production of proteins that interfere with viral messenger RNA activity. Complement is a group of more than a dozen serum proteins that react with antibody in a cascading manner and are able to disrupt the cell membrane of gram-negative bacteria. Properdin is a serum protein that stabilizes C3 convertase [C3bBb] generated by the alternative pathway of complement activation.

Lysozyme is a mucopeptidase that hydrolyzes the bacterial cell wall, rendering the cell susceptible to osmotic lysis.

9. The answer is E [III H 2 c (2); Table 1-4]. Leukotriene B_4 is produced from arachidonic acid via the lipoxygenase pathway during inflammatory reactions. It is able to increase vascular permeability and activates and attracts (ie., is chemotactic for) neutrophils and eosinophils. Fibronectin is an adhesive glycoprotein that is important in connective tissues where it cross links collagen. One form of fibronectin circulates in plasma and acts as an opsonin; another is a cell surface component that mediates cellular adhesive interactions. C3a is an anaphylatoxin that reacts with a specific receptor in the membrane of mast cells and basophils and causes them to degranulate and release their vasoactive contents. Lysozyme is a mucopeptidase that hydrolyzes the bacterial cell wall, rendering the cell susceptible to osmotic lysis. It is found in secretions and in the granules of phagocytic cells. IgG1 is an immunoglobulin produced by B cells and plasma cells that functions as an opsonizing and complement activating antibody.

Chapter 2

Immunogens and Immunizations

Vignette

Anh, a refugee from Vietnam, received all of her immunizations in that country before immigrating to the United States. These included immunization with the polysaccharide capsule of *Haemophilus influenzae* to prevent meningitis. Upon arrival in the United States it was found that her immunization records had been lost, and she was re-immunized with all her previous vaccines. When an outbreak of *H. influenzae* meningitis developed in the community a few weeks later, her parents thought it best to have all her immunizations boosted. Two months later, at the age of 3½ years, Anh developed meningitis due to *H. influenzae.*

1. Why had these repeated immunizations failed?
2. What is immunologic tolerance and how does it develop?
3. Do infants produce a good response to polysaccharide antigens?
4. What are T-cell dependent and T-cell independent antigens?
5. How could the polysaccharide antigen of H. *influenzae* be converted to a T-cell dependent antigen?

I. **IMMUNOGENICITY** refers to the inherent ability of a substance (an **immunogen**) to induce an immune response. An immune response is characterized by an induction of B lymphocytes to produce immunoglobulins (antibodies) and an activation of T lymphocytes to enter their specific responses leading to the secretion of lymphokines. Antigenicity refers to the capacity of a substance, termed an **antigen,** to induce the immune response and to react with the receptors for antigen produced by B cells (the antibodies) and T cells (antigen receptors on their surface). Immunogenicity and antigenicity are used almost interchangeably in the discussion of the immune response.

A. **The degree of immunogenicity** of a molecule is influenced by several factors.

1. **Foreignness.** An antigen must be foreign or alien to the host with which it makes contact. The greater the phylogenetic distance between the source of the antigen and the animal being immunized, the greater the chance of success in the immunization. Thus, horse serum is more immunogenic in humans than is serum from primates, such as baboons.

2. **Chemical complexity.** The chemical complexity of a molecule contributes significantly to its immunogenicity. Chemical diversity enables the formation of numerous different structures, called **epitopes,** that are the units to which antibodies are directed. The more varied the epitope composition of an antigen, the more likely an individual will respond to one or more of its epitopes.

   a. **Proteins are the most potent immunogens** because proteins are built from 20 or more separate amino acids and thus can include many individually distinct **epitopes.** Conjugates of proteins with other molecules of biologic origin (e.g., glycoproteins) are all good antigens.

   b. **Most polysaccharides are weak antigens** or even nonantigenic. Because polysaccharides often are constructed of only a few monosaccharides, they do not possess sufficient chemical diversity for full immunogenicity.

    c. **Nucleic acids** in their pure form are considered to be **nonimmunogenic.** However, when combined with basic proteins, nucleic acids can act as immunogens.

3. **Antigen size.** The size of a molecule is important in determining its ability to induce an immune response. Usually, the larger the molecule, the better the immunogen, because this provides the opportunity for more molecular complexity (i.e., a more diverse epitope population).

4. **Degradability.** Molecules that are not biodegradable, such as polystyrene particles or asbestos, are nonimmunogenic because they cannot be processed by phagocytic cells of the body.

5. **Route of immunization.** As a general rule, the subcutaneous or intramuscular routes of antigen injection are best for inducing an antibody response. Intravenous injections may thwart or minimize the immune response.

6. **Nature of the host.** Immature animals or those with a limited spectrum of responses to antigens because of their genetic make-up may not respond to certain antigens especially to the weaker antigens such as polysaccharides.

7. **Antigen dose.** It is reasonable to expect that minimal doses of antigen may not engender an immune response, but it is equally true that excessively large or repeated doses of antigen may impair the immune response. This is especially true of polysaccharide antigens.

B. **Antigen nomenclature.** Antigens are given many names according to their origin (such as capsular antigen, blood group antigen, transplantation antigen) or chemical composition. The functional names of antigens as T-cell dependent or T-cell independent antigens and their description as superantigens are perhaps more useful in explaining their role in the immune response.

1. **T-cell dependent and independent antigens.** Although most antigens may rely to some extent on T cell assistance to engender an immune response, antigens having a proteinaceous component are the prototypical **T-cell dependent (TD)** antigens, meaning that the B cell that actually synthesizes the antibody cannot do so effectively in the absence of assistance from the T lymphocytes. This help comes in the form of **cytokines** secreted by the T cell after it comes in contact with antigen. In contrast, polysaccharides and other molecules with a limited number of determinant sites stimulate B cells to make antibodies without the cooperation of T cells and are thus **T-cell independent (TI)** antigens. **TI antigens exist in two forms, TI 1 and TI 2.** TI 1 antigens such as bacterial lipopolysaccharide function like mitogens and activate many B cells (i.e., they are polyclonal B-cell activators), even those that are not committed to make antibody to the TI 1 antigen. TI 2 antigens have multiple repeats of their epitopes and cross link numerous antigen receptors on the B cell surface, thus signalling proliferation of that specific B-cell population. TI antigens can be converted to a T-cell dependent state by coupling them to an existing T-cell dependent antigen. One advantage of this is that booster injections of a T-cell dependent antigen stimulate a pronounced boost in antibody levels, the **anamnestic response,** whereas booster injections of T-cell independent antigen fail to do this. Characteristics of thymus-dependent and independent antigens are summarized in Table 2-1.

2. **Superantigen.** These unique molecules are extremely potent T-cell mitogens that would perhaps be more correctly called **supermitogens.** They can trigger mitosis of CD4+ T cells in the absence of antigen processing (remember that thymus-independent antigens were mitogenic for B cells). Superantigens bind to the variable region of the beta chain of the T-cell receptor and simultaneously bind to the class II MHC molecule outside of its epitope-presenting cleft. This cross-linking is a powerful signal for mitosis. As these molecules react with many different T-cell receptor beta chains, they are able to activate a large population of T cells (up to 20% of all peripheral blood T cells may be activated by a single superantigen). Examples of superantigens include enterotoxins and toxic shock syndrome toxins produced by *Staphylococcus aureus*. These molecules are able to induce the release of large quantities of cytokines such as interleukin-1 and tumor

TABLE 2-1. Thymus-Dependent and Thymus-Independent Antigens

Characteristic	Dependent	Independent TI1	TI2
Chemical nature	Protein	Polysaccharide Lipopolysaccharide (LPS)	Polymeric polysaccharides
Immunoglobulin (Ig) class	All	IgM only	IgM and IgG
Anamnestic response	Yes	No	No
Delayed-type hypersensitivity	Yes	No	No
B-cell mitogen	No	Yes	No

necrosis factor from T cells, which in turn contribute to the local tissue pathology seen in these staphylococcal diseases.

3. **Heterophile antigen.** Sometimes used synonymously with **heterogenetic antigen,** a heterophile antigen is one that is found widely distributed throughout the phylogenetic tree. Such antigens often are the basis for serologic cross reactions, which occur when an antibody to one antigen reacts unexpectedly with a seemingly unrelated antigen when in fact both contain the same shared epitopes.

II. **IMMUNOGENS** and antigens possess unique clusters of chemical groupings that serve as the B- and T-cell stimulating sites in the molecule. These sites, mentioned earlier, are called **epitopes.**

A. An **epitope (also known as an antigenic determinant)** is that portion of an antigen with which antibodies and T-cell receptors react.

1. **Structure**
   a. **Size.** Epitopes consist of four or five amino acids of a protein or an equal-size area of a polysaccharide. These are the sites with which antibodies combine.
   b. **Conformation.** Epitopes may be linear (i.e., continuous within the amino acid sequence of a protein) or conformational (i.e., containing amino acids that are adjacent in the folded structure of the antigen but which are not sequential in the amino acid sequence.) (Figure 2-1).
   c. **Site.** Some antibody-binding sites (i.e., epitopes) are on the antigen's surface (e.g., **topographic epitopes**), whereas others are internal. Internal epitopes are exposed only after the antigen has been partially degraded in vivo by antigen-processing macrophages.

2. **Function**
   a. Epitopes determine the specificity of the antigen molecule. Antigens that share one or more identical or similar epitopes are said to be **cross-reactive antigens.**
   b. All epitopes of an antigen are not equally effective in stimulating an immune response. **Immunodominant epitopes,** those that dominate the antibody response, have been identified at the terminus of the blood group polysaccharide antigens. However, such determinants are not always situated at the end of a molecule.

3. **Valence of an antigen.** Antigens are multivalent, that is, an antigen molecule carries a number of different epitopes. Each antibody molecule reacts with a single epitope; therefore, an antigen initiates the production of numerous antibody molecules, each with its own specificity. The valence of an antigen is **equal to the total number of epitopes the antigen possesses.**

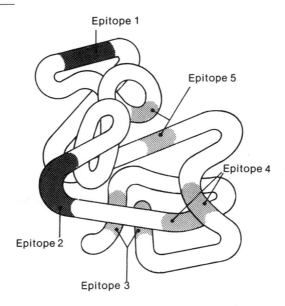

FIGURE 2-1. Model of epitopes on lysozyme. The *shaded areas* are the specific epitopes. They are composed of chain segments that are either linear (epitopes 1 and 2) or conformational (epitopes 3–5). (Adapted from Klein J: *Immunology: The Science of Self–Nonself Discrimination.* New York, Wiley, 1982, p 356.)

4. **Altering antigenicity.** Antigen molecules can be artificially altered, and the antibody with which it is associated also becomes altered. Epitopes can be deleted, added, or changed.

5. **Haptens.** A common method of increasing the number of epitopes is by adding a compound described as a hapten to an existing antigen. Haptens are small, nonimmunogenic molecules that can add a new epitope (i.e., a new specificity) when combined to an existing antigen. The antibody directed against the new epitope will react with the free hapten as well as the hapten—epitope site in the altered antigen.

III. ADJUVANTS. Nonspecific stimulation of the immune response can occur with the use of adjuvants. The mechanisms by which adjuvants exert their biologic effect are multiple.

A. Adjuvants may act as **depots** and **prolong the period of exposure** to the immunogen by releasing small quantities of the antigen into the physiologic milieu of the animal. This is equivalent to series of small booster injections.

B. Some adjuvants may **amplify** the proliferation of **antigen processing cells,** whereas others amplify the proliferation of immunologically reactive cells, the **B and T cells.**

C. The **mechanisms of action** of various immunopotentiating adjuvants are presented in Chapter 5, Table 5–3.

IV. IMMUNIZATION

A. **Types of immunization.** Agents used for immunization can be divided into two categories based on the **type of immunity** they induce.

1. **Active immunization** (immunoprophylaxis) uses vaccines (i.e., killed or attenuated microorganisms or their products) to initiate immunity. Upon active immunization:
   a. The immunized individual's **own cells** contribute to their immunity. The immunization is not complete until these cells are fully activated.
   b. The immunity is **long lasting** and is easily **re-activated** by booster injections of antigen.
   c. This re-activation is relatively free of such dangers as serum sickness (see Chapter 7), which can hamper the usefulness of passive immunization.
   d. **Both B-cell and T-cell based immunity are activated.**
   e. Active immunization is a prophylactic procedure.

2. **Passive immunization** consists of the injection of antibodies from a donor animal into the person to be immunized.
   a. This provides **humoral (antibody-based) immunity** but no T-cell based immunity.
   b. This type of immunity is present immediately after the injection but lasts only as long as the in vivo life span of the antibodies, which is **approximately 3 weeks** for the most protective form of immunoglobulin (IgG).
   c. There is danger of causing anaphylaxis or serum sickness when reactivating passive immunity with antisera from lower animals.
   d. Passive immunization may be either prophylactic or therapeutic but is least successful as a therapy. Depending on the content and purity of these antisera, the preparations may be called antitoxins, immune globulin, or specific immune globulin, if developed against a specific pathogen.

B. **Routes of administration**

1. **Injection** by the intramuscular or subcutaneous routes are the most common for both active and passive immunization. Immunoglobulins are injected intravenously in the treatment of patients with some antibody-mediated immune deficiencies (e.g., Bruton's hypogammaglobulinemia).

2. **Oral administration** is used for immunization with the oral polio vaccine (OPV; Sabin vaccine) because this consists of an attenuated strain of a virus that reproduces in cells of the intestinal tract.

3. **Herd immunity** is illustrated by the oral polio vaccine because the immunized individual sheds virus, which may be spread to others, thereby immunizing them.

4. **Intranasal** immunization stimulates an immune response that mimics the response induced by natural exposure to airborne pathogens and may benefit the secretory immunoglobulin A (sIgA) response.

V. **ACTIVE IMMUNIZATION (IMMUNOPROPHYLAXIS).** Routine immunization for children and adults in the United States differs from recommendations in other countries. In addition, the recommendations for immunocompromised individuals, individuals in certain age groups, pregnant women, and other groups (e.g., day care or health care workers, military personnel, food handlers, travelers) may differ from those listed below.

A. **Bacterial vaccines**

1. **Diphtheria, pertussis, and tetanus (DPT).** This is a **polyvalent** product containing the toxoids of *Corynebacterium diphtheriae* and *Clostridium tetani* plus killed bacteria of *Bordetella pertussis,* which is the causative agent of whooping cough. **Toxoids** are toxins that have been treated to preserve their antigenicity but which have lost their toxicity. The pertussis organism is of Phase I, which is the most virulent form of this bacterium. A newer preparation contains soluble antigens of the pertussis organism, and is referred to as DPaT, Pa meaning acellular pertussis. The major components of the acellular vaccines (there are two formulations) are the pertussis toxoid and the filamentous hemagglu-

tinin (an adhesion organelle). This preparation is less toxic than the whole cell vaccine. Each of these products is available for booster injections, although pertussis boosters are seldom recommended. **Td** is the combination used to boost immunity to tetanus and diphtheria every 10 years after the primary immunization.

2. *Haemophilus influenzae* **type b (Hib)** polysaccharide conjugated to bacterial toxoids or outer membrane proteins (OMP) from the meningococcus is used to prevent meningitis from serotype b of *H. influenzae.* These vaccines do not provide protection against infection by nonencapsulated strains of *H. influenzae.* The purified carbohydrate (polyribitol phosphate) is very poorly immunogenic in children younger than 2 years and acquires immunogenicity only when it is chemically linked to a carrier protein.

3. *Neisseria meningitidis* **vaccine** is used to prevent meningococcemia and meningococcal meningitis in military recruits. The vaccine is composed of the capsular carbohydrates from four meningococcal strains: A, C, Y, and W-135.

4. **Pneumococcal polysaccharide vaccine** is prepared from the polysaccharide capsule of 23 antigenic types of *Streptococcus pneumoniae.* This vaccine is advised for special groups of individuals: those older than 65 years, those with chronic lung conditions, or those who are asplenic. The vaccine protects against 90% of the pneumococcal strains that affect humans.

5. A vaccine against **Lyme disease,** caused by a spirochete acquired from the bites of infected ticks, has recently been approved in the United States. The vaccine is composed of purified outer surface protein A from *Borrelia burgdorferi.*

6. **Bacille Calmette-Guérin (BCG) vaccine** is a live attenuated strain of *Mycobacterium bovis* that is used as a vaccination against human tuberculosis in most parts of the world. BCG is NOT used routinely in the United States because it invalidates the skin test that is used to verify exposure to the tubercle bacillus.

B. **Viral vaccines**

1. **Rubella (German measles) vaccine** contains live attenuated virus of a single antigenic type grown in animal tissue cultures or human diploid cell lines.

2. **Influenza virus vaccine** consists of whole type A and type B influenza viruses or disrupted (split) virus grown in chick embryos and inactivated by formalin or propiolactone. The composition of the vaccine is adjusted annually to account for antigenic shift and drift of the influenza viruses.

3. **Measles vaccine** is a live attenuated virus vaccine of a single antigenic form grown in chick embryos.

4. **Mumps vaccine** is also a live attenuated vaccine of a single antigenic type of the virus recovered from infected chick embryos. MMR is a combination of the measles, mumps, and rubella viruses combined into a single injectable mixture. The combination of antigens from different sources or of multiple antigenic forms of a single agent creates a polyvalent vaccine. The individual component parts do not interfere with the immunogenicity of the other components.

5. **Poliomyelitis vaccine** is available in two forms; each is a polyvalent vaccine of the three antigenic types of the virus.
   a. **Inactivated polio vaccine (IPV; Salk vaccine)** is made from virus grown in tissue culture (e.g., monkey kidney) then inactivated with formalin or ultraviolet light. This vaccine provides immunity to paralytic or systemic disease but not to intestinal infection by the polio virus.
   b. **Oral polio vaccine (OPV; Sabin vaccine)** is made from a virus grown in tissue culture (e.g., monkey kidney, human diploid cells). This live attenuated vaccine provides protection against intestinal infections as well as paralytic disease.

6. **Hepatitis B vaccine** composed of inactivated, alum-adsorbed **hepatitis B surface antigen (HbsAg)** particles purified from the plasma of human hepatitis carriers is no longer

manufactured in the United States but is still available commercially. The **recombinant HbsAg (rHbsAg) vaccine** is produced by a genetically engineered strain of *Saccharomyces cerevisiae* containing a plasmid that carries the gene for the HbsAg antigen.

7. **Varicella vaccine** has been available in the United States since 1995 for the prevention of chicken pox. This is a live attenuated product that, like the MMR vaccine, is usually not given to children until all passively acquired maternal IgG is cleared from the body (approximately 15 months of age).

8. **Hepatitis A vaccine** is a newly available product that consists of inactivated virus. This virus is one of the picornaviruses and is therefore related to the polio virus, whose inactivated vaccine has been very successful.

9. **Rotavirus vaccine** is also newly available and should help to prevent infant death due to diarrhea. This vaccine contains all four of the antigenic types of this virus involved in human disease. This vaccine has been associated with obstructive bowel disease in a small number of recipients, and its continued use in the United States is uncertain at this time.

10. **Rabies vaccine** is available in two forms: killed virus preparations are used in humans, and live attenuated viral agents are used to immunize domestic animals. There are two human vaccines. One is grown in duck embryos and has some encephalitogenic side effects, whereas the other is a human diploid cell-derived virus, which is much safer.

C. **Dangers of active immunization**

1. **Adverse reactions to vaccines** may depend on an **allergy** to a component of the vaccine (e.g., egg proteins found in measles, influenza, and mumps vaccines prepared from viruses grown in chick embryos; antibiotics used in tissue culture–grown agents) or to preservatives in the vaccine.

2. Vaccines containing live but attenuated pathogens should never be administered to **immunocompromised** individuals. This could be a life-threatening mistake because such persons cannot control even the most **attenuated organisms** and clinical disease may result. This is why the current recommendation for polio immunization is two injections with IPV followed by a single OPV exposure.

VI. **PASSIVE IMMUNIZATION (IMMUNOTHERAPY).** Passive immunizations are not given routinely. They are used in specific circumstances, such as: (1) exposure of a patient to an agent that could be particularly dangerous in that individual or (2) as a long-term therapeutic regimen in antibody-deficient individuals. Passive immunization is based on the injection of either antitoxins or antiviral sera (Table 2-2).

A. **Antitoxins** consist of toxin-neutralizing antibodies (**antiserum**) that are specific for a given toxin. These are produced by the immunization of human volunteers, horses, or cows. Antitoxin efficacy is related to the half-life of the antibodies in vivo.

1. **Botulism antitoxin** is a polyvalent antitoxin made against three types of toxin (types A, B, and E) produced by *Clostridium botulinum* (see Table 2-2). Animal-derived antitoxin also is available but not preferred because of the risk of serum sickness. (see Ch. 7 IV C2)

2. **Diphtheria antitoxin** is prepared in horses by injection of toxoid of *Corynebacterium diphtheriae.*

3. **Tetanus antitoxin** consists of human-derived immune globulin specific for the toxin of *Clostridium tetani.* Animal-derived antitoxin also is available but not preferred because of the risk of serum sickness.

B. **Gamma globulin,** also referred to as immune globulin **(IG),** is used for passive immunization against various diseases or for maintenance of immunodeficient people.

TABLE 2-2.   Immunoglobulins Used in Passive Immunization

Human Immunoglobulins	Animal Immunoglobulins*
Source: Pooled gamma globulin	
Hepatitis A	
Hepatitis B	
Measles	
Varicella	
Source: Immunized donors	
Hepatitis B (HBIG)	Tetanus
Rabies (HRIG)	Rabies
Tetanus (HTIG)	Botulism
Varicella-Zoster (HVIG)	Diptheria
Botulism	Snake and spider antivenins

*Animal, usually horse, antiserum should be used only if no human-derived product is available. This decreases the incidence of adverse reactions such as serum sickness and anaphylaxis.

1. **Preparation.** Prepared from pooled, healthy adult human plasma or serum, IG contains a variety of different antibodies to several microorganisms, depending on the experience of the persons contributing to the pool.

2. **Human-derived gamma globulin** may be used in the prevention or treatment of **hepatitis A** and **measles.**

C. **Specific immune globulin (SIG)** is a gamma globulin preparation obtained from a group of people who have recently recovered from a specific infectious disease, or from hyperimmunized human volunteers. Representative preparations include the following:

1. **Hepatitis B immune globulin (HBIG)** is pooled human plasma that has a high titer of antibody to HBsAg.

2. **Human-derived rabies immune globulin (HRIG)** is prepared from the serum of humans who have been hyperimmunized against rabies (usually veterinary students or veterinarians). HRIG may be used in conjunction with rabies virus vaccine to treat people exposed to rabid animals.

3. **Human-derived varicella-zoster immune globulin (HVIG),** is selected for its high titer of antibody to varicella-zoster virus. This product is used prophylactically in immunodeficient children to prevent chickenpox, but it is of no benefit to people with active varicella or herpes zoster (shingles).

4. **Rh_o(D)-immune globulin (RhoGAM)** is a human-derived preparation given to Rh-negative women within 72 hours of delivery, miscarriage, or abortion of an Rh-positive infant or fetus. The objective is to prevent sensitization of the mother to possible Rh-positive fetal red blood cells. It is also given during the last trimester (week 26) to prima gravida Rh-negative women.

5. **Antisera to cytomegalovirus** is routinely given to those receiving bone marrow transplants to minimize reactivation of this virus when immunosuppressive drugs are used to reduce the possibility of graft rejection.

6. **Equine antivenin** is used to treat people who have been bitten by poisonous creatures (e.g., certain snakes or spiders; scorpions). The danger of serum sickness is present in these individuals.

VII. EXPERIMENTAL IMMUNIZATION PROCEDURES. Concern about the safety and efficacy of current immunizations has prompted the search for improved methods and products for immunization.

A. **Immunopotentiation.** See Chapter 5 XI for a discussion of this topic.

B. **Specific immunization.** New vaccines under consideration are those for Group A streptococcal infections, Group B streptococcal infections, gonorrhea, cholera, and traveler's diarrhea due to *Escherichia coli*. Two new vaccines for typhoid fever are being developed; a live, attenuated strain of *Salmonella typhi,* which is administered orally, and a purified capsular carbohydrate (the Vi antigen), which is administered parenterally. **HIV vaccines against AIDS** are in experimental development. Included among the products being tested are mutated HIV viruses that are unable to reproduce normally in tissue cultures, and the gp120 and gp41 surface proteins of the virus essential for its attachment to host cells.

C. **Immunization routes.** New interest has developed in the percutaneous method of immunization with a "gun" that forces the vaccine through the skin without the use of needle or syringe. Recent success with the intranasal spray administration of the influenza virus vaccine to increase the secretory IgA response may soon result in its preference, in part because it is less toxic than the intramuscular method now used.

D. **DNA vaccines.** It has been demonstrated that DNA corresponding to an antigen can be injected intramuscularly and induce an antibody response to the antigen. This DNA combined with colloidal gold favors phagocytic ingestion of the DNA. Details of this are still unclear, but experimental results have been very promising and practical applications are anticipated. Apparently the DNA is taken up by cells of the host and is transcribed. The resultant messenger RNA (mRNA) is translated producing the vaccine immunogen in vivo.

E. **Recombinant vaccines.** The use of the vaccinia virus as a carrier for genes of extraneous bacterial or viral origin is a future prospect for immunizations via recombinant DNA technology. One advantage of the vaccinia virus as a vector is its size; it is large enough to transport the genes for several antigens. Plasmids already have been used to transport genes for important antigens into bacteria or yeasts, which then produce the antigen (e.g., rHBsAg)

F. **Anti-idiotypic antibody vaccines.** Immunoglobulin idiotypes represent unique amino acid sequences in the variable region associated with the antigen-binding capability of the molecule. Idiotypic sites are capable of inducing antibody production (i.e., anti-idiotypic antibody) when the globulin is injected into a foreign species. The anti-idiotypic antibody represents a reflection of the antigen and can substitute for it. Anti-idiotypic vaccines are not yet available for human use.

Vignette Revisited

1. Anh had been immunized repeatedly with the polysaccharide antigens of *Haemophilus influenzae*. Polysaccharide from capsular type b of this bacterium is one form of the antigen used to immunize against infection by this organism. However, this has the risk of creating an immunotolerant state if repeated or large doses of the antigen are given. During experiments conducted in the 1940s, large doses of pneumococcal polysaccharides were discovered to be less efficient in provoking an immune response than intermediate or low doses. This was the origin of the concept of immunotolerance (then labeled immunoparalysis), which lead to the current understanding of how B and T cells become unresponsive to antigens, particularly polysaccharides. This seems to be a logical explanation for Anh's contraction of meningitis due to *H. influenzae*. It is also possible that Anh received the purified capsular vaccine, which would not have been immunogenic prior to the age of 2 years.

The recognition that polysaccharide antigens are T-cell independent antigens and that the IgM response to these antigens fades quickly due to the short half-life of IgM prompted a modification of this and other T-independent antigens by covalently coupling them to proteins. This converts these antigens to T-cell dependent antigens, a condition that favors an IgG response and other protective attributes of that immunoglobulin.

2. Immunologic tolerance is the inability of an antigen to induce the expected immune response in an individual. This may be due to a failure of either B or T cells to respond. B-cell tolerance is noted to develop after large doses of antigen are given. B cells develop an anergy to the antigen through mechanisms that remain unclear, possibly even by cell death of the potentially responding B-cell clone. T-cell anergy is more easily induced by lower doses of the antigen (sometimes called the toleragen) and is of a longer duration. (see Ch. 5 X B 2 a)

3. Infants of all species studied are poor responders to polysaccharide antigens. Tolerance to antigens is more easily developed in young rather than adult animals. Immunization schedules for human or animal vaccines should keep this in mind.

4. T-cell independent antigens are almost exclusively polysaccharides, but some synthetic polymers also fall into this grouping. It is believed that the simple chemistry of these molecules results in numerous repetitions of a single or limited number of epitopes. The cross-linking by antigen of many surface antibody molecules with the same epitope specificity is presumed to relate to the ease by which tolerance in B cells can be developed. In more complex antigens, in which epitope repetition is unlikely, only two antigen receptor molecules on the B-cell surface are cross linked, and tolerance is not favored.

5. Polysaccharide antigens of *H. influenzae* used for immunization are now commercially available in a T-cell dependent form. One preparation consists of the capsular saccharide of the type b organism linked to tetanus toxoid and provides immunity to both Haemophilus infections and tetanus. Diphtheria toxoid has also been used as a carrier protein. Another product has outer membrane proteins of the meningococcus as the carrier to stimulate T cells. These products are equally effective in preventing meningitis caused by *H. influenzae*.

Questions 1-5

Karen E., an 11-year-old girl, was given booster immunizations with tetanus-diphtheria booster (Td), nonconjugated *Haemophilus influenzae* b (Hib), and oral polio vaccine (OPV) before leaving on a 2-week camping and hiking trip with her church youth group.

1. For which of the following diseases is Karen given a nonidentical but cross-reacting antigen with the main virulence factor of the pathogen(s)?

(A) Tetanus and poliomyelitis
(B) Diphtheria and poliomyelitis
(C) Tetanus and diphtheria
(D) Poliomyelitis
(E) Meningitis due to *H. influenzae*

2. Which one of the antigens given Karen is T-independent?

(A) Hib
(B) OPV
(C) T of Td only
(D) d of Td only
(E) Both T and d of Td

3. Which one of the antigens given Karen is expected to give a strong secretory IgA response?

(A) Hib
(B) OPV
(C) T of Td only
(D) d of Td only
(E) Both T and d of Td

4. Which one of the antigens given Karen is expected to give the most feeble anamnestic response?

(A) Hib
(B) OPV
(C) T of Td only
(D) d of Td only
(E) Both T and d of Td

5. Which one of the antigens given to Karen is viable and would be dangerous if given to a person with AIDS?

(A) Hib
(B) OPV
(C) T of Td only
(D) d of Td only
(E) Both T and d of Td

6. An immigrant child from Moscow is encountered at the immigration services at J. F. Kennedy airport with symptoms of diphtheria. The child's parents explained that immunizations against diphtheria had been reduced in Russia because of the economy. The preferred vaccine against diphtheria consists of

(A) heat-killed *Corynebacterium diphtheriae*
(B) attenuated *Corynebacterium diphtheriae*
(C) precipitated or adsorbed toxoid
(D) capsular polysaccharide
(E) capsular polysaccharide covalently coupled to meningococcal protein

7. A genetically engineered yeast is used as the source of the vaccine against

(A) rubella
(B) measles
(C) poliomyelitis
(D) hepatitis B
(E) mumps

8. A superantigen is best described by which one of the following statements?

(A) It stimulates a large number of B-cell clones
(B) It is viable and reproduces in the immunized person to create a larger dose of antigen than that actually given
(C) Macrophages do not fully degrade it, thereby leaving many epitopes in a fully immunogenic state
(D) It is presented to a T cell after macrophage processing
(E) It stimulates a large number of T-cell clones

9. A feature of large protein antigens is their

(A) relatively high content of different epitopes compared to polysaccharide antigens of the same size
(B) failure to be presented to B cells destined to produce immunoglobulin M (IgM)
(C) ability to be combined with antigen presenting cells bearing IgD but not those bearing IgM
(D) inability to stimulate IgM synthesis
(E) failure to produce an enhanced immune response when combined with an adjuvant

10. A substance that reacts with an antibody but will not stimulate antibody formation in its native state is called a(n)

(A) antigen
(B) immunogen
(C) hapten
(D) adjuvant
(E) allergen

11. Which one of the following is an example of artificial passive immunization?

(A) Injection of adjuvant alone
(B) In utero infection
(C) Transplacental passage of antibody
(D) Injection of pooled human gamma globulin
(E) Injection of DNA from a bacterium into a human

12. Which of the following is a polyvalent vaccine?

(A) *Haemophilus influenzae* type b (Hib) vaccine
(B) Rabies vaccine
(C) Mumps vaccine
(D) Hepatitis B vaccine
(E) Oral polio virus (OPV) vaccine

13. A 13-year-old boy is seen in the emergency department with a heavy nasal discharge, cough that brought up a rusty sputum, consolidation of the lower left lobe of the lung, and fever. Proper use of the multivalent polysaccharide vaccine could have prevented this infection by

(A) *Bordetella pertussis*
(B) *Corynebacterium diphtheriae*
(C) *Salmonella typhi*
(D) *Streptococcus pneumoniae*
(E) *Clostridium tetani*

14. Passive immunization relies upon the use of

(A) bacterial polysaccharides
(B) toxoids
(C) vaccines
(D) antitoxins
(E) attenuated pathogens

1. The answer is C [V A 1]. Virtually all the symptoms of tetanus and diphtheria are caused by the exotoxins they produce. Antibody to these toxins is protective against these diseases. The toxins are easily converted to toxoids by treatment with formaldehyde or glutaraldehyde. This preserves their immunogenicity while destroying their toxicity. The toxoids differ in structure from the toxins by having formyl or glutaryl groups attached to their free amino groups. Thus, toxoids are not identical to toxins but are cross-reactive with them because they share the nonmodified epitopes.

2. The answer is A [I B 1, V A 2]. The Hib vaccine consists of the polysaccharide capsule of *Haemophilus influenzae* type b. This is a simple polymer of ribitol phosphate and, like many other polysaccharides, is able to initiate an antibody response without the participation of T cells.

3. The answer is B [V B 5 b]. The oral polio vaccine (OPV) is successful because the active virus in the vaccine reproduces in the intestinal tract and develops an intestinal immunity against poliomyelitis. Mucosal tissues of the gut, as with other mucosal tissues, are well equipped to produce secretory immunoglobulin A (sIgA). The other vaccine choices are given by injection, which leads to an IgG or IgM response, depending on the chemical nature of the antigen.

4. The answer is A [V A 2]. Polysaccharide antigens stimulate an immunoglobulin M (IgM) response, and little if any of the other immunoglobulins are produced. All the choices listed except Hib have proteins as the dominant antigens. Hib is polyribitol phosphate; it stimulates an IgM response, and the IgM titer of the secondary or anamnestic response is little changed from the primary titer. Anamnesis will also not be induced by the Hib vaccine unless it is conjugated to a protein carrier molecule.

5. The answer is B [V B 5]. The oral polio vaccine (OPV) is a mixture of three antigenic varieties of the poliomyelitis virus in an attenuated but active state. Exposure of any immunocompromised individual to a living, active bacterial, viral, or other vaccine is a potentially life-threatening act and must be avoided because these agents can "revert to virulence" in immunologically deficient patients.

6. The answer is C [V A 1]. The preferred vaccine for diphtheria is fluid toxoid precipitated with potassium alum or adsorbed onto aluminum hydroxide or phosphate. Because diphtheria results primarily from the action of the toxin formed by *Corynebacterium diphtheriae* rather than from invasion by the organism, resistance to the disease depends on specific neutralizing antitoxin such as that induced by vaccination.

7. The answer is D [V B 6]. The only genetically engineered vaccine currently available is that against the hepatitis B virus. The vaccine consists of hepatitis B surface antigen (HbsAg), which is produced by yeasts containing a plasmid bearing the DNA coding for the surface antigen of the hepatitis B virus.

8. The answer is E [I B 2]. Superantigens cross link T-cell receptor molecules on CD4+ cells with the class II major histocompatibility complex (MHC) protein on the antigen presenting cell. This is a signal for mitosis and a large number (2%–20%) of CD4+ T cells will respond and release cytokines such as interleukin-1 and tumor necrosis factor.

9. The answer is A [I A 2a]. Proteins are composed of approximately 20 different amino acids, and these are irregularly distributed along the peptide chain. This provides an opportunity to create numerous epitopes. In contrast, polysaccharides often are composed of a limited number of monosaccharides, and this limits the variability in epitope formation.

10. The answer is C [II A 5]. By definition, haptens are nonantigenic substances that, when conjugated to an existing antigen, can create or alter an antigenic determinant. The antibody to this determinant reacts with the haptenic molecule in its original state.

11. The answer is D [IV A 2]. Passive immunization is based on the contribution of immunity from one individual to another—by antibodies or cells. "Artificial" refers to a man-made circumstance, basically an injection in reference to immunity. Transplacental passage of antibody is considered a natural phenomenon.

12. The answer is E [V B 5]. A polyvalent vaccine can be defined as one with two or more antigenic varieties of the same immunogen. In this instance, the oral polio vaccine (OPV) contains the three antigenic types of the polio virus and is thus polyvalent. Polyvalent vaccines could also be defined as a vaccine containing more than one antigen. On this basis all answers would be correct because none of the vaccines listed consists of a single antigenic molecule. Because single, molecularly pure antigens seldom are used for human immunization, the first definition is the most practical.

13. The answer is D [V A 4] This child has symptoms consistent with a diagnosis of pneumonia. Of the choices listed, *Streptococcus pneumoniae* is the organism most consistently associated with pneumonia. Twenty-three antigenic types of the capsule of this bacterium are incorporated into a multivalent vaccine to provide protection against this pathogen. A conjugated vaccine similar to that used for *H. influenza* infections has been developed to protect infants from pneumococcal meningitis.

14. The answer is D [IV A 2]. Passive immunization consists of the donation of immunity from a donor to a recipient. Only antitoxins represent a form of protection from a donor. Bacterial polysaccharides, toxoids, vaccines, and attenuated pathogens are agents used to induce an active immunity in the recipient.

Chapter 3

Immunoglobulins

Vignette

Nina M., a 6-month-old infant, was awake crying most of the night, much to her mother's distress. The infant was healthy until now, with no illness of any kind. But now, Nina was experiencing her first infection, if her fever and crying were any indication.

1. How is the resistance of many infants to infectious disease during the first months of their life explained?
2. What property of immunoglobulins contributes to this immunity of infants?
3. It is not given that Nina's mother breastfed her daughter. How could this contribute to Nina's health?
4. At what age do infants develop the ability to synthesize antibodies?
5. Which antibodies are formed earliest by infants?

I. **IMMUNOGLOBULINS (Ig), OR ANTIBODIES (Ab),** are glycoproteins present in the gamma-globulin fraction of serum.

A. **The concentration of immunoglobulins in the body** is divided between the intravascular and extravascular (primarily lymphatic) compartments. Every day, 25% of the antibody concentration exchanges as the tissues are bathed in plasma proteins.

B. **Immunoglobulins are produced by B lymphocytes (B cells) or plasma cells** in response to exposure to an immunogen. Therefore, immunoglobulins are a part of the adaptive immune response (specifically, humoral immunity). They react with the corresponding epitope of the antigen that induced their production.

II. **GENERAL IMMUNOGLOBULIN STRUCTURE.** The basic structural unit of an immunoglobulin molecule consists of four polypeptide chains linked covalently by disulfide bonds (Figure 3–1). The four-chain, monomeric immunoglobulin structure is composed of two identical heavy (H) polypeptide chains and two identical light (L) polypeptide chains.

A. Heavy (H) and light (L) chains

1. **H chains** have a molecular weight of **50 to 75 kilodaltons** (kDa), which is approximately twice that of L chains. H chains contain approximately **400 amino acids,** which is twice the number in L chains.
   a. **Amino acid differences** in the carboxy-terminal portion of the H chains identify five antigenically distinct H-chain **isotypes,** which form the basis for the five **classes** of immunoglobulin molecules (Table 3–1).
   b. H-chain classes γ and α are subdivided into **subclasses** (see Table 3–1). The subdivision is based on the greater similarity of amino acid sequence shown by subclasses within the same class compared to that of other classes. H-chain differences determine the immunoglobulin subclasses; γ1 corresponds to IgG1; α1 to IgA1, and so forth.

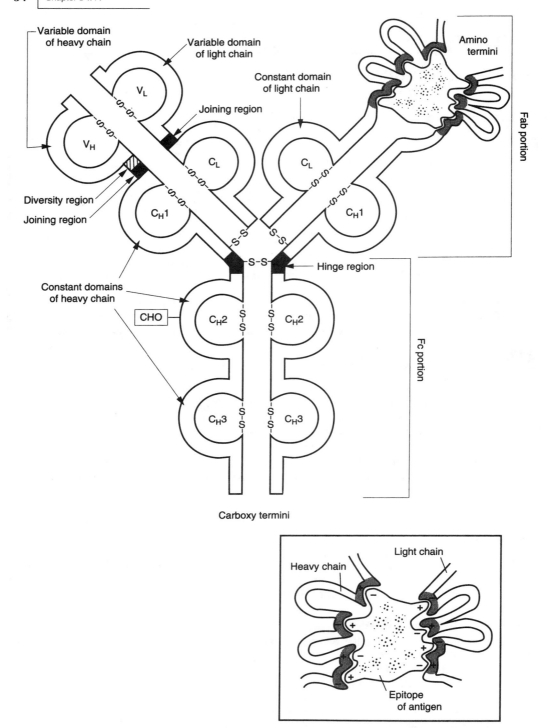

FIGURE 3-1. Basic unit (monomer) of the IgG molecule, consisting of four polypeptide chains linked covalently by disulfide bonds (S-S), with intrachain disulfide linkages as well. The loops correspond to domains within each chain. V = variable domain; C = constant domain; L = light chain; H = heavy chain; CHO = carbohydrate side chain. The *inset* shows the hypervariable complementarity-determining regions as *shaded.* The framework regions of each variable domain in the paratopic region are not shaded. Similar hypervariable regions are found in the α and β chains of the T-cell receptor for antigen.

TABLE 3-1. Properties of Human Immunologlobulins

	IgG	IgA	IgM	IgD	IgE
H-chain	γ	α	μ	δ	ϵ
H-chain subclasses	$\gamma_1, \gamma_2, \gamma_3, \gamma_4$	α_1, α_2	—	—	—
H-chain allotypes	Gm	Am	—	—	—
J chain	—	+	+	—	—
Carbohydrate (%)	3	7	12	13	11
Serum concentration (mg/dl)	1200	200	120	3	0.05
Serum half-life (days)	21[†]	6	10	3	2

H chain = heavy chain; J chain = joining chain.

[†]IgG3 has a half-life of 7 days.

    2. L chains are composed of approximately 200 amino acids. They are of two types—κ or λ—based on their structural (antigenic) differences.
        a. All immunoglobulin classes have both κ and λ chains. However, a given immunoglobulin molecule will contain either two identical κ chains or two identical λ chains, but never a κ chain and a λ chain combined.
        b. λ chain subtype. There is no isotypic variation in κ chains. However, there are four distinct λ chains, giving rise to four distinct subtypes (so called to avoid confusion with the H-chain subclasses that distinguish immunoglobulin isotypes).

B. **Disulfide (-S-S-) bonds** hold together the four polypeptide chains in immunoglobulin molecules. There are **two types** of disulfide bonds.
    1. Interchain bonds occur between H chains (H-H), between H and L chains (H-L), and between L chains (L-L).
        a. Disulfide bonds between heavy chains occur primarily in the hinge region of the immunoglobulin molecule (see II G).
        b. Only one disulfide bond connects H and L chains.
        c. Single light-chain bonds occur in IgA2m(1) and in the Bence Jones protein seen in the urine of patients with multiple myeloma.
    2. Intrachain bonds occur within an individual chain. The number of intrachain disulfide bonds varies depending on the number of **domains** in the molecule (see II D).

C. **Each H chain and each L chain has a variable (V) and one or more constant (C) regions.** The V region shows a wide variation in amino acid composition, whereas the C region demonstrates a much more uniform (constant) amino acid sequence.
    1. The V regions associate with appropriate constant regions, so that a variable H-chain region (V_H) does not occur in an L chain, and vice versa. During **class switching** in an immune response, such as when B cells change their production from μ to γ heavy chains (i.e., from producing IgM to IgG), only the constant portion of the H chain changes and the antibody specificity remains the same.
    2. Hypervariable regions are particular areas within the variable regions that are highly variable in amino acid sequence. These hypervariable regions, often called complementarity-determining regions (CDRs), occur at similar amino acid positions in an otherwise relatively invariant molecule.
        a. The hypervariable regions are important in the structure of the antigen-binding site (i.e., the paratope).
        b. There is extreme variability in the amino acids found in the hypervariable regions (Figure 3–2). However, the peptide sequences that intervene between the hypervari-

able regions, called **framework regions (FRs),** are relatively constant in amino acid composition.

D. Each immunoglobulin chain consists of a series of globular regions, or domains, enclosed by disulfide bonds (see Figure 3–1).

1. **Domains consist of approximately 110 amino acid residues.**

2. **Each H chain has four or five domains:** one in the variable region (V_H) and three or four in the constant region (C_H1, C_H2, C_H3, and C_H4). The γ, α, and δ H chains have four domains. The μ and ϵ H chains have five domains.

3. **Each L chain has two domains:** one in the variable region (V_L) and one in the constant region (C_L).

E. **The paratope is the area of the immunoglobulin molecule that interacts specifically with the epitope of the antigen.** The paratope is formed by a very small portion of the entire immunoglobulin molecule. Folding of the polypeptide chains brings the hypervariable regions of the V_H and V_L domains into close proximity. This folding creates a three-dimensional structure that is complementary to the epitope (see Figure 3–1).

F. The **hinge region** is the portion of the H chain between the C_H1 and C_H2 domains (see Figure 3–1). Its sequence is unique for each immunoglobulin type and subclass. IgM and IgE do not possess a hinge but have an additional C_H domain. The hinge region is **highly flexible** and allows for movement of the Fab arms in relation to each other.

G. **Fab and Fc fragments.** Early studies of immunoglobulin structure used proteolytic enzymes to degrade immunoglobulin molecules into definable fragments.

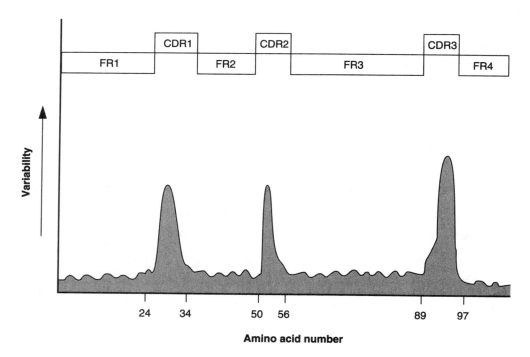

FIGURE 3-2. Amino acid variability in the variable region of the light chain of an immunoglobulin molecule. The variability index used is an arbitrary scale of the number of different amino acids found in each position if 100 different light chains were analyzed. *FR* = framework region; *CDR* = complementarity-determining region.

1. **Papain** splits the monomeric basic unit at the hinge region into three fragments of approximately equal size. It breaks the heavy chains above (i.e., on the amino-terminal side) the interchain disulfide bonds (see Figure 3–1).

   a. Two **Fab fragments** (**f**ragment **a**ntigen-**b**inding) each contain an entire L chain and the amino-terminal half of the H chain. An Fab fragment is monovalent; that is, it possesses only one antigen-binding site.

   b. One **Fc fragment** (**f**ragment **c**rystallizable) comprises the carboxy-terminal portion of the H chain. The two heavy chains are held together by disulfide bonds. The Fc portion of the molecule has several properties:

      (1) It binds the C1q component of complement and **activates the complement cascade** (see Chapter 4 I A 1).

      (2) It contains carbohydrate.

      (3) It reacts with Fc receptors on various cells of the body; therefore, it **dictates biologic activities** of the molecule [e.g., whether a given immunoglobulin can cross the placenta, sensitize mast cells to degranulate when they contact allergen, or opsonize bacteria and other cellular elements for phagocytosis (Table 3–2)].

2. **Pepsin** digests away most of the Fc fragment below (on the carboxy-terminal side) the interchain disulfide bonds in the hinge region (see Figure 3–1), leaving one large piece termed the F(ab')2 fragment, which consists of two Fab fragments joined by disulfide bonds. This fragment has two antigen-binding sites.

H. **Immunoglobulins are glycoproteins.** From 3% to 13% of the immunoglobulin molecule is composed of oligosaccharides, which usually are attached to the immunoglobulin at one or more locations in the C_H regions (i.e., the C_H2 or C_H3 regions). **N-Glycosidic bonds** usually link an N-acetylglucosamine in the carbohydrate moiety to an asparagine residue in the polypeptide chain at the C_H region.

I. **J (joining) chains** are small glycoproteins that are covalently linked to the carboxy-terminal portions of the alpha and mu heavy chains of polymeric immunoglobulins.

TABLE 3-2. The Distribution of Receptors on Various Cells of the Body and the Biologic Significance of Their Presence

Receptor	Immuno-globulin specificity	Cellular presence	Biologic significance
Fcα R	IgA	Neutrophils Macrophages	Opsonization; protection of body surfaces by inhibition of adherence of microbes; neutralization of toxins and enzymes
Poly-IgR	J chain	Mucosal epithelial cells	Serves as a receptor for dimeric IgA and facilitates passage through the cell and secretion of IgA dimers in sIgA form; also reacts with IgM
Fcε R	IgE	Basophils Mast cells	Involved in atopic allergies; cross-linking in cell membrane by allergen triggers degranulation and release of vasoactive compounds
		Eosinophils	Kills metazoan parasites
Fcγ R	IgG	Neutrophils (+) Monocytes (+ +)	Opsonization; different receptors react with varying avidity with individual antibodies, thus Fc_γ RII reacts with IgG1, 3, & 4, but not 2
		Natural killer cells	Antibody-dependent cytotoxic cells
		Trophoblasts	Responsible for IgG transport across the placenta

Fc = fragment crystallizable; Ig = immunoglobulin; R = receptor. There are different receptors for many of these (identified by Roman numerals, e.g., Fcγ RI, Fcγ RII, and so forth).

J. **Membrane immunoglobulins.** Presumably all immunoglobulins exist in both membrane and secreted forms. IgM and IgD are found in the membrane of mature B lymphocytes. After the cell interacts with antigen, it proliferates and matures into a cell that is actively **secreting** immunoglobulin. The switch from membrane-bound monomeric IgM to secreted polymeric IgM is accompanied by an increase in J-chain synthesis. Membrane forms of IgG and IgA are thought to function as antigen receptors on memory B cells. The membrane forms of these immunoglobulins are larger than their serum counterparts because of the presence of transmembrane and cytoplasmic components attached to the carboxy-terminal end of the heavy chain.

K. **Immunoglobulin superfamily.** The immunoglobulin molecule is a member of a very large family of proteins that share a similarity of structure and function.

1. Structure. Structurally, all members of the family have significant amino acid sequence homology and contain at least one **domain** (see II D).

2. Function. The members of this superfamily are involved in **cellular interactions.** Most occur in cell membranes and serve as **recognition molecules.** Some of the members of the family are the T-cell receptor, MHC and some CD molecules.

III. STRUCTURE AND FUNCTION OF SPECIFIC IMMUNOGLOBULINS

A. **Isotypic variation.** Immunoglobulins fall into five classes (isotypes), based on certain structural differences (see Table 3–1). Each class also has certain unique biologic and chemical properties.

1. IgG is the major immunoglobulin in human serum. It is the major antibody produced in the secondary immune response. Most serum IgG is IgG1.
  a. Structure. IgG is a **monomer** consisting of identical pairs of H and L chains linked by disulfide bridges (see Figure 3–1). Four subclasses of IgG have been identified, based on H-chain differences: subclasses IgG1, IgG2, IgG3, and IgG4, which correspond to H chains $\gamma 1$, $\gamma 2$, $\gamma 3$, and $\gamma 4$.
  b. Function. IgG is the only immunoglobulin that crosses the placenta; therefore, maternal IgG provides most of the protection of the newborn during the first months of life. (Secretory IgA in colostrum protects a newborn's gastrointestinal tract.) In addition, IgG is the major opsonizing immunoglobulin, and it activates complement by the classical pathway. The binding site for complement component C1q is in the $C_H 2$ domain.

2. IgA is present in two forms: one in the serum (serum IgA) and the other in various body secretions [secretory IgA (sIgA)]. The dominant subclass in secretions is sIgA2.
  a. Structure. The sIgA molecule consists of two monomeric units plus a J chain and secretory component (Figure 3–3).
  b. Secretory component is a polypeptide synthesized by exocrine epithelial cells that enables dimeric IgA to pass through the mucosal tissues into secretions.
    (1) The epithelial cells bear a receptor for serum immunoglobulins called the poly-Ig receptor. It has a very high affinity for IgA dimer, but other polymeric immunoglobulins also may react. For example, some IgM is synthesized in secretory tissues. Secretory IgM, like sIgA, contains secretory component.
    (2) After binding IgA, the receptor–IgA complex is internalized by endocytosis, transported across the cell cytoplasm, and extruded into the external secretions. As the complex is extruded, proteolytic cleavage of the receptor leaves a fragment—the secretory component—attached by a disulfide bond to the IgA dimer.
    (3) Secretory component appears to protect IgA from mammalian proteases.
    (4) Secretory IgA protects mucosal surfaces by reacting with adhesion molecules on the potential pathogens and interfering with their adherence and colonization of the host. It also may opsonize foreign particles because polymorphonuclear neu-

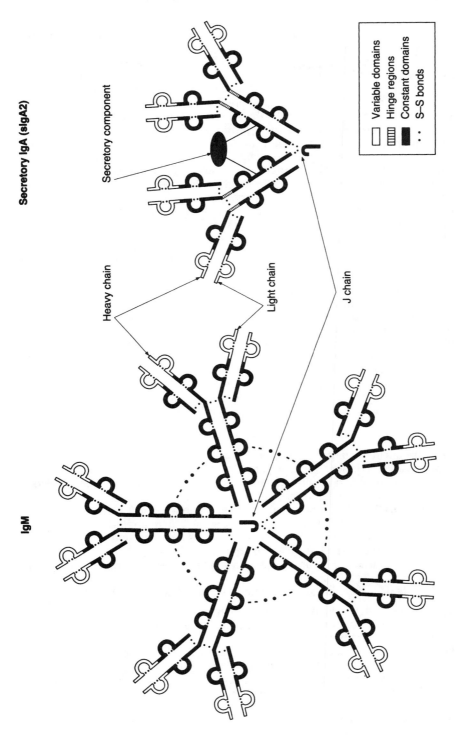

FIGURE 3-3. Structural models of IgM and secretory IgA (sIgA). IgM has a pentameric structure linked by the J chain at the Fc fragment. The sIgA molecule has a dimeric structure plus joining (J) chain plus secretory component.

trophils (PMNs) monocytes, and alveolar macrophages have a receptor for the Fc portion of IgA (i.e., FcαR) on their membranes.

3. IgM has a pentameric structure (see Figure 3–3) consisting of five monomeric units linked by a J chain and by disulfide bonds in the Fc fragment. It is easily dissociated by reducing agents, forming five monomeric units.

   a. IgM is the **first antibody** that an immunologically committed B lymphocyte can produce. Monomeric IgM appears in the B-cell membrane (followed shortly by IgD) before an encounter with its homologous epitope.

   b. IgM is the predominant antibody in the primary immune response to most antigens. IgM also is the **predominant antibody produced by the fetus.** An elevated IgM level in the cord blood of a newborn may indicate that the fetus was infected before birth.

   c. IgM is the major antibody made to thymus-independent antigens (see Chapter 2 I B 1).

   d. IgM is the **most efficient immunoglobulin in activating complement** because it has more of the CH units required for this function than the other immunoglobulins. IgM is not intrinsically opsonic because phagocytic cells do not possess a receptor for the Fc portion of the μ chain. However, IgM markedly enhances phagocytosis by causing complement activation and C3b deposition onto the target cell surface where the IgM antibody resides.

4. IgD represents less than 1% of the total immunoglobulin pool. It occurs in large quantities on the B-cell membrane and may be involved as an antigen receptor in B-cell activation.

5. IgE is present in trace amounts in normal serum. It is associated with atopic diseases (e.g., asthma and anaphylaxis).

   a. IgE is homocytotropic; that is, it has an affinity for cells ("cytotropic") of the host species that produced it ("homo"). This affinity is particularly strong for tissue mast cells and blood basophils. Fixation to these cells occurs via a cell-membrane-bound FcεR (i.e., receptor for the Fc portion of the ε chain of IgE) reacting with the Fc fragment (C_H3 and C_H4 domains).

   b. On combining with allergens, IgE antibodies trigger the release of histamine and other mediators of atopic disease from the cells. IgE also may be important in immunity to certain helminthic parasites.

B. | **Allotypic and idiotypic variation** also are displayed by immunoglobulins.

1. Allotypes are allelic variants of isotypes. They exist in different individuals within the same species and are inherited in a Mendelian manner.

   a. Allotypes are identified by **allotypic markers** [i.e., structural (antigenic or epitopic) differences] found in the constant regions of H and L chains.

   b. Nomenclature for allotypic markers has been established for γ, α, and κ chains.

   (1) **Markers on γ H chains** are designated **Gm,** and there are more than 20 antigenically different markers of this type. All markers are not found on all IgG molecules; they seem to be restricted to certain subclasses.

   (2) **Markers on α H chains** are designated **Am,** and there are only two alleles at this locus (i.e., m1 and m2).

   (3) **Markers on κ L chains** are designated **Km,** and there are four alleles at this locus.

2. Idiotypes represent the antigen-binding specificities of immunoglobulins. They are unique structural determinants in the V region that are associated with the antigen-binding capability of the antibody molecule.

   a. Idiotypic variability pertains to the generation of the antigen-binding site in the hypervariable regions of the H and L chains. **Variability in amino acid sequence** in these regions is concentrated in three to four hypervariable regions surrounded by relatively invariant (framework) residues. These hypervariable regions are the areas that make contact with the epitope of the antigen.

   b. Idiotopes and idiotypes

   (1) **Idiotopes** are epitopes that occur in the variable region of the Fab portion of an antibody molecule.

   (2) The **idiotype** of a particular immunoglobulin is the sum of the idiotopes.

   c. Anti-idiotypic antibodies. If an antibody is used as an immunogen, it is possible to in-

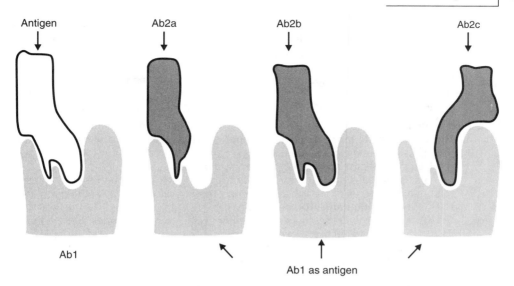

FIGURE 3-4. The first antibody *(Ab1)* is made to the original antigen and contains an idiotype associated with its hypervariable region. Ab1 can then be used as an immunogen in a different group of animals. Ab2 is produced and can react with different areas of the hypervariable region of Ab1; that is, it is an anti-idiotypic antibody. Among anti-idiotypic antibodies are molecules that react with idiotopes within the paratope and therefore mimic the epitopes of the original antigen (e.g., Ab2b). When Ab2b molecules are injected into "naive" animals, they act as surrogate antigens for the original antigen. The immunized animals respond by producing antibodies that can bind the original antigen because they carry the Ab1 idiotype.

duce the production of antibodies that structurally resemble the original epitope (Figure 3–4). These second-generation anti-idiotypic antibodies could be used in artificial vaccines as an immunizing antigen to induce the original antibodies in a "naive" recipient.

IV. ANTIBODY DIVERSITY

A. Genetics of immunoglobulin diversity

1. **Overview**
   a. **Similarity.** Immunoglobulin gene organization is remarkably similar, whether in H or L chains or in the different H-chain classes. The genetics of the T-cell receptor also has a pattern of locus clusters that resembles very closely that of immunoglobulins, although different genes are involved.
   b. **Diversity.** The human immune system is capable of producing a vast number of different antibody molecules, each with its own antigenic specificity. This vast diversity is possible because immunoglobulin genes undergo an unusual type of interaction.
      (1) Embryonic DNA contains a great many genes for the variable regions of the H and L chains. The process of **somatic recombination** (i.e., DNA rearrangement and deletion), followed by RNA splicing, results in a large variety of plasma cell lines that encode different H and L chains.
      (2) A fairly high rate of **somatic mutation** in H and L chains adds to the diversity.
      (3) A similar process of DNA rearrangement gives the T-cell receptor its epitope-binding specificity.
2. **Exons, introns, and gene rearrangements**
   a. **Exons and introns.** As in other genes, **coding sequences (exons)** in the DNA code for

the amino acid sequences in immunoglobulin molecules. The exons are separated by **intervening, noncoding nucleotide sequences (introns).** Both exons and introns are transcribed into RNA, but RNA splicing then removes the introns, leaving the exons joined together.

    b. Gene rearrangement. The exons that code for variable domains are split into smaller segments of DNA along the chromosome. Making proper exons from these segments requires rearranging and rejoining the segments to form immunoglobulin gene sequences.

3. L-chain gene organization

    a. Three genes code for each immunoglobulin L chain; the human κ L chain (Figure 3–5) is used here as an example.

        (1) Two gene segments encode the variable domain.

            (a) The initial gene segment, the **variable (Vκ) segment,** encodes the first 95 amino acids of the variable-region protein. More than 200 Vκ region genes exist on human chromosome 2.

            (b) A second gene segment, the **joining (Jκ) segment,** encodes the remaining 13 amino acids of the V exon (this joining segment is unrelated to the J chain found in IgM and IgA). There are five genes at this locus.

        (2) The third gene dictates the amino acid sequence of the constant region. There is only one **Cκ region** on this final segment.

    b. The **λ L chains** arise from a similar gene complex on chromosome 22. However, there are several slightly different copies of the Cλ region gene, which correspond to the various subtypes of λ protein.

4. H-chain gene organization. The **H chain of IgM** (Figure 3–6) is used as an example.

    a. Although it is similar to that of L-chain genes, H-chain gene organization is more complex. Whereas an L-chain gene region encodes only one constant domain, the H-chain gene region must code for three or four constant domains. Also, the H-chain constant gene region must code for each of the five immunoglobulin classes and for four IgG and two IgA subclasses as well. Furthermore, the exon coding for the variable portion of the H chain is composed of three, not two, segments of DNA.

        (1) All of the H-chain immunoglobulin classes are coded at one site on chromosome 14.

        (2) The λ-chain gene complex is at one site on chromosome 22.

        (3) The κ-chain gene complex is at one site on chromosome 2.

    b. Assembly of the V/D/J exon. The additional variable-region DNA segment is designated the **diversity (D_H) gene region.** The D_H gene region accounts for the third hypervariable region of the H chain; it comprises only two or three amino acids. Gene rearrangements link a D_H to a J_H segment, and then join these to a V_H to produce the **V/D/J exon.**

    c. There are more than 200 V_H genes, at least 20 D_H genes, and 6 J_H genes. This enormous gene pool, with its large number of potential combinations, underlies the great diversity of the H-chain variable region.

5. The 12/23 spacer rule provides a mechanism for joining immunoglobulin gene segments (Figure 3–7).

    a. Each gene segment is flanked by noncoding **recombination signal sequences (RSSs)** that specify the direction of joining the segments.

    b. Each RSS consists of a highly conserved sequence containing three parts:

        (1) A **heptamer** (seven DNA bases)

        (2) A **spacer** containing either 12 nucleotides equaling one turn of the DNA helix or 23 nucleotides (two turns)

        (3) A **nonamer** (nine DNA bases)

    c. Joining of immunoglobulin genes. One RSS is located 3' to each V-gene segment, 5' to each J-gene segment, and on both sides of each D-gene segment. Each RSS contains a conserved palindromic heptamer and a conserved AT-rich nonamer sequence separated by an intervening 12/23 base pair spacer sequence. These recognition signals are the result of base-pairing reactions similar to that seen in DNA-and RNA-dependent polymerase reactions. They function to hold the DNA strand together so the recombinase enzymes can effect the joining of these individual exons.

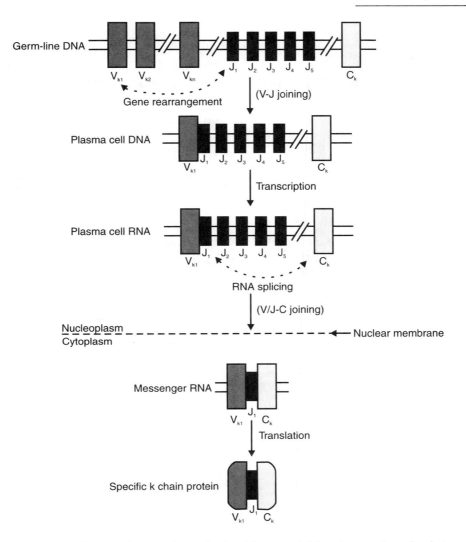

FIGURE 3-5. Human κ light (L)-chain gene organization. The potential for a large variety of κ chains exists because of random recombination in the DNA, and RNA splicing. As the B-cell precursor differentiates into a mature B cell, DNA deletion brings one of the variable ($V_κ$) genes next to one of the joining (J) genes—in this example, $V_κ$ and J_1. This unit and the remaining J genes are separated from the constant ($C_κ$) region by an intervening sequence (intron) of DNA. The $V_κ 1 / J_1$ unit codes for one of the numerous possible κ chain variable exons. The plasma cell DNA is transcribed into nuclear RNA, which is spliced to form messenger RNA (mRNA), with $V_κ$, J_1, and $C_κ$ messages joined and ready for translation into the κ chain.

6. **VJ and VDJ recombinases.** The cleavage and rejoining of the DNA strands are presumed to be carried out by **endonucleases and ligases,** respectively. These enzymes recognize the heptamer and nonamer RSSs when they are separated by one or two turns of the DNA helix. Recently, two genes that function in immunoglobulin gene recombination have been identified in mouse pre-B cells. It is not known whether these **recombination-activating genes 1 and 2 (RAG-1 and RAG-2)** code for enzymes or for other regulatory proteins. Cleavage and rejoining are active only in the early stages of B-and T-lymphocyte maturation, during the development of immunologic commitment.

7. **T-cell receptor gene organization**

   a. The T-cell receptor for antigen (see Chapter 5 IV A 1 b) is similar to the immunoglob-

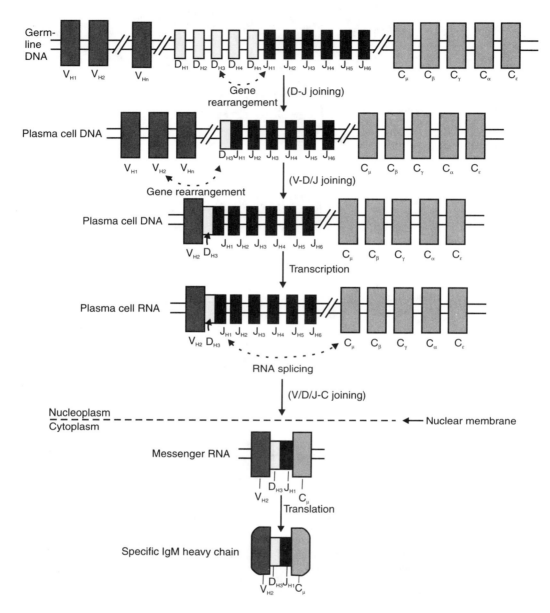

FIGURE 3-6. Human μ heavy (H)-chain gene organization. The potential for variety in H chains, as in L chains, is due to random recombination in the DNA and to RNA splicing. As the B-cell precursor differentiates into a mature B cell, DNA deletion brings one of the variable (V_H) genes, one of the diversity (D_H) genes, and one of the joining (J_H) genes together—in this example, V_{H2}, D_{H3}, and J_{H1}. This unit and the remaining J genes are separated from the constant (C) region by an intervening sequence of DNA. The plasma cell DNA is transcribed into nuclear RNA, which is spliced to form messenger RNA (mRNA). In this process, the C_μ gene is selected and joined to the $V_{H2}/D_{H3}/J_{H1}$ complex, and the entire unit is ready for translation into a μ chain. Each C_H gene is presented as a single box; however, in reality, it is composed of several exons corresponding to C_H1, hinge region, C_H2, C_H3, and so forth.

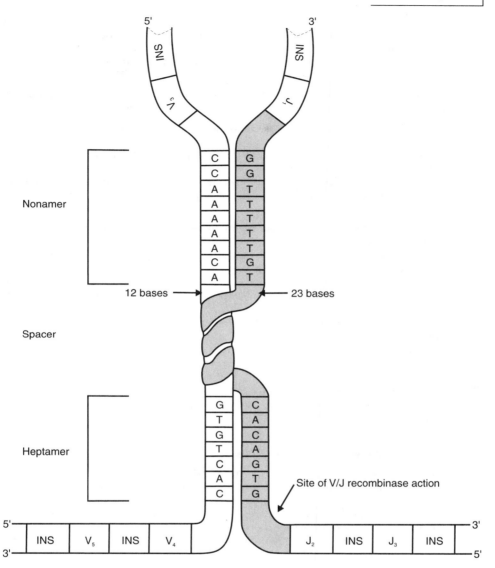

FIGURE 3-7. A schematic representation of the joining of immunoglobulin κ chain variable (V) and joining (J) gene segments. The alignment of the heptamer and nonamer components of the DNA strand is essential for gene recombination. The 23-base strand makes one full turn around the 12-base strand, which brings the recombination signal sequences together. Then, the enzymatic cleavage and ligation of the DNA strand occurs and the two genes are joined. A = adenine; C = cytosine; G = guanine; INS = intervening non-coding sequences (introns); T = thymidine.

ulin molecule in gene organization as well as in molecular structure and biologic function.

    b. During T-cell development in the thymus, the genes for the T-cell receptor undergo **DNA rearrangements** much like those for the immunoglobulin molecule.

B. Mechanisms contributing to antibody diversity

    1. Chance recombination creates a large amount of antibody diversity.

a. If all events occurred randomly, somatic recombination in the DNA followed by RNA splicing (see Figures 3–5 and 3–6) could produce more than 1000 varieties of κ and λ L chains plus perhaps as many as 20,000 varieties of H chains.

b. The random combining of H and L chains greatly expands the immunologic repertoire.

2. **Imprecise joining of the V, D, and J genes** can also be a source of immunoglobulin diversity. Whenever genes join, imprecision in joining can occur.

3. **N-region additions** can produce changes in the specificity and reactivity of the immunoglobulin molecule.

   a. N regions are very short peptides of variable sequence, often found near the third hypervariable region of the H chain.

   b. Immature lymphoid cells contain an enzyme, **terminal deoxynucleotidyl transferase,** which catalyzes the generation of N regions by the addition of nucleotides at the 3′ end of the DNA strands.

4. **Extensive mutation involving variable-region genes produces even further diversity after antigen exposure.**

   a. Mutations can occur by several **mechanisms** including **point mutations** and **recombination events.**

   b. The antibodies produced by mutations in variable-domain genes may confer a **selective advantage** to the lymphocyte if they possess a **higher affinity** (i.e., stronger attraction) for the antigen. Cells coated with high-affinity antibody are better able to capture the immunogen and perpetuate the immune response. A characteristic of prolonged immunization is the increase in antibody affinity for the antigen as the duration of exposure to the antigen increases, because the longer time of exposure increases the chance that a "good" mutation will occur.

C. **Immunoglobulin class switching (isotype switching)**

1. During the immune response, plasma cells switch from producing **IgM to IgG** or to another immunoglobulin class.

2. There is no alteration in the L chain or in the variable portion of the H chain; thus, there is **no change in antigen-binding specificity.**

3. The switch involves a change in the **H-chain constant domains** (C_H).

   a. When constant-region genes loop out during immunoglobulin switching, the cell loses its ability to produce earlier immunoglobulin class(es). Thus, a cell that has switched to IgG will not be able to revert to IgM synthesis, but it could switch again to IgA or IgE because these gene loci are downstream from the IgG loci.

   b. In the process, DNA rearrangement and RNA splicing place the remaining C_H gene sequence adjacent to the V/D/J exon (see Figure 3–7).

D. **Nonproductive rearrangements**

1. **The H or L chains are formed during the pre-B-cell phase of immunologic maturation.** In the formation of a functional gene, **DNA segments must be joined properly** to ensure that the correct reading frame is maintained.

   a. If the joining is erroneous, the downstream sequences are out of frame, preventing translation into a functional polypeptide. Such erroneous rearrangements occur frequently, and in this case the cell continues to rearrange and join its immunoglobulin gene segments until a functional immunoglobulin is made; rearrangement then ceases.

   b. The appearance of an intact H chain in the cytoplasm seems to be the signal for the end of H-chain gene shuffling. It is also the signal for commencement of L-chain gene rearrangement. The trial-and-error process is repeated until a functional L chain, either κ or λ, is produced.

2. The pre-B cell then enters the **B-lymphocyte stage** of development, in which the H and L chains are joined by disulfide bonds and are expressed in the B-cell membrane. It is

likely that many lymphocytes have nonproductive rearrangements and are of no value to the immune system. This appears to be the price that must be paid to preserve the generation of immunologic diversity by such an elaborate system.

E. **Allelic exclusion and clonal restriction.** These phenomena are peculiar to antibody-producing cells.

1. **Allelic exclusion** is the expression, in a single cell, of only one allele at a particular immunoglobulin gene locus. The process of allelic exclusion results in the synthesis of molecules with identical variable regions because the expressed messenger RNA (mRNA) is derived from a single chromosome. Therefore, the antibodies produced by each B lymphocyte are identical in their specificity.

2. **Clonal restriction.** On its surface, each B cell expresses multiple identical copies of an antibody that is specific for a single epitope. When a B cell divides, the chromosomes in its progeny cells bear the selected allelic genes, and these genes do not undergo any further V/J or V/D/J rearrangements. This is why all of the immunoglobulin molecules produced by a given clone (a B lymphocyte and its progeny) are identical in epitope specificity and in κ or λ L-chain isotype.

V. **PLASMA CELL DYSCRASIAS** represent a group of diseases characterized by the overproduction of immunoglobulins (or their fragments) by a single clone of plasma cells. The abnormal monoclonal product is called **M component (paraprotein).**

A. Overview

1. **Clinical effects.** The most important of the plasma cell dyscrasias is multiple myeloma. Also notable are Waldenström's macroglobulinemia, benign monoclonal gammopathy, primary amyloidosis, and heavy chain disease. These diseases cause **malfunction of the immune system** with resultant increases in susceptibility to infectious disease.

2. **Therapy** for a plasma cell dyscrasia includes the following:
   a. Administration of **prednisone,** with or without cytotoxic drugs
   b. Removal of the excess protein (e.g., IgM in Waldenström's macroglobulinemia) via plasmapheresis

B. **Multiple myeloma.** This plasma cell tumor in bone marrow overproduces a single class of immunoglobulin; most cases involve IgG.

1. **Characteristics**
   a. The most characteristic feature of multiple myeloma is the demonstration of **M component** in the blood, urine, or both. The M component consists of intact monoclonal antibodies, H chains, or L chains, alone or in any combination.
   b. In some cases, a substance called **Bence Jones protein,** which is a dimer of L chains, is found in the urine. This abnormal immunoglobulin fragment is a **pyroglobulin** and can be irreversibly precipitated by heating urine to 56°C.

2. The **clinical features and complications** of multiple myeloma vary widely. Some of the more common manifestations include fatigue and weakness, bone pain and pathologic fractures, bone marrow infiltration by abnormal plasma cells with resultant normochromic, normocytic anemia, and renal abnormalities, which can result in chronic renal failure.

C. **Waldenström's macroglobulinemia** is a lymphocytic lymphoma characterized by overproduction of lymphocytes and plasma cells.

1. **Characteristics.** The most distinguishing feature of this disorder is a high level of **monoclonal IgM** in the serum. Bence Jones proteins also may be seen in the urine.

2. **Clinical features and complications.** Because of the high serum IgM, patients have a hy-

perviscosity of the blood, which may be severe. Anemia, lymphadenopathy, and chronic lymphocytic leukemia also are common clinical features.

D. **Amyloidosis** is a disease characterized by deposition of an abnormal protein (i.e., amyloid) in the vascular endothelium of various organs of the body. The clinical features depend on the site and extent of amyloid deposition.

E. **Heavy chain diseases**

1. **Characteristics.** These rare malignancies are characterized by a serum paraprotein consisting of incomplete H chains without L chains; γ, α, and μ heavy chain diseases have been described.

2. **Clinical features.** The abnormal H chain shows deletion of the hinge region, or partial deletion of the Fd portion (i.e., the heavy chain component of Fab), or a combination of these abnormalities.

F. **Errors in immunoglobulin gene rearrangement are thought to contribute to the genesis of several B-cell malignancies.**

1. **Follicullar lymphoma**
   a. In many patients with follicular lymphoma—the most common B-cell cancer—a putative proto-oncogene (called *bcl*-2) on chromosome 18 is translocated into the H-chain gene region on chromosome 14.
   b. It is thought that the close proximity of *bcl*-2 to the active H-chain gene region enhances the expression of the proto-oncogene and, thus, contributes to malignant transformation.

2. **Burkitt's lymphoma**
   a. In the malignant cells of this B-cell cancer, a portion of chromosome 8 containing the cellular proto-oncogene c-*myc* is translocated into chromosome 14 so that c-*myc* lies right next to the H-chain gene region.
   b. The c-*myc* proto-oncogene is thought to be activated as a result of this proximity to the genetically active H-gene region.

Vignette Revisited

1. The first level of resistance to infections by infants depends on the activity of the phagocytic cell system. It is known that this system matures slowly, and properties such as antigen processing by macrophages are not fully developed at birth. Most of the antigen-specific resistance of infants is directly related to the immunoglobulin-based immunity of their mother. Prior to pregnancy, it is advisable for expectant mothers to receive booster immunizations with the common vaccines. For example, it has been proven that immunization of pregnant women with tetanus toxoid protects infants against umbilical tetanus neonatorum, a condition estimated to take 500,000 lives each year worldwide.

2. Immunoglobulin G is able to pass the placental barrier, and levels of IgG in an infant is a reflection of the maternal level. IgG is considered the most protective antibody for several reasons. First, it is typically present in higher amounts in blood than any of the other antibodies. Second, IgG tends to bind avidly with antigen so that once bound the antigen (virus, toxin, or other) cannot easily dissociate to create further host damage. Third, IgG does activate the complement system, thereby marshaling the protective functions of that system, and finally, it is a very efficient opsonizing antibody.

3. Immunoglobulin A in its secretory form is present in mother's milk, and breastfed infants have the benefit of this antibody for protection of their upper respiratory and intestinal tracts against infection.

4–5. Fetuses are able to produce IgM in utero from approximately the middle of the second trimester until birth. These immunoglobulins usually are in low titer unless an in utero infection is present. After birth, as the infants become exposed to antigens in their environment, the titers of all immunoglobulins steadily increases. Adult levels of the antibodies are approached gradually and are achieved at about the time of puberty.

1. In a study of IgA synthesis and blood levels in infants, one population of infants had normal levels of circulating IgA but an unexpected high level of respiratory disease. These infants probably

(A) could not synthesize J chain
(B) lacked J genes
(C) came from mothers who did not synthesize IgG
(D) had a paraproteinemia
(E) had antibodies that lacked an Fab unit

2. If a person is unable to join H and L immunoglobulin chains together with disulfide bonds, which one of the following normal immunoglobulins would be found in their blood?

(A) IgA
(B) IgD
(C) IgE
(D) IgG
(E) IgM

3. Chromosomal analysis of an abortus was performed to determine if any genetic problem had been responsible for the failed pregnancy. Both parents insisted on this examination because this was their first effort to have a child, and they wanted assurance that it was reasonable for them to expect normal pregnancies and children in the future. The pediatric genetics expert found that chromosome 22 was missing and advised the parents that, among other serious defects associated with this missing chromosome, this chromosome was needed to produce immunoglobulin

(A) H chains
(B) J chains
(C) lambda chains
(D) of any class
(E) kappa chains

4. When describing the hinge region of an antibody molecule, one of the first facts to mention would be that the hinge region

(A) contains two disulfide linked domains of 80 amino acids
(B) is present in all L chains
(C) contains the V, J, and D genes
(D) is the same size in all antibody molecules
(E) lies between the CH1 and CH2 domains

5. A child was identified in the pediatrics department that could synthesize only one class of immunoglobulin. This immunoglobulin had four C domains in its H chain and was a potent activator of the complement cascade. These facts identify the immunoglobulin as

(A) IgA
(B) IgD
(C) IgE
(D) IgG
(E) IgM

6. A 55-year-old male had been losing weight slowly over the past 2 months. A medical examination 5 months ago had revealed only a slight anemia. During the physical examination today, a general lymphadenopathy was noted, and his physician requested blood studies. The report was returned 2 days later with a description of anemia and excessive lymphocytes characteristic of a low-level leukemia. The man was recalled to his physician's office for consultation and was informed that he might have a plasma cell abnormality called Waldenströms macroglobulinemia. The physician said that one finding that would indicate this diagnosis was

(A) immunoglobulins having an incomplete H chain
(B) lymphocytes devoid of immunoglobulin on their surface
(C) elevated levels of IgM in the blood
(D) failure to synthesize any antibodies except IgE
(E) the presence of amyloid in the patient's lymph glands

7. A child in the pediatric intensive care unit had been ill since he was 5 months old. He was subjected to a complete immunologic work-up, during which it was found that he was making small amounts of IgD and IgM but none of the other immunoglobulins. The pediatric genetics division chief suggested this was due to

(A) failure of the *myc* gene to move normally to chromosome 14
(B) a failure in the antibody switch mechanism
(C) an inability to synthesize L chains
(D) an inability to synthesize lymphocytes
(E) a chromosomal abnormality of chromosome 2

8. Digestion of a patient's IgG with papain produced the expected fragments, except when the IgG was combined with its specific antigen. One explanation for this is

(A) blocking of the hinge region by antigen
(B) inactivation of papain by antigen
(C) the presence of IgE in the patient because of an allergy to papain
(D) that the IgG has no hinge region
(E) the hinge region lacks the disulfide bonds that papain attacks

9. If a plasma cell that is making IgA antibody could be analyzed at the molecular level, which one of the following genetic sequences would be found?

(A) A DNA sequence for variable (V), diversity (D), and joining (J) genes translocated near the gamma DNA exon
(B) Messenger RNA (mRNA) specific for both the κ and λ light chains
(C) mRNA specific for J chains
(D) mRNA specific for secretory component
(E) A DNA sequence for the secretory component

10. A culture of plasma cells that was synthesizing IgA was given to a professor in the molecular biology unit. The professor was asked to analyze the DNA and RNA of the cell, which was done with the finding that

(A) the DNA sequence for the V, D, and J genes were located near the gamma chain DNA exon
(B) messenger RNA was found for both kappa and lambda L chains
(C) messenger RNA was present for J chains
(D) messenger RNA was present for secretory component
(E) introns were found in the final transcript for IgA

ANSWERS AND EXPLANATIONS

1. The answer is A [II I]. The J chain is essential to the completion of the structure of secretory IgA and IgM. Secretory IgA is a significant contributor to the antibody activity found on mucosal surfaces. Therefore, in this case, the absence of secretory IgA was responsible for the increased susceptibility of this child to respiratory disease.

2. The answer is A [II B 1]. Disulfide bonding between H and L chains occurs in all immunoglobulin molecules except IgA2m(1). In this unique immunoglobulin molecule, the two light chains share a single disulfide bond. This type of bonding is also seen in some pathologic conditions, such as the Bence Jones pyroglobulin, which is found in the urine of patients with multiple myeloma.

3. The answer is C [IV A 3 b]. The genes that encode the lambda light chain are located on human chromosome 22. Similar genetic information is located on the chromosome 16 in mice. Kappa light chain genes are located on chromosome 2 in humans. All of the heavy chain genes are on chromosome 14.

4. The answer is E [II F; Figure 3–1]. The hinge region is found in all immunoglobulin molecules except IgM and IgE. These two isotypes have an extra constant heavy domain, and their flexibility is a function of the CH2 domain. The hinge region has no homology with other immunoglobulin domains and is rich in proline and cysteine. The large number of proline residues confers an extended polypeptide conformation to the molecule, making it particularly vulnerable to proteolytic enzymes such as papain and pepsin. The cysteine residues form interchain disulfide bonds that hold the two heavy chains together.

5. The answer is E [III A 3]. IgM is the first immunoglobulin that is made in the immune response. It is a pentamer of immunoglobulin molecules of approximately 190,000 daltons each. The molecule has five domains in its heavy chain, one variable domain, and four constant domains. There is no hinge region. Constant heavy domain 2 assumes the function of the absent hinge region, and it provides flexibility to the molecule. IgM is the most ac-

tive immunoglobulin at activating the complement cascade due to the presence of five Fc fragments. C1q binds to the CH2 domain and activates C1r, thus initiating the esterase activation that culminates in the generation of the vasoactive split products and opsonins, which are products of the classical pathway of complement activation.

6. The answer is C [V C]. Waldenström's macroglobulinemia is characterized by excessive quantities of IgM in the blood. This is a plasma cell dyscrasia that disregulates production of this important antibody. The high molecular weight of IgM coupled with the high quantities in blood places an unusual stress on the cardiovascular system—more so than with the other forms of plasma cell disease.

7. The answer is B [IV C]. The child has a B-cell deficiency and is unable to change isotypes. The IgM and IgD molecules are produced in a normal manner but the change to other heavy chains is defective. This disease is known as X-linked hyper-IgM (XHM) syndrome. Children with XHM syndrome suffer recurrent infections, especially infections caused by *Pneumocystis carinii*. The genetic defect is in the gene encoding the CD40 ligand (CD40L). T-helper 1 cells from patients with this disease fail to express functional CD40L in their membranes. Because an interaction between CD40 on the B cell and CD40L on the helper cell is required for B-cell activation, the absence of this co-stimulatory signal inhibits B-cell response to thymus-dependent antigens. The response to thymus-independent antigens is unaffected, so IgM and IgD are present in the serum.

8. The answer is A [II G 1]. When an immunoglobulin molecule reacts with its homologous antigen, the tertiary structure of the antibody is altered. The hinge is the flexible portion of the molecule, and it bends to allow the two molecules to achieve the appropriate spatial configuration for optimal interaction. This change blocks the access of the papain enzyme to its catalytic target and also expresses the second constant heavy domain complement-reactive area, thus permitting its reaction with C1q with resultant activation of the complement cascade.

9. The answer is C [III A 2 b]. The plasma cell makes joining (J) chains to join monomers of IgA; thus, there is a J-chain messenger RNA (mRNA). The DNA sequence for the variable (V), diversity (D), and J genes is translocated near the alpha exon; the gamma exon is spliced out. Only a single light-chain type is produced, and thus mRNA for κ or λ chains would be found. Secretory component is synthesized in mucosal epithelial cells.

10. The answer is C [III A 2]. The plasma cell that is secreting IgA will be synthesizing alpha heavy chains, either kappa OR lambda light chains, and the J chain which links the monomers together to make the dimers and trimers. Secretory component is a portion of the poly immunoglobulin receptor found on exocrine gland epithelial cells.

Chapter 4

The Complement System

Vignette

Timmy is a 4-year-old boy who is at the eighth percentile in weight for his age group. He has been plagued with infections since infancy. His grandfather, a physician, has suggested that an evaluation of his immunologic status be performed. The results indicate that he has responded normally to his childhood immunizations and has intact antibody and T-cell responses. His phagocytic cells also are found to be normal, but his serum is unable to lyse erythrocytes that have been sensitized to complement-induced lysis by antibody specific to antigens in the RBC membrane. This observation suggests a defect in the complement system, which is a complex group of plasma proteins that interact with each other in a cascading fashion to protect against infectious agents.

1. How does this happen? What protective products are generated during the cascade, and what effects do they have in the body?
2. Can this protective action cause damage if it is uncontrolled? How? What occurs in vivo to provide protection from a complement system gone awry?

I. COMPLEMENT

A. **The complement system plays a major role in host defense and the inflammatory process.** Complement consists of a complex **series of at least 20 proteins** that normally are functionally inactive in plasma. Once activated, the complement system becomes a part of the **innate immune defenses** of the body.

1. **Complement cascade.** Complement is activated sequentially in a cascading manner, each protein activating the protein that directly follows it in the sequence.

2. Activation of the complement cascade has widespread **physiologic and pathophysiologic effects.** It causes lysis of erythrocytes in hemolytic anemias, sensitizes foreign particles to phagocytosis, and causes release of histamine from mast cells (see I D).

3. **Synthesis.** The **liver** is the major site of synthesis of complement proteins; tissue macrophages and fibroblasts can synthesize some complement proteins as well.

4. Inflammation increases the synthesis of complement components, presumably through the action of interleukin-1 (IL-1) and gamma interferon.

B. Nomenclature of complement proteins

1. The nine major complement components (Table 4-1) are designated by "C" followed by an identifying numeral from 1–9 (e.g., C1, C2). The numerals indicate the order in which components are activated, except that component C4 is activated out of numeric order; it is activated before C2.

2. **Cleaved peptides** from fragmented peptide chains are denoted by lowercase letters (e.g., C3a).

TABLE 4-1. Properties of Complement Components

Component	Serum Concentration (µg/ml)	Activation Products
Classic Pathway		
C1q	70	
C1r	50	$\overline{C1r}$
C1s	50	$\overline{C1s}$
C4	500	C4a, $\underline{C4b}$
C2	25	C2a, $\underline{C2b}$
C3	1200	C3a, C3b
Alternative pathway		
Factor B	200	Ba, $\overline{Bb}$
Factor D	1–5	$\overline{D}$
Properdin	25	
Membrane attack (common) pathway		
C5	75	C5a, C5b
C6	60	
C7	55	
C8	55	
C9	60	
Regulatory proteins		
$\overline{C1}$ INH	200	
Factor 1	25	
C4bBP	250	
Factor H	500	
S protein	500	
Anaphylatoxin inactivator	30	

$\overline{C1}$ INH = C1 esterase inhibitor; C4bBP = C4 binding protein.

3. If further proteolysis results in loss of fragment activity, an "i" is added to indicate **inactivation** (e.g., i C 3 b).

4. A horizontal bar over the numeral of a component (e.g., $\overline{C1}$) indicates that the complement protein is in an activated state.

5. Components of the **alternative pathway** are designated by a capital letter (e.g., factor B, factor H).

C. **Genetics.** Most complement proteins have been found to have polymorphic genetic variants. Most variants are specified by autosomal codominant genes.

1. Genes for several **complement proteins** (e.g., factor B, C2, C4) are located in the major histocompatibility complex (MHC) on human chromosome 6 in a region called class III.

2. **Congenital deficiencies** of each of the component proteins except factor B (of the alternative pathway) have been observed in humans.
   a. **Heterozygous** individuals have approximately half the normal amount of the protein in question, and usually suffer **no ill effects.**
   b. Many of those with **homozygous** deficiency suffer from **immune complex diseases** or from **increased susceptibility to bacterial infections.**

D. **Activation of the complement system generates a wide range of biologic activities.** These can be grouped into three major functions.

1. **Opsonic function.** Opsonization occurs when activated complement components coat pathogenic organisms or immune complexes, facilitating the process of phagocytosis.

2. **Inflammatory function.** Activation of the complement system results in the release of histamine from mast cells and basophils, and it also stimulates the inflammatory response.

3. **Cytotoxic function.** In the final stage of the complement cascade, the membranes of target cells (e.g., bacteria and red blood cells) are attacked, leading to cell destruction.

II. PATHWAYS OF COMPLEMENT ACTIVATION. The activation of complement components takes place in a cascading sequence, each component activating its successor protein in the cascade.

A. **Complement activation may occur by two pathways: the classical pathway and the alternative pathway.** Comparisons between both pathways are listed in Table 4-2. Both pathways can be divided into three phases:

1. **Initiation phase.** This phase consists of a recognition event, which initiates the complement cascade. The classical and alternative pathways differ at this phase.

2. **Amplification phase.** During this phase, activation of early complement components culminates in activation of C3, which is a critical component. As in the initiation phase, the classical and alternative pathways also differ at this phase.

3. **Membrane attack phase.** This phase culminates in target cell lysis. **The classical and alternative pathways share a common final pathway for this phase.**

B. The **classical pathway** is activated through antigen–antibody complexes.

1. Classically, an **antigen–antibody complex** is designated EA, where E is the antigen (erythrocyte in the original historical observations), and A is the antibody.
   a. Other antigens can substitute for E, and EA might not represent an antigen–antibody complex but an antibody-coated bacterial cell, a tumor cell, or a lymphocyte.
   b. Complement components bind to EA in an orderly sequence to form a macromolecular complex, **EAC142356789.** The numerals are arranged in the order in which components bind to the complex.

2. Activation follows the binding of complement component C1 to a site on the Fc fragment of the immunoglobulin. The site is the C_H2 domain on IgG or C_H3 on IgM.

3. Native IgG and IgM molecules do not interact with C1q and activate the complement

TABLE 4-2. Comparisons Between the Classical and Alternative Pathways

Classical Pathway	Alternative Pathway
Specific adaptive immunity	Nonspecific innate immunity
Initiated by antibody, usually bound to antigen	Initiated by bacterial cell walls
Requires interaction of all nine major complement components	Does not require complement components C1, C4, and C2
Three phases: 　Initiation phase—different in both— 　Amplification phase—different in both— 　Membrane attack phase—final common pathway—	Three phases: 　Initiation phase 　Amplification phase 　Membrane attack phase

cascade. The site of interaction is obstructed and unavailable in uncomplexed immunoglobulin molecules. Once the antibody reacts (complexes) with an antigen, the tertiary structure of the molecule changes, exposing the C1q-reactive site on the heavy chain. The complement cascade then can be initiated.

4. The immunoglobulins that are most efficient in reacting with complement are **IgG (mainly IgG1 and IgG3) and IgM.**
   a. Only one molecule of pentameric IgM is required, whereas at least two adjacent molecules of the monomer IgG are needed. Thus, the antibody density (i.e., the number of molecules in close proximity) is a limiting factor in IgG activation of complement. It is estimated that 1000 IgG molecules must be on a membrane before any two will be in close enough proximity to activate C1q.
   b. **IgG4, IgA, IgD, and IgE** do not activate the classic complement cascade at all in their native configuration. IgG2 binds complement weakly.
   c. In the laboratory, aggregated and denatured immunoglobulins also have been shown to activate complement.

5. **Components and steps** of the classical pathway (Figure 4-1)
   a. **C1 (the recognition unit)** is a trimolecular complex. That is, it contains **three polypeptides—C1q, C1r, and C1s**—held together by calcium ions. With the removal of the calcium, C1 breaks down into its three subunits and loses activity.
      (1) **C1q** is the portion of the C1 molecule that attaches first to immunoglobulin and initiates complement activation.
         (a) C1q has six binding sites, globular structures extending on stalks from a central core (see Figure 4-1).
         (b) Because of its multivalency, C1q can cross-link multiple immunoglobulin molecules, which is a requirement for activation.
         (c) To initiate the process of complement activation, two or more of the six globular domains of C1q interact with the C_H domains of at least two immunoglobulin monomers.
         (d) C1q binding breaks a peptide bond and activates C1r proenzyme to an active serine protease.
      (2) **C1r,** when activated, cleaves the proenzyme C1s.
      (3) **C1s,** when activated, becomes another serine protease, referred to as C1 esterase (C1s) because of its esterase activity.
         (a) C1s mediates the cleavage of native C4, the next component in the complement cascade.
         (b) One molecule of C1s can cleave several C4 molecules, thus serving as one of the sites in the amplification process.
   b. **C1s cleaves C4 into C4a and C4b.**
      (1) **C4a,** the weakest of the three **anaphylatoxins,** is released into the surrounding medium (i.e., the fluid phase). An anaphylatoxin is a complement fragment that has the ability to stimulate mast-cell degranulation and the release of vasoactive amines.
      (2) **C4b** can bind to cell membranes. The binding is rather inefficient, but several C4b molecules may cluster around C1s on the membrane surface.
   c. Once bound to the C4b molecule, the next component becomes **susceptible to enzymatic attack by the C1s serine protease.**
      (1) **C2b** is activated to become the third serine protease in the cascade. Its substrates are C3 and C5 (Table 4-3).
      (2) C2b remains linked to the cell-bound C4b, thus forming the enzymatically active bimolecular complex **C4b2b.**
         (a) Formation of the C4b2b complex requires **magnesium ions.**
         (b) C4b2b is referred to as classical pathway **C3 convertase** because it cleaves C3.
         (c) **C2b** is the enzymatic molecule in the C4b2b and C4b2b3b complexes. The other molecules in the complex serve as docking, or attachment, vehicles, which hold the substrates in position for enzymatic attack.

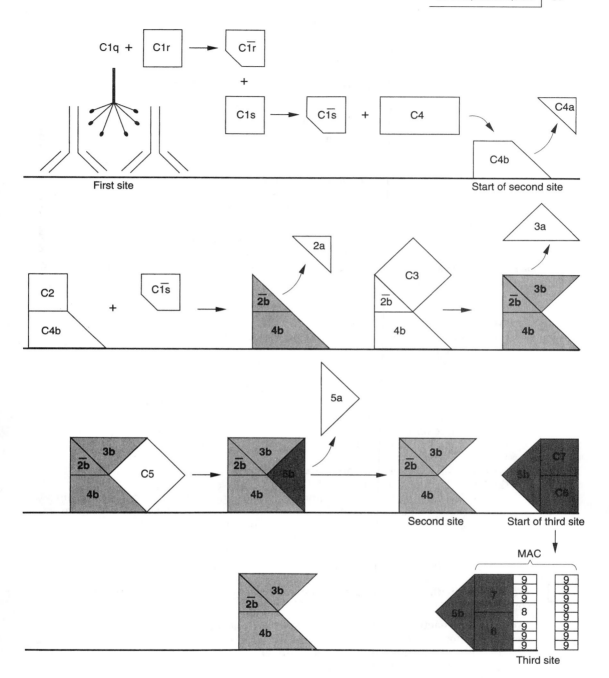

FIGURE 4-1. The classical pathway of complement activation. A *line over a component* indicates the activated form. These molecules are deposited on an activating surface at three distinct sites. The antibody molecules react with the C1q molecule, which then binds C1r and C1s; C1s becomes activated and cleaves C4. The C4b fragment attaches to the surface at a second site; C2 and C3 then interact. The membrane attack complex (MAC) portion of the cascade occupies a third site when C5 is cleaved, and the C5b molecule attaches to the membrane. The different locations are shown in the figure by changes in the shading of the complexes: The second site is *shaded lightly* and the third site is *shaded darkly*.

TABLE 4-3. Serine Proteases Generated During Complement Activation

Protease	Substrate	Comments
C1r	C1s	These molecules are part of the calcium-dependent trimolecular $C1q/C1r_2/C1s_2$ complex
C1s	C4, C2	C4 is the first cleaved; it binds C2 and helps to position it for efficient cleavage into C2a and enzymatically active C2b
C2	C3	Protease is active as $\overline{C2b}$ in the $\overline{C4b2b}$ complex; C4b binds and positions C3 for cleavage
	C5	Protease is active as $\overline{C2b}$ in the $\overline{C4b2b3b}$ complex; C3b binds and positions C5 for cleavage
D	B	B is bound by C3b on the activator surface and is cleaved by $\overline{D}$ to yield enzymatically active $\overline{Bb}$
B	C3, C5	Needs stabilization by properdin; protease is active as $\overline{\overline{Bb}}$ in C3bBbP and C3bBb3BP; in the latter complex, first C3b binds and positions B; second C3b positions C5

C designates a component of the classic pathway; D, B, and P (properdin) are proteins of the alternative pathway.

    (3) The smaller peptide, designated **C2a,** is released into the fluid phase.
    (4) The nomenclature of the split products of C2 is cumbersome in that, by convention, the portion that binds to the membrane is termed C2a, whereas the peptide split product is termed C2b. This is the opposite usage of the letter designations for the rest of the complement proteins. [For simplicity and consistency in this book, the **"b"** designation will be used for all products that **bind** to a membrane, and **"a"** will be used for the peptide split products that diffuse **away,** most of which have **anaphylatoxin** activity.]
  d. **The substrate for C3 convertase is C3.** Circulating C3 binds to the C4b portion of the C4b2b complex. This binding renders C3 subject to cleavage by C2b into two fragments, C3a and C3b.
    (1) **C3a** is an anaphylatoxin and remains unbound.
    (2) **C3b** is a major component in the complement system, with several key roles:
      (a) The C3b bound to the membrane in the vicinity of the C4b2b complex forms the trimolecular enzymatic complex C4b2b3b (i.e., convertase). This complex acts on C5, which is the first component of the membrane attack pathway.
      (b) C3b binds the C5 molecule and positions it for cleavage by C2b.
      (c) C3b initiates the alternative complement pathway.
      (d) C3b has several other important biologic properties (see IV B 2).

C. The **alternative pathway** is considered to be a primitive defense system; a bypass mechanism that does not require C1, C4, and C2 (Figure 4-2).

  1. **Activation by bacterial products** has immense biologic significance: It represents a primitive defense mechanism by which the body can activate inflammatory processes and opsonize pathogens for phagocytic destruction.
    a. **Substances capable of activating complement by the alternative pathway include:**
      (1) **Polysaccharides of microbial origin**
        (a) Lipopolysaccharides of gram-negative bacteria (e.g., endotoxins)
        (b) Teichoic acids of gram-positive bacteria (e.g., adhesion molecules of some pathogens)
        (c) Zymosan from yeast cell walls
      (2) **Surface components of some animal parasites** (e.g., *Schistosoma mansoni* larvae)
    b. These cell wall components (polysaccharides) appear to protect C3b from inactivation by the regulatory proteins H and I (i.e., factors H and I) [see V A 1; B 2].

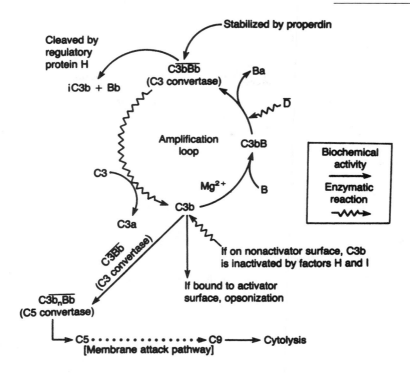

FIGURE 4-2. The alternative pathway of complement activation.

2. **Activation by immunoglobulins** occurs when antibodies that are unable to interact with C1q in their native state are aggregated, either chemically or by mild heating. The biologic significance of this pathway of activation is unclear.

3. The **initial recognition event** for alternative pathway activation is the presence of C3, specifically **C3b,** which is continuously present in very small amounts in normal serum.
   a. **Factor B (the C3 proactivator)**
      (1) The surface-bound, protected C3b interacts with factor B to form C3bB, a **magnesium-dependent complex.**
      (2) Factor B is analogous to C2 of the classical pathway.
   b. **Factor D** is a serine protease resembling C1s.
      (1) Factor B, when bound to C3b is susceptible to enzymatic cleavage by factor D.
      (2) Two fragments are formed, Ba and Bb.
         (a) The Ba fragment is released; it is chemotactic for neutrophils.
         (b) An active site is exposed in the Bb fragment, which remains bound to C3b, forming the enzymatically active C3bBb complex.
            (i) C3bBb is the **alternative pathway C3 convertase.**
            (ii) The C3b molecule serves to bind substrate, which may be either more C3 molecules or C5 molecules, and hold it for enzymatic action of the activated serine protease, Bb.
   c. **Properdin (P)** is a protein that stabilizes the C3bBb complex.
      (1) In the presence of properdin, the dissociation of Bb is slowed, stabilizing the C3bBb complex.
      (2) When stabilized by properdin, the C3bBb complex becomes a C3 convertase that cleaves C3 and generates more C3b.
      (3) As more C3b is generated, the complex expands, with numerous C3b molecules attached to a single Bb (C3b$_n$Bb, where n > 1), and becomes a C5 convertase capable of cleaving C5 and thereby **initiating the membrane attack pathway.**

    d. Inhibition. Initiation by C3b is prevented by interaction with factors H and I.

        (1) If C3b binds to a nonactivator (i.e., nonprotected) surface, it reacts with factor H and becomes inactivated through the combined actions of factors H and I.

        (2) If C3b binds to an activator (i.e., protected) surface, its ability to bind to factor H is diminished, and it can activate the alternative pathway.

D. **Many of the components of the complement system are enzymes; therefore, the potential for self-amplification is tremendous.** When activated, several of the components of the complement cascade become serine proteases or serine esterases (see Table 4-3).

    1. The substrates for these serine proteases are not hydrolyzed by the enzymes until they are bound into the complex by a "positioning" molecule.

    2. For example, C4b holds C3 so that $\overline{C2b}$ can hydrolyze it. Similarly, C3b holds C5 so that $\overline{C2b}$ can act on it.

III. THE MEMBRANE ATTACK PATHWAY (THE COMMON PATHWAY).

The convergence of the classical and alternative pathways occurs at the point of C5 activation.

A. **Activation of the membrane attack pathway is initiated by C5 convertase.**

    1. C5 convertase is:

        a. $\overline{C4b2b3b}$ in the classical pathway

        b. $C3b_nBb$ in the alternative pathway

    2. These C5 convertases are the only components in the attack pathway that have enzymatic activity.

        a. Thus, substrate cleavage of C5 into C5a and C5b occurs only once in the attack sequence.

        b. Subsequent steps involve spontaneous binding and polymerization of intact proteins.

B. There are **five components** in this portion of the pathway.

    1. C5 convertase cleaves C5 into a smaller C5a fragment and a larger C5b fragment.

        a. C5a, an anaphylatoxin and chemotactic factor, is released into the surrounding fluid medium.

        b. C5b is the first component of the membrane attack complex. As such, it is the receptor for C6 and C7, and it initiates assembly of the terminal components, C8 and C9.

    2. Unstable C5b binds to C6 to form a stable C5b6 complex. C5b6 then binds to C7 to form the metastable trimolecular C5b67 complex, which attaches to the target cell membrane without inflicting any damage.

    3. Formation of the membrane attack C8 and C9 complex (MAC) begins when C8 attaches to the membrane-bound C5b67 complex to form C5b678. The addition of C9 to the complex forms **C5b6789,** the MAC.

    4. C9 shares a great deal of amino acid homology with the perforin molecule. Perforin causes membrane damage when it is released from the cytoplasmic granules of T lymphocytes and NK cells. Because C9 is homologous to perforin, C9 also can cause the same type of membrane damage.

    5. Cell lysis can occur when the C5b678 complex forms. In the absence of C9, tiny (3 nm) pores form in the membrane, and the cells become somewhat leaky.

        a. The polymerization of C9 greatly accelerates cell lysis.

        b. The C9 polymer forms a **cylindrical transmembrane channel** (Figure 4-3 inset). Attached to the channel is the C5b678 complex.

        c. The hollow cylindrical channels of the MAC are in the lipid bilayer of the cell membrane.

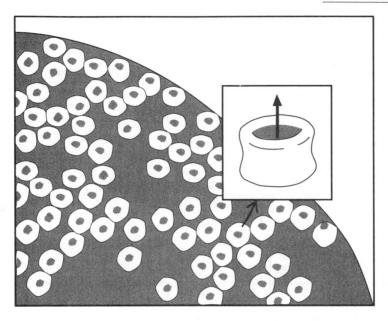

FIGURE 4-3. Effect of membrane attack complex (MAC; C5b6789) on cell membrane. *Inset* shows a schematic diagram of the transmembrane channel formed by polymerized C9 molecules, which allow water and ions to cross the cell membrane, leading to cell lysis. The top of the C9 polymer cylinder is hydrophilic and is capped by a ring that remains outside the cell. The other end of the cylinder is lipophilic and forms the transmembrane channel.

    d. The channels coalesce into leaky patches, and the surface of the membrane is covered with craters and looks like the surface of the moon (see Figure 4-3).
    e. **The channels allow the passage of electrolytes and water across the membrane, leading ultimately to osmotic lysis of the target cells.** Thus, the process of cell lysis is nonenzymatic.

IV. BIOLOGIC CONSEQUENCES OF COMPLEMENT ACTIVATION (Table 4-4)

A. Overview

1. During complement activation, a number of materials with important biologic activities are generated.
    a. The **cleavage products (split products)** of C3, C4, and C5 appear to be the most important complement components in terms of **biologic functions** associated with the inflammatory response.
    b. **C8 and C9** play a major role in membrane attack and the lytic process.

2. **Cell receptors** that have complement fragments for their homologous ligands have significant biologic roles (Table 4-5).
    a. Some receptors (e.g., CR3) react with larger fragments (e.g., C3b) and promote opsonization and, therefore, phagocytosis.
    b. Other receptors (e.g., C3aR) are specific for the smaller "a" fragments that play a role in inflammatory processes.
    c. The CR1 receptor on human erythrocytes provides an important mechanism for clearing immune complexes from the circulation. They bind the complexes and transport them to the liver and spleen, where they are engulfed by phagocytic cells.

TABLE 4-4. Principal Inflammatory Activities of Activated Complement Proteins and Their Fragments

Component	Activity
C3a, C5a	Anaphylatoxin—releases histamine, and other vasoactive compounds from basophils and mast cells, increasing capillary permeability
C3b, iC3b, C4b	Immune adherence and opsonization—binds antigen—antibody complexes to membranes of macrophages and neutrophils, enhancing phagocytosis; also binds complexes to erythrocytes, facilitating removal by the liver and spleen
C5a	Chemotaxis and chemokinesis—attracts phagocytic cells to sites of inflammation and increases their overall activity
C8, C9	Membrane damage—transmembrane channels form, permitting flux of cytoplasmic constituents. Mammalian cells swell and burst; bacterial cells become leaky and lose vital intracellular metabolites, but usually do not burst
Ba	Neutrophil chemotaxis
Bb	Macrophage activation—causes macrophages to adhere to surfaces and spread on them

TABLE 4-5. Complement Receptors of Human Cells

Receptor	Ligands	Cell Types	Functions
CR1	C4b, C3b, iC3b	Erythrocytes, phagocytes, B cells, eosinophils	Opsonin: cofactor in factor 1 cleavage of C3b to C3dg; clearance of antigen–antibody complexes*
CR2	iC3b, C3d, C3dg, C3b	B cells, some T cells, NK cells	Immunoregulatory; attachment site for Epstein-Barr virus
CR3	iC3b	Phagocytes	Opsonin; cofactor in iC3b degradation
CR4	C3b, iC3b, C3dg	Phagocytes	Not established; presumably an opsonin
C3aR	C3a	Mast cells, basophils, eosinophils, smooth muscle, phagocytes	Release of histamine and other mediators
C4aR	C4a	Mast cells, basophils	May be same as C3a receptor; same effects as C3a
C5aR	C5a	Mast cells, basophils	Same effects as C3a

NK cell = natural killer cell; PMN = polymorphonuclear neutrophil.

*Immune complexes bind rapidly to erythrocytes (by immune adherence) and are tansported to the liver and spleen, where macrophages strip the complexes from the cell surface and return the erythrocyte to the circulation.

B. **Cleavage products of C3 and C5**

   1. **C3a and C5a** are **anaphylatoxins.**
      a. **Shared characteristics**
         (1) C3a and C5a **react with specific receptors** (i.e., C3aR and C5aR) on basophil and mast cell membranes.
            (a) This reaction causes the **release of pharmacologic mediators of inflammation** (e.g., histamine) in a manner that is similar to mediator release by IgE.
            (b) The mediators cause **smooth muscle contraction and increased vascular per-**

meability, which are effects that can be counteracted by antihistamines and anaphylatoxin inactivator.

    (2) C3a and C5a also appear to have the ability to **contract smooth muscle and increase capillary permeability** directly (i.e., without the mediation of mast cells and basophils).

  b. C5a is much more active than C3a on a molar basis and, in addition to anaphylatoxin activity, has a **wider range of biologic activity,** including the following:

    (1) C5a is the major complement-derived chemotactic factor in serum.

      (a) Chemotaxis. C5a causes neutrophils and macrophages to migrate toward the site where C5a is generated (i.e., chemotaxis).

      (b) Chemokinesis. C5a also increases the overall activity of phagocytic cells (i.e., chemokinesis).

    (2) C5a **causes neutrophils to adhere** to the endothelium of vessels and to one another, which leads to cell diapedesis into inflammatory sites.

    (3) C5a **activates neutrophils,** which triggers a bactericidal oxidative burst and degranulation.

    (4) C5a **stimulates the production of leukotrienes** [e.g., slow-reacting substance of anaphylaxis (SRS-A)] by mast cells.

  c. C5a-des-arg is C5a without the carboxy-terminal arginine, which is removed by anaphylatoxin inactivator. C5a-des-arg lacks the anaphylatoxin activity of C5a, but it retains chemotactic and neutrophil- activating ability.

2. The generation of C3b and the coating of target cells by C3b are perhaps the major biologic functions of complement.

  a. The role of C3b in the **activation of the alternative complement pathway** was described in II C.

  b. C3b is a major factor in **opsonization.**

    (1) Several cell types have **surface receptors** for C3b and iC3b, including neutrophils, eosinophils, monocytes, macrophages, B cells, basophils, and primate erythrocytes.

    (2) In the case of **phagocytic cells,** a coating of C3b on particles such as bacteria or antigen–antibody complexes promotes the attachment and ultimate ingestion of the particles.

    (3) Clinical importance. Individuals who have low levels of C3 or whose phagocytic cells do not bear a C3bR molecule suffer from **recurrent pyogenic infections.**

3. C3 nephritic factor (C3NeF) is an antibody against C3 converlase of the alternative pathway. It is found in the circulation of patients with mesangiocapillary glomerulonephritis.

C. **C4 and its cleavage products**

  1. Activated C4 molecules attach to membranes in proximity to the C1 site. The binding of C1 and C4 by a virus–antibody complex can **neutralize virus activity.**

  2. C4a has weak **anaphylatoxin** activity.

  3. C4b receptor sites exist on several cell types (e.g., phagocytic cells), which suggests that C4b is involved in opsonization.

D. **C2.** C2 cleavage has been reported to be linked to the production of a kinin-like molecule that increases vascular permeability and contracts smooth muscle. C2a is thought to be involved in the symptoms seen in hereditary angioneurotic edema (HANE; see V B 1 b).

E. **Ba and Bb.** These two factors are generated exclusively by the alternative pathway.

  1. Ba has been reported to have chemotactic activity.

  2. Bb activates macrophages and causes them to adhere to and spread on surfaces.

F. **C8 and C9**

  1. Function. C8 and C9 are responsible for the membrane damage that causes the lysis of bacteria and other cells.

2. **Clinical importance.** Absence of C8 is accompanied by an increased incidence and/or severity of *Neisseria meningitidis* and *Neisseria gonorrhoeae* infections.

G. **Interaction of the complement system with other systems is a common characteristic of the complement cascade.**

1. **Complement activation, kinin generation, blood coagulation, and fibrinolysis** all are physiologic processes that occur through the sequential activation of enzymes in cascading fashion. These cascades interact with each other, sharing some activators, inhibitors, and cell membrane receptors.

2. **Tissue injury can initiate each of the cascades.** For example, neutrophils are attracted to the site of injury by the chemotactically active C5a that is cleaved from C5 by proteases released from lysosomes (Figure 4-4).

3. Cascade-initiating factors can be activated by contact with **negatively charged surfaces,** such as heparin or lipid A of the lipopolysaccharide from gram-negative bacteria. **Hageman factor** (HF; coagulation factor XII) is thereby activated, producing HFa, which has serine protease activity.

4. Three proteins—HFa, prekallikrein, and high–molecular-weight kininogen—are also the initiating factors required for the **intrinsic blood coagulation and fibrinolytic pathways.**
   a. **HFa,** by activating coagulation factor XI, **initiates the blood clotting cascade.**
   b. HFa also activates prekallikrein to kallikrein, which in turn activates plasmin.
      (1) Plasmin can activate HF and can initiate the complement cascade.
      (2) Plasmin also releases chemotactic and vasoactive fibrinopeptides from fibrin.

5. **Inhibiting factors**
   a. **C1 esterase inhibitor ($\overline{C1}$ INH)** of the complement system is an important control mechanism in various cascading processes (see V B 1).
   b. In addition to inhibiting the serine protease activity of $\overline{C1s}$, $\overline{C1}$ INH inhibits HF, factor XI, plasmin, and kallikrein.

V. **REGULATORY MECHANISMS.** Complement activation is associated with potent biologic functions that, if left unchecked, exhaust the complement system and can cause sig-

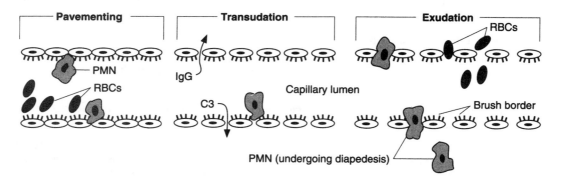

FIGURE 4-4. Biologic activities of component split products that contribute to an acute inflammatory response. This response is usually protective, but if exaggerated it may lead to tissue destruction. The inflammatory response, spurred on by microbial invasion or tissue damage, occurs in three stages. In *pavementing,* the endothelial cells become sticky, and the polymorphonuclear cells (*PMNs*) adhere. C5a is active in this stage. In *transudation,* proteins leave the lumen of the capillaries. C5a and C3a act on mast cells during this stage to cause mediator (e.g., histamine) release. In *exudation,* cells [e.g., PMNs and red blood cells (*RBCs*)] leave the capillaries via diapedesis. Once the cells leave the capillaries, opsonization and phagocytosis can occur.

nificant damage to the host. Uncontrolled activation of the complement system is prevented by several types of protein–complement interactions.

A. **Some serum proteins enzymatically attack complement components, thereby inactivating them.**

1. **Factor I,** the C3b inactivator, is a serine protease that degrades C3b into a product that is incapable of functioning in the C4b2b3b complex.

2. **Anaphylatoxin inactivator** (i.e., serum carboxypeptidase N) enzymatically destroys the biologic activity of C3a, C4a, and C5a by removing the carboxy-terminal arginine.

B. **Some serum proteins bind to, and thus inhibit, complement components.**

1. **$C\bar{1}$ INH**
   a. **Inhibitory effects.** $C\bar{1}$ INH inhibits the enzymatic activity of $C\bar{1}$ esterase by dissociating the subunits C1q, C1r, and C1s. It also inhibits plasmin, kallikrein, activated HF, and coagulation factor XIa.
   b. **Clinical importance.** Deficiency of $C\bar{1}$ INH results in hereditary angioneurotic edema **(HANE),** which is an inherited defect characterized by transient but recurrent episodes of local edema due to uncontrolled C1s activity.

2. **Factor H** acts with factor I to bind C3b and to allow factor I to cleave the α chain of C3b. This leads to formation of cleavage product iC3b, which does not interact with the alternative pathway components.

3. **S protein (vitronectin)** protects the target cell from lysis by binding to the developing fluid-phase C5b67 complex. It does not stop the MAC from forming, but prevents it from penetrating the lipid layer of the cell membrane.

C. **Regulatory proteins in cell membranes**

1. **Decay-accelerating factor (DAF)** has the same function as factor H; it inactivates membrane-bound C3b and C4b, whereas factor H acts on C3b and C4b in solution.
   a. **Function.** DAF prevents assembly of the two C3 convertases by promoting dissociation of C2b from C4b and Bb from C3b.
   b. **Clinical importance.** DAF is deficient or absent from cells in people with **paroxysmal nocturnal hemoglobinuria (PNH).** The red blood cells of these patients have increased sensitivity to complement-mediated lysis.

2. **Membrane cofactor protein** is an integral membrane protein that serves as a cofactor for the proteolytic inactivation of C4b and C3b by factor I.

Vignette Revisited

1. The classical pathway is activated via antigen–antibody complexes. The alternative pathway may be triggered either immunlogically, when antibodies that are unable to interact with C1q in their native state are aggregated, or nonimmunologically, by certain cell products such as lipopolysaccharides of gram-negative bacteria, teichoic acids of gram-positive bacteria, or zymosan from yeast cell walls.

   The biologic functions of complement include the following: membrane attack complex (C5–C9) formation promotes lysis of cells and kills microorganisms; C3b or iC3b on the surface of microorganisms binds to CR1 (and CR3, CR4) on neutrophils and macrophages, promoting phagocytosis; C5a, C3a, and C4a stimulate mast cell histamine release and smooth muscle contraction; C5a is a chemoattractant for neutrophils and activates neutrophil oxidative metabolism; complement activation on immunoglobulin molecules inhibits immune complex formation; C3b on immune complexes binds to CR1 on erythrocytes, and the immune complexes are cleared from the circulation as the erythrocytes traverse the liver and spleen (Table 4-6).

2. Even when properly regulated and activated, the complement system can cause sig-

TABLE 4-6. Summary of the Biologic Functions of the Complement System

Inflammation
    Mast cell granulation
    Chemotaxis
    ↑ Vascular permeability
    PMN margination and diapedesis
    Smooth muscle contraction
    PMN, NK, and macrophage activation

Clearance of immune complexes

Cell lysis
    Gram-negative bacteria
    Protozoa
    Enveloped viruses

Viral neutralization

Opsonization

These functions are activated by either the alternative (antibody-independent) or classic pathways (antibody-mediated) and hence are part of the innate as well as the acquired immune systems. In most instances the participation of antibody will accentuate the effect.

nificant tissue damage, especially in people with immune complex diseases. Immune complex glomerulonephritis and systemic vasculitis may result from the deposition of antigen–antibody complexes in glomeruli and blood vessel walls. Complement activated by the immunoglobulin in these deposited immune complexes initiates the acute inflammatory responses that destroy the glomeruli or vessel walls, leading to thrombosis, ischemic damage to tissues, and scarring.

A variety of deficiencies in many of the complement proteins have been described and are mostly attributable to genetic mutations. Defects in classical pathway activation have been associated with systemic lupus erythematosus, glomerulonephritis, pyogenic infections, and vasculitis. Alternative pathway activation defects most commonly result in pyogenic infections. Abnormalities in membrane attack complex formation are associated with disseminated *Neisseria* infections, systemic lupus erythematosus, and glomerulonephritis.

Deficiencies in complement regulatory proteins are associated with abnormal complement activation and a variety of related clinical abnormalities. Hereditary angioneurotic edema (HANE) is an autosomal dominant deficiency in C1 inhibitor manifested by acute, intermittent attacks of skin and mucosal edema. Paroxysmal nocturnal hemoglobinuria is a complement-mediated intravascular hemolysis caused by deficiencies in the integral membrane protein regulators decay-accelerating factor (DAF), homologous restriction factor (HRF), and protectin (CD59). Abnormalities in factor I or factor H result in deregulated classical pathway activation, with consumption of C3, and are associated with pyogenic infections, vasculitis, and glomerulonephritis.

1. A patient is admitted to the hospital with a history of multiple bacterial infections. Laboratory results indicate that he is devoid of the third complement component. Which of the following complement-associated events would still be present in such a patient?

(A) Bacteriolysis
(B) Bacterial opsonization
(C) Chemotaxis
(D) Hemolysis
(E) Hereditary angioneurotic edema (HANE)

2. The patient presents with anorexia, malaise, puffy eyelids, and abdominal pain. Significant laboratory data include marked proteinuria and a unique protein, C3 nephritic factor (C3NeF), in the patient's serum. C3NeF is an antibody against

(A) C3bBb
(B) glomerular antigens
(C) C5b6789
(D) C3a
(E) C3b

3. Which of the following is a potent opsonizing protein of the complement system?

(A) C1r
(B) C1s
(C) C2b
(D) C3b
(E) Bb

4. Antibody is the major serum factor that neutralizes virus activities; however, some complement proteins have also been ascribed such a role. Which of the following has such an antiviral activity?

(A) C2
(B) C4
(C) C5b6789
(D) C3bBb
(E) C3b

5. An otherwise apparently healthy 12-year-old girl presents to the emergency department with a grossly swollen lower lip. Pertinent historically is the fact that she had a canine tooth extracted earlier in the day. A tentative diagnosis of hereditary angioneurotic edema is made. Which protein listed below is associated with this genetic disease?

(A) C2
(B) C9
(C) C3bBb
(D) Decay accelerating factor
(E) Factor I

6. Which of the following proteins activates macrophages and also causes them to become sticky and adhere to the vascular endothelium?

(A) C3b
(B) C4b
(C) C3a
(D) C4a
(E) Bb

7. Systemic anaphylaxis is a life-threatening allergic reaction that kills hundreds of people in the United States each year. One of the proteins in the body that protects humans from this reaction is anaphylatoxin inactivator, a serum enzyme that destroys the biologic activity of

(A) C1a
(B) C2a
(C) C2b
(D) C3b
(E) C5a

8. Complement regulatory proteins that are active in the cell membrane include

(A) C1q
(B) C1 esterase inhibitor (C1 INH)
(C) Factor I
(D) Decay-accelerating factor (DAF)
(E) Factor H

9. Which of the following complement components are required exclusively in the classical pathway?

(A) C1, C2, C4
(B) C5, C6, C7
(C) C3
(D) C8, C9
(E) Properdin

10. The lipopolysaccharide in the outer membrane of gram-negative bacteria can serve as a protective surface and activate complement. The protein in the alternative cascade that is stabilized by properdin is

(A) C5b6789
(B) C1q
(C) C3bBb
(D) C3a
(E) C3b

11. Which of the following proteins activate neutrophils and also causes them to become sticky and adhere to the vascular endothelium?

(A) C3a
(B) C4b
(C) C3bBb
(D) C5a
(E) C5b6789

1. The answer is E [II C; IV B; V B 1]. The third complement component (C3) is the junction for both the classical and the alternative pathways of complement activation. Most of the biologic activities are expressed after this point in the cascade. Thus, lytic phenomena, such as bacteriolysis and hemolysis, are the result of membrane damage caused by the terminal membrane attack complex of the cascade. The major opsonin, C3b, would obviously be absent in a C3-deficient individual, as would the inability to generate the chemotaxins C3a and C5a. There might be slight chemotactic activity because of C4a, but this would be minimal at best. The propensity to develop immune complex diseases is accentuated in individuals who lack the early components C1, C2, and C4. Hereditary angioneurotic edema (HANE) occurs in individuals who are deficient in the inhibitor of C1 esterase. This disease is characterized by swelling of the face, neck, genitalia, and extremities that is accompanied by abdominal cramps and vomiting. Laryngeal swelling can be life-threatening. Attacks occur after surgical trauma and severe stress. C1 esterase is activated and splits C2, releasing the C2a peptide that causes increased capillary permeability with resultant edema. Because C1, C4, and C2 all participate in the complement cascade before the entry of C3, a deficiency in the latter molecule would not interfere with the development of HANE.

2. The answer is A [IV B 3]. C3 nephritic factor (C3NeF) is a pathologic component of the alternative complement pathway that is found in the circulation of patients with mesangiocapillary glomerulonephritis. C3NeF is an antibody against the C3bBb complex and leads to significant nephrotic disease accompanied by a marked hypocomplementemia. Antibodies against glomerular antigens are seen in Goodpasture's disease (the specific antigen is type IV collagen). There are no autoimmune diseases characterized by antibodies against classical pathway complement proteins.

3. The answer is D [IV B 2 b; Table 4-3] C3b is a potent opsonin that sensitizes bacteria and other foreign particles to phagocytosis. Neutrophils and macrophages have on their membranes a receptor (CR3) that reacts with C3b and holds the microbe in close proximity to the phagocytic cell, thus enhancing the engulfment process. Five serine proteases become activated in the complement cascade: C1r, C1s, C2b, and factors D and B (as Bb). These serine proteases are proteolytic enzymes that cleave the next components in the cascade.

4. The answer is B [IV C 1]. The binding of C1 and C4 by a virus–antibody complex can neutralize virus activity; it is probable that the C4 prevents viral attachment to target cells. In the alternative pathway, the C3bBb complex is cleaved by factor D. The Ba fragment is released, and the C3bBb complex, stabilized by properdin, becomes a C3 convertase. C2 is thought to be involved in the symptoms of hereditary angioneurotic edema, a disease caused by uncontrolled C1 esterase activity. C2 cleavage has been reported to be linked to the production of a kinin-like molecule (C2a) that increases vascular permeability and contracts smooth muscle. C3b plays an important role in opsonization. C5b6789 is the membrane attack complex generated by either the alternative or the classical pathways while C3bBb is the C3 convertase of the alternative pathway.

5. The answer is A [IV D]. C2 is involved in the symptoms of hereditary angioneurotic edema, a disease caused by uncontrolled C1 esterase activity. C2 cleavage has been reported to be linked to the production of a kinin-like molecule that increases vascular permeability and contracts smooth muscle. C9 is the protein that polymerizes in the membrane and causes leakage of cytosol from the cell. C3bBb is the C3 convertase of the alternative pathway that is stabilized by properdin. Decay accelerating factor is one of the control proteins that down regulates the complement cascade. Factor I is a serine protease that inactivates C3b.

6. The right answer is E [IV E 2]. Factor B of the alternative pathway is cleaved by factor D. The larger fragment, Bb, activates macrophages and causes them to adhere to vascular endothelium and other body surfaces. C3B is the major opsonic product of the complement system. The other peptide derived from proteolysis of C3 (C3a) is an anaphylotoxin that causes histamine release from mast cells and basophils. C4b is a split product of C4 that binds to membranes and serves to position other complement proteins for proteolysis by the esterases of the classical pathway cascade. C4a is a weak anaphylotoxin that may be involved in local edema such as that seen in hereditary angioneurotic edema.

7. The answer is E [V A 2]. C5a is destroyed by anaphylatoxin inactivator. C5a, and also C3a and C4a, are referred to as anaphylatoxins. They cause the release of vasoactive amines from mast cells and basophils; the amines, in turn, cause smooth muscle contraction and increased vascular permeability. Anaphylatoxin inactivator (serum carboxypeptidase N) removes the carboxy-terminal arginine residue from the anaphylatoxins, destroying their biologic activity.

8. The answer is D [V C 1]. Decay-accelerating factor (DAF) is found on the surface of many cells of the body. It prevents the assembly of C3 convertases by promoting dissociation of the enzymatically active fragments C2b and Bb from their membrane-associated ligands, C4b and C3b, respectively. DAF is not an integral membrane protein but is anchored to the membrane by attachment to phosphatidylinositol. C1 esterase inhibitor (C1 INH) controls the generation of vasoactive compounds from proteolysis of C2 and C4; a deficiency of this protein is associated with hereditary angioedema. Factor H and I are serum proteins that act in concert to cleave C3b.

9. The answer is A [II C]. The alternative pathway of complement activation does not re-

quire C1, C4, and C2, whereas the classical pathway cascade starts with these three proteins. The alternative pathway, also referred to as the properdin pathway, is considered to be a primitive defense system, a mechanism that bypasses components C1, C4, and C2. The initial requirement for the alternative pathway is the presence of C3, specifically C3b.

10. The answer is C [II C 3 c]. Properdin stabilizes the C3bBb complex. This is the C3 convertase of the alternative pathway. C5b6789 is the membrane attack complex. C1q is the complement component that reacts with the CH2 domain of IgG and IgM immunoglobulin molecules to initiate the classical cascade. C3 is proteolytically cleaved to C3a (anaphylotoxin I) and the potent opsonin, C3b.

11. The answer is D [IV B 1 b]. C5a is the peptide split product of C5 that has both anaphylactic and chemotactic activities. It also activates neutrophils to greater antimicrobial activity and causes the cells to express intercellular adhesion molecules that enhance neutrophil margination in the vascular system. Another anaphylotoxin, C3a, is also generated during complement activation; however, it does not have the wide variety of actions on neutrophils that C5a exhibits. C4b is a split product of C4 that binds to membranes and serves to position other complement proteins for proteolysis by the esterases of the cascade. C3bBb is the C3 convertase of the alternative pathway that is stabilized by properdin. C5b6789 is the membrane attack complex.

Chapter 5

The Immune Response System and Its Regulation

Vignette

An acutely ill 3-year-old boy was brought to the emergency department by his aunt. His breathing was extremely labored, and he had hemoptysis (i.e., blood-tinged, rust-colored sputum). Gram's stain of the sputum revealed numerous polymorphonuclear neutrophils and gram-positive cocci in grapelike clusters. A tentative diagnosis of staphylococcal pneumonia was made, and the child was hospitalized and placed on intravenous oxacillin. The aunt revealed that the child had experienced several similar episodes. She has been the child's daytime caretaker and had been able to control his previous infections successfully with antibiotics that she had in her medicine cabinet. The child also had problems with skin infections, such as boils, and had recently recovered from poison ivy. He contracted measles approximately 6 months before being admitted to the hospital and had recovered normally.

1. On the basis of the information obtained from the aunt, the physician was able to exclude what type of immune deficiency diseases from the differential diagnosis?

Laboratory data:

Leukocytes	14,800/mm^3
Platelets	200,000/mm^3
Hemoglobin	12 g/dl
Hematocrit	49%
Neutrophils	69%
Lymphocytes	21
Monocytes	5
Eosinophils	4
Basophils	1

2. Which, if any, of the above values seem abnormal?
   Leukocyte function studies also were performed. Chemotaxis, phagocytosis, and intracellular killing activities were all within normal limits. An immunoglobulin profile was ordered. The child had no detectable immunoglobulin A or M (IgA or IgM) in his serum. A small amount (30 mg/dl) of IgG was detected when the assay was repeated with low-level radial immunodiffusion plates.
3. From these additional laboratory data, what immunodeficiency is suspected?
4. What prophylactic measures would the physician likely recommend to prolong the life expectancy of this child?

I. HEMATOPOIESIS is the development of blood cells from the bone marrow.

A. **Myeloid cells.** An undifferentiated stem cell gives rise to the myeloid precursor cell. Myeloid precursor cells differentiate into progenitor cells of the **erythrocytic, granulocytic, and monocytic cell lines.** Of these, the monocytic line, which includes **monocytes and macrophages,** is directly involved in the adaptive immune response.

B. **Lymphoid cells.** The undifferentiated stem cell also gives rise to the **lymphoid precursor**

cell. The precursor cell further matures into three different types of lymphocytes. The **T and B lymphocytes** both contribute to the adaptive aspects of the immune response. A third type of lymphocyte, the **natural killer (NK) cell,** contributes to the innate (nonadaptive) side of the immune response.

II. MACROPHAGES

A. **Development.** Monocytes are found predominantly in the blood, and macrophages are primarily in tissues. Several chemical modulators assist in the conversion of the myeloid precursor cell into monocytes and macrophages. Notable among these are **granulocyte–monocyte colony stimulating factor (GM-CSF), monocyte colony stimulating factor (M-CSF), and interleukin3 (IL-3),** which assist in the production and maturation of the monocytic cells.

1. **GM-CSF** is produced by bone marrow stromal cells, lymphocytes, and other cells to foster the production of monocytes from bone marrow.

2. **M-CSF** released from these same cells, endothelial and epithelial cells, and lymphocytes stimulates the production of monocytes as well.

3. **IL-3** derived from lymphocytes also stimulates bone marrow to produce monocytes and other blood cells, thus accounting for its description as the **multi-lineage CSF.**

B. **Macrophage markers.** Macrophage surface molecules and secreted products—the monokines—regulate macrophage functions.

1. **Surface molecules**
   a. The **class I and II MHC proteins** assist in the presentation of epitopes to different subsets of T lymphocytes. This is presented below after a description of the separate categories of T cells.
   b. **Complement receptors 1 and 3 (CR 1 and 3)** bind complement component C3b in various forms. CR3 also acts as an integrin and binds leukocyte functional antigen 1 (LFA 1) on T cells.
   c. **Receptors** for the **Fc portion of immunoglobulin G** also are found on the macrophage surface.

2. **Monokines**
   a. **Interleukin 1 (IL-1)** derived from macrophages exists in two molecular forms, IL-1 alpha and IL-1 beta, which differ slightly in size but have identical activities. These activities include the stimulation of both T and B cells, immunoglobulin synthesis, activation of other macrophages, sensitizing cells to IL-2 and interferon (IFN), and contributing to fever and the inflammatory response. IL-1 is also known as endogenous pyrogen.
   b. **Tumor necrosis factor alpha (TNF-α)** is very similar in function to IL-1 but its major source is the helper T cells (Th cells) rather than the macrophage.
   c. **Interleukin 8 (IL-8)** is chemotactic for neutrophils and T cells and is secreted by activated macrophages and other cells. **Chemotactic cytokines** are now **called chemokines** and most share paired cysteines in a common relationship to each other. The attraction of T cells to the macrophage enhances the cellular interactions necessary for an efficient immune response.
   d. **Interleukin 12 (IL-12)** promotes induction of Th1 cells but inhibits Th2 cells. Acting synergistically with IL-2 produced by Th1 cells, IL-12 enhances cell-mediated immunity by enhancing differentiation of cytotoxic T cells and stimulating proliferation of NK cells.
   e. **Interferon (IFN)** exists in three molecular forms: **alpha, beta, and gamma.** Macrophages and other leukocytes are the source of the first of these. The alpha and beta IFNs activate host cells to an antiviral state by inducing enzymes that inhibit protein synthesis needed for viral replication (see Chapter 1, IV B 3 c). Also, class I major histocompatability complex (MHC) expression (see Chapter 10 I B 3) on host cells is increased, and NK cells are activated, as are both T cells and other macrophages.

3. Other secreted products

    a. Eight separate proteins of the complement system (see Chapter 4) are secreted by macrophages.

    b. Numerous other proteins are secreted by macrophages, including blood clotting factors, prostaglandins, transferrin, and erythropoietin.

C. Macrophage functions

1. Macrophages present certain epitopes in company with class II MHC proteins (see Chapter 10 I B 3 d). This is accomplished by regular endocytosis by the macrophage, degradation of the antigen in the phagolysosome, and preservation of its epitopes. The epitope is coupled with the MHC class II protein and moved to the cell surface where contact with the T-cell receptor occurs.

2. Other epitopes are presented with MHC class I proteins. In this instance, the antigens are intracellular parasites that are degraded in proteasomes of macrophages rather than in phagolysosomes. Unique peptides of the proteasome of macrophages allow coupling of the epitope to special **transporters associated with antigen processing (TAP) molecules 1 and 2** that carry the epitope and MHC class I protein to the cell surface and protect epitopes from phagocytic destruction.

3. Phagocytosis of foreign substances that enter the body is a property of phagocytic cells. Through the action of lysosomal enzymes and the generation of toxic forms of oxygen, phagocytes kill living organisms, which are then digested (see Chapter 1 III E). Sparing of antigenic epitopes that are then distributed on the cell membrane is what initiates the immune response.

4. Monokines are secreted by macrophages (see II B 2).

III. THE LYMPHOID SYSTEM. The lymphoid system consists of **lymphocytes** and the **organs and tissues** in which these cells originate, differentiate, and mature. The lymphoid precursor is the source of the lymphoid cells, which reside in special tissues as well as circulating through the blood.

A. Primary and secondary lymphoid tissues (Figure 5-1).

1. The **primary lymphoid tissues** are the **thymus** and the **bone marrow.** Precursor stem cells of the lymphoid system originate in the yolk sac, pass through the liver and the spleen, and mature in the thymus and bone marrow of mammals.

2. The **secondary (peripheral) lymphoid organs** are the **lymph nodes, spleen, diffuse lymphoid tissues,** and lymphoid follicles. Upon maturation, the primary lymphoid tissues seed the secondary tissues with lymphocytes.

B. Circulation of lymphatic cells

1. Mature lymphocytes bind to specialized endothelial cells in the postcapillary venules of lymph nodes or in the marginal sinuses of the spleen.

    a. These cells then leave the venules through **diapedesis** and move into the deep cortex of the lymph nodes or the white pulp of the spleen. Here they remain for 10–20 hours before leaving via the efferent lymphatics.

    b. After traveling in the lymphatic channels, lymphocytes eventually reach the thoracic duct and are returned to the peripheral blood.

2. The **high endothelial venule (HEV)** is a specialized section of the postcapillary venule where diapedesis occurs.

    a. Recirculating lymphocytes interact with the cells of the HEV and migrate through them in a process referred to as **emperipolesis** (lymphocyte penetration of, and movement within, another cell).

    b. Specialized adhesion molecules (called **integrins, selectins,** or more generally, **adhesins**) are present on the surface of lymphocytes and the endothelial cells of the

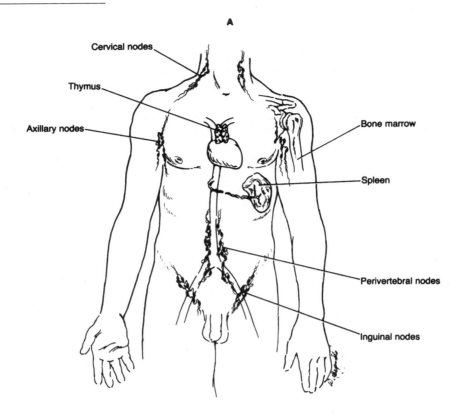

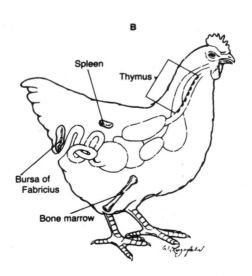

FIGURE 5-1. Tissues, organs, and cells of the lymphoid system in humans *(A)* and in birds *(B)*. In *(A)*, the primary, or central, lymphoid organs are the bone marrow and the thymus. The *bone marrow* is the source of the stem cells, which serve as postpartum progenitors of immunocytes. B cells originate and mature in the bone marrow. The *thymus* supplies the body with T cells that are involved in cell-mediated immunities. The secondary lymphoid organs, such as the lymph nodes, contain mature T and B cells as well as antigen-presenting cells, which initiate immune responses. Part *(B)* shows the location of the *bursa of Fabricius* and thymus in birds. These central lymphoid organs can be extirpated, allowing examination of the separate arms of the immune response. T cells mature in the thymus, and B cells develop in the bursa of Fabricius.

HEV. These allow **selective homing** and emigration of cells into particular lymphoid tissues or tissues where an infection is in process. Some lymphocytes home to gut-associated lymphoid tissues (**GALT**) and others to different mucosal-associated lymphoid tissues (**MALT**).

    (1) Integrins are composed of two peptides: the alpha, existing in at least 15 varieties, and the beta, existing in 7 or more forms. This heterogeneity allows the different integrins to bind to several different molecules on the blood vessel walls, including intercellular adhesion molecules 1 and 2 (**ICAM-1 and ICAM-2),** vascular adhesion molecule (V-CAM), collagen, and fibrinogen.

    (2) **Selectins** function like the integrins but bind to different ligands, especially carbohydrates and mucins on blood vessel walls.

3. One to two percent of the available lymphocyte pool recirculates every hour, thereby providing an ample opportunity to encounter foreign molecules.

C. **There are two major lymphocytic facets of the immune response system—the T-cell (thymic) and B-cell (bursal)** systems.

    1. The **T-cell system** controls the **cell-mediated (cellular) branch** of the immune system.
        a. The immunocompetent cells produced in the thymus are called **T lymphocytes (T cells).** T cells live for months or years.
        b. Epithelial cells of the thymus produce soluble **thymic hormones,** small peptides that regulate the differentiation and maturation of T cells. Thymic hormones include **thymosin, thymopoietin,** and **thymic humoral factor.**
        c. Both **positive and negative selection of T cells** occurs in the thymus. T cells that recognize self antigens are eliminated (**negative selection**) to prevent later self-destructive autoimmune reactions. These cells die through a process termed **apoptosis,** a programmed event in which steps leading to cell death occur in a regulated order. T cells that recognize self MHC markers are expanded (**positive selection**) because they will be needed for subsequent responses to antigens that require association with MHC proteins.
        d. Selection of T cells with specific CD markers (see below) also occurs in the thymus.

    2. The **B-cell system** controls the **humoral (antibody) branch** of the immune system.
        a. Discovery of the need for B cells in the immunoglobulin arm of the immune system resulted from the observation that a lymphoid organ in chickens known as the **bursa of Fabricius** (see Figure 5-1) played a role in the production of circulating antibodies. The immunocompetent cells that develop in the bursa are called **B lymphocytes (B cells).** Most B cells have a shorter life span than T cells and survive for only 5–7 days.
        b. Mammals lack a bursa but have a **functional equivalent in** the **bone marrow.**

    3. A third set of lymphoid cells, the **NK cells,** also are derived from the lymphocytic stem cell. These cells are empowered on their first exposure to kill foreign cells and host cells that express antigens of infectious agents on their surface.

D. **Lymph nodes and the spleen show an anatomic division between the two branches of the immune system.**

    1. **Lymph nodes** (Figure 5-2)
        a. The **B-cell—dependent regions** of the lymph nodes are the sites of antibody production. These anatomic sites (follicles) are found in the **cortical area** of the lymph node. The primary follicles contain small B lymphocytes, whereas the secondary follicles, which develop after antigenic stimulation, contain many large, dividing lymphocytes and plasma cells. These dividing cells allow the term **germinal center** to be applied to the secondary follicles.
        b. The **thymus-dependent regions** of the lymph nodes are the paracortical areas, also referred to as the juxtamedullary region.

    2. **Spleen.** The **B cells** are located in the white pulp of the spleen. The **T cells** ensheath the trabecular arteries before these vessels enter this region.

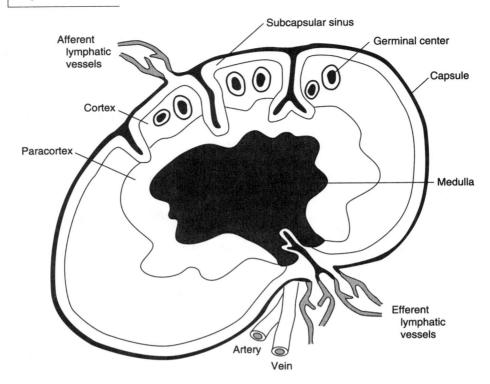

FIGURE 5-2. Compartmentalization of immune functions in a lymph node. The *subcapsular sinus* is lined with phagocytic cells. Antigens and lymphocytes from adjacent tissues enter the node via the *afferent lymphatic vessels,* and lymphocytes from the blood enter through the paracortical venules. B cells are located in the *cortex* in aggregates called primary follicles. If active proliferation of B cells occurs, the area is called a *germinal center* or secondary follicle. The *paracortex* of the node contains primarily T cells in intimate association with antigen-presenting dendritic cells. The *medulla* contains both B and T cells, as well as most of the lymph node's plasma cells.

IV. GENERAL CHARACTERISTICS OF T CELLS

A. T-cell surface markers

1. Molecules on the T-cell membrane that function in epitope acceptance are the **CD proteins,** and **the T-cell receptor (TCR) for antigen.**

   a. **CD (cluster of differentiation) antigens.** As a thymocyte matures, it acquires certain CD antigens in its membrane and loses others, eventually allowing an identification of T-cell subsets by its complex of these proteins (Table 5-1).

      (1) **CD2, CD3,** and **CD5** are found on most peripheral blood T cells.

         (a) **CD2** is an adhesion molecule that reacts with LFA-3 in the membrane of many different cells of the body, including the cells of the immune response.

         (b) **CD3** is a heteropolymer of at least five polypeptide chains that is closely associated with T-cell receptors (TCRs) (Figure 5-3). It is not directly involved in antigen recognition but is important in intracellular signaling to initiate an immune response once the cell's TCR has interacted with a homologous epitope. Molecular details of T-cell activation are discussed below (see IV D).

TABLE 5-1. The Functional Heterogeneity of T Cells

T-Cell Subtype	Symbol	Identifying Surface Antigen	MHC Restriction	Target Cell	Function
Cytotoxic	Tc	CD8	Class I	Tumors* Virally infected cells Allografts*	Kills foreign cells or cells with new surface antigens
Helper	Th	CD4	Class II	B cells Tc cells	Interleukin secretion
Inducer	Th	CD4	Class II	B cells Tc-cell precursors Macrophages	Interleukin secretion
Suppressor	Ts	CD8	Class I	B, Th, Tc cells	Down-regulates cell growth
Delayed-type hypersensitivity	Tdth	CD4	Class II	Langerhans cells Macrophages Tc cells	Releases MAF, MIF, and other lymphokines
Memory	Tm	CD8; CD4†	Both	B cells T cells	Anamnesis

MAF = macrophage-activating factor; MHC = major histocompatibility complex; MIF = migration-inhibiting factor.

*Not subject to MHC restriction.

†Depends on function.

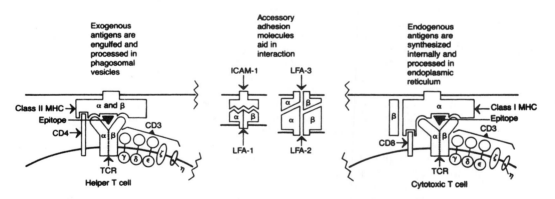

FIGURE 5-3. Interaction between the T-cell receptor (TCR)–CD3-CD4/CD8 complex and the major histocompatibility complex (MHC)-restricted antigen-presenting cell. The TCR is a heterodimer with disulfide-linked α and β chains, which functions as the antigen recognition site. On the T-cell surface, the TCR is associated with clusters of differentiation antigen (CD4 or CD8), depending on the T-cell subset, and with five invariant chains (γ, δ, ε, ζ, and η) referred to collectively as the CD3 complex. CD4 or CD8 binds the MHC molecule during epitope presentation to the T cell. CD3 is not directly involved in epitope recognition but is important in intracellular signaling to initiate an immune response once the T cell has interacted with antigen. The accessory adhesion molecules are important in strengthening the interaction between cells. They come into play after the antigen fragment has interacted with the TCR. The integrin molecules on the T cell interact with specific receptors in the membrane of the antigen-presenting cell. *ICAM* = intercellular adhesion molecule; *LFA* = lymphocyte function-associated antigen [LFA-1 is a dimer of CD11a and CD18; LFA-2 (CD2) and LFA-3 (CD58) are dimeric molecules composed of α and β chains].

(c) **CD5** is expressed on all T cells and on a subset of B cells seen in chronic lymphocytic leukemia.

(2) **CD4** and **CD8** are present on different subclasses of mature T cells (see Table 5-1). These receptors react with the MHC molecule on the macrophage and control T cell activation (see Chapter 10 I B 3 d). CD4 and CD8-positive T cells are end cells of the T-cell lineage.

(3) **CD 4 and CD 8 T lymphocytes** originate from cells that were positive for both markers but which diverge to produce the singly positive cells. The doubly positive CD4/CD8 cell in turn originated from cells doubly negative for these two markers.

(4) **CD 45 and CD 28** are discussed below under T-cell activation.

b. **TCRs.** T cells have an antigen-specific receptor that bears close structural homology with the Fab portion of an antibody molecule (see Figure 10-4).

(1) **Structure and function**

(a) TCRs are heterodimers, consisting of two nonidentical polypeptide chains, which are linked together by disulfide bonds (see Figure 10-4). Two different TCR molecules, **TCR1 and TCR2,** are known.

(i) More than 95% of T cells express the αβ heterodimer (TCR2), which is a member of the immunoglobulin superfamily of molecules.

(ii) TCR1 is composed of γ and δ chains.

(iii) Both chains of each TCR are variable in their amino acid sequence much as in the structure of immunoglobulins, thus providing specificity for antigen.

(b) The TCR contains **idiotypic determinants** similar to those of immunoglobulin molecules. **Hypervariability** occurs in particular areas of each polypeptide chain in a manner analogous to the **complementarity-determining regions (CDRs)** of immunoglobulin molecules (see Chapter 3 II C 2).

(c) The TCR heterodimer is noncovalently associated with the γ, δ, and ε chains of the CD3 molecule (see Figure 5-3). This TCR–CD3 complex apparently makes contact with both the antigen and a portion of the MHC molecule. Different portions of the hypervariable regions of the α and β chains interact with both the epitope and the MHC protein (see Figure 5-3).

(d) The γ chain of CD3 is situated almost entirely within the T-cell membrane.

(2) **Genetic composition.** Genetically, the construction of the TCR is remarkably similar to that of the immunoglobulins (see Chapter 3 IV).

(a) Three gene segments are involved in the synthesis of the α chain: multiple variable (V), multiple joining (J), and a single constant (C) gene segment.

(b) In addition, the β chain has diversity (D) gene segments.

(c) As with immunoglobulins, rearrangements of the V, J, and D gene segments mediate the vast immunologic diversity of the TCR. Two of the receptor's hypervariable regions are encoded in the V gene segment, and one region is encoded in the VJ (α chain) or VDJ (β chain) segment.

c. The **major histocompatibility complex (MHC)**

(1) The MHC proteins are determined by a large number of genes (more than 800 in humans) distributed among six or more loci. Some of these genes are extremely polymorphic; that is, many genes may occur at a single locus but only one is expressed per locus (per chromosome). A gene map for the MHC region of the human chromosome is presented in Chapter 10 (see Figure 10-1) with a fuller description of the MHC proteins and their role in transplantation and tumor immunology.

(2) Three sets of molecules are encoded within this region: the **class I, II, and III proteins (antigens).** Class I and II proteins on macrophages are involved in the presentation of antigenic epitopes to T cells, specifically the class II protein and epitope to CD4+ T cells and the class I protein and epitope to CD8+ T cells. Class III products are not involved in epitope presentation.

B. **Cytokines.** T cells secrete numerous cytokines, the majority of which come from Th2 cells.

1. Interleukin 2 (IL-2) from Th1 cells has several regulatory roles, including a proliferative influence on antigen-primed T cells; it was originally called T-cell growth factor. IL-2 also heightens cell killing by NK cells and some Tc cells.

2. Interleukin 4 (IL-4), originally called B-cell growth factor, is a major regulator of the heavy chain class switch. For example, it stimulates **B cells to switch to IgE synthesis** and thus is an important contributor to the immediate-type hypersensitivities. The stimulation of IgE is of interest because IL-4 also stimulates mast cell and eosinophil proliferation, and these cells are also important in immediate hypersensitivities. IL-4 also enhances the activities of cytotoxic T cells, macrophages, and Th2 cells.

3. Interleukin 5 (IL-5) from Th2 cells is another cytokine with influence on the growth of eosinophils. It is also important in class switching and induces synthesis of IgA.

4. Interleukin 6 (IL-6) is produced by Th2 cells, antigen-presenting cells, fibroblasts, and other cells of the body. Its major targets are B cells, where it promotes terminal differentiation into plasma cells and stimulates antibody secretion, and hepatocytes, where it induces synthesis of acute phase proteins such as C-reactive protein. It acts synergistically with IL-1 and TNF in this latter activity and also acts in the induction of fever, activation of phagocytic cells, and other proinflammatory effects.

5. Interleukin 10 (IL-10) from Th2 lymphocytes **inhibits synthesis of cytokines** by Th1 cells and antigen-presenting cells. Although best known as a downregulator of the immune response, it does stimulate B-cell growth.

6. Other lymphokines and their functions include:
   a. IL-3 is a stimulator of stem cell proliferation.
   b. IL-7, produced by bone marrow and thymic stromal cells, induces differentiation of stem cells into B- and T-cell progenitors.
   c. IL-8 is also described as a chemokine because of its chemoattractant property for T cells and granulocytes.
   d. IL-12, which is a product of antigen-presenting cells (e.g., Langerhans cells in the skin), stimulates Th1 and NK cells. It acts synergistically with IL-2 to enhance development of cell-mediated immune responses (Tdth and Tc).
   e. IL-13–IL-18, whose roles are varied and whose functions in immune regulation are still incompletely understood (although IL-16, by virtue of its attraction of CD4+ T cells, monocytes, and eosinophils can be listed as a chemokine).

C. **Functional classes of T cells.** Subpopulations of T cells have been defined according to their particular function and their CD membrane markers (see Table 5-1).

1. Cytotoxic T (Tc) lymphocytes [also called **cytolytic T lymphocytes (CTLs)**] cause lysis of target cells. Tc cells are **CD8+** (i.e., they carry the CD8 surface marker).
   a. Tc cells rid the body of foreign cells that express non-self antigens. Tc cells are induced by, and are active against, tumors, virus-infected cells, and transplanted allogeneic tissue (i.e., tissue transplanted from a genetically different member of the same species).
   b. Tc cells are usually subject to **MHC restriction** and recognize the foreign epitope in association with **class I MHC** molecules except during graft rejection.
   c. CTLs destroy their target cells by releasing **perforin and granzymes** (see Chapter 1, Table 1-9).
      (1) Perforin embeds and polymerizes in the lipid membrane of the target cell to create pores through which the cell cytoplasm escapes.
      (2) The granzymes are a group of serine esterases and nucleases that harm target cells by degrading these essential macromolecules.
      (3) TNF also is released from the CTL; it depresses protein synthesis.

(4) Fas ligand in the CTL membrane reacts with the Fas protein in the target cell membrane to initiate apoptosis.

2. **Helper T (Th) lymphocytes** are **CD4+** and recognize a specific epitope in association with a homologous **class II MHC molecule.**
   a. The cells collaborate with B cells and macrophages in the immunoglobulin response and with other T cells to facilitate the production of Tc cells.
   b. **Subsets of Th cells**
      (1) **Th1 cells** mediate several functions associated with the lymphokines they secrete. Th1 cells secrete **gamma interferon, interleukin 2, and tumor necrosis factor.**
      (2) **Th2 cells** secrete several interleukins, including 4, 5, 6, and 10.
      (3) Both subsets secrete IL-3 and GM-CSF.
      (4) The Th subsets **downregulate one another** as follows:
         (a) Gamma interferon suppresses the development of Th2 cells.
         (b) IL-10 suppresses Th1 production.

3. **Inducer T lymphocytes** are **CD4+** and recognize epitopes associated with **class II MHC molecules** also. They activate Th cells, Tc cells, and macrophages, in contrast to CD4+ Th cells, which primarily activate B cells.

4. **Delayed-type hypersensitivity effector cells (Tdth, or TD, cells)** are **CD4+** lymphocytes and are subject to **class II MHC restriction** (see Chapter 7 V B 2).

5. **Memory T (Tm) lymphocytes** are induced during the primary immune response; they recognize the specific antigen and participate in the anamnestic response. Most Tm cells have Th functions and are **CD4+**, and, like Tdth cells, they are **subject to class II MHC restriction.** The lifespan of Tm cells may be as long as 40 years, but effective anamnesis probably cannot function much beyond 10 years; booster immunizations extend this time period. Some **memory T cells** are induced to differentiate and proliferate to form mature helper or cytotoxic T cells, which, when they contact antigen a second time, are triggered to release biologically active metabolites.

D. **T-cell activation**

1. **Th and Tdth-cell activation**
   a. This process requires two signals, each of which is mediated by **macrophages** (Figure 5-4).
      (1) The **first signal** is the **presentation of antigen** with class II MHC molecules.
      (2) The **second signal** is the synthesis and release of **IL-1** from macrophages.
   b. The membrane reaction with **IL-1 induces** the synthesis of a second distinct interleukin, **IL-2,** by Th1 cells. It is the action of IL-2, in concert with other interleukins (see Table 5-2), that allows full T-cell activation to proceed.
   c. The responding T lymphocytes synthesize more **IL-2 receptors** (CD25 molecules), thus forming an **autocatalytic (autocrine) cycle.**

2. **Tc-cell activation**
   a. Once again, the T cell must be stimulated by antigen that is associated, in this instance, with class I MHC molecules on the macrophage surface.
   b. The **CD38 molecule** in the Tc-cell membrane may be important in this because cells bearing this membrane marker will release cytotoxins. Killing of virus-modified target cells can occur only **if the target cell (virus infected or tumor cell) has in its membrane a homologous class I MHC molecule** recognized by the CD8+ cytotoxic cell.
   c. In **graft rejection,** allogeneic MHC antigens are targets recognized directly by Tc cells, and the process of MHC restriction is not involved.

E. **Chemistry of T-cell activation. Cell activation occurs after interaction of the TCR with its homologous epitope.** The epitope must be associated with a groove in the class II MHC

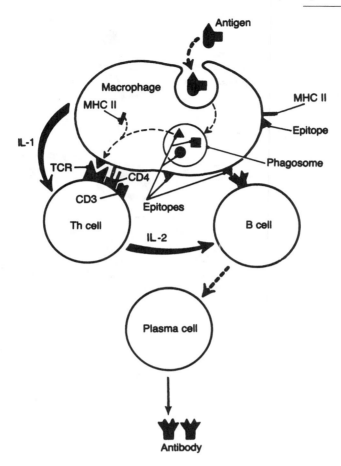

FIGURE 5-4. Cellular interactions in the humoral immune response. *CD3, CD4* = cluster of differentiation antigens 3 and 4; *IL-1, IL-2* = interleukins 1 and 2; *MHC II* = major histocompatibility complex class II protein; *TCR* = T-cell receptor for antigen.

molecule to create the **antigen-specific activation signal.** It may be necessary to have 10–100 such signals for cell activation (Figure 5-5).

1. **Antigen-independent costimulation** also occurs.
   a. Interaction of **CD28 on T cells** and **B7 on antigen-presenting cells** is required to in-duce proliferation of antigen-primed T cells.
   b. Accessory **adhesion molecules** such as ICAM-1 and the leukocyte functional antigens (e.g., LFA-1) enhance intercellular interactions by holding the T and B cells together.
   c. **Cytokines,** such as **IL-1, IL-2, and IL-6,** also participate in the activation process.
   d. The intracellular domains of the proteins are important in intracytoplasmic signaling.

2. The intracellular pathways of activation involve a **complex series of enzymatic steps** that lead to gene expression and biosynthetic events.
   a. Ligation of the MHC-epitope complex with its specific T-cell receptor activates a **ty-rosine kinase** (associated with the intracytoplasmic tails of CD3 and CD4 or CD8). This enzyme then phosphorylates **phospholipase C,** which generates **inositol triphos-phate** (IP_3) and **diacylglycerol** (DAG) from **phosphatidylinositol biphosphate (PIP_2).**

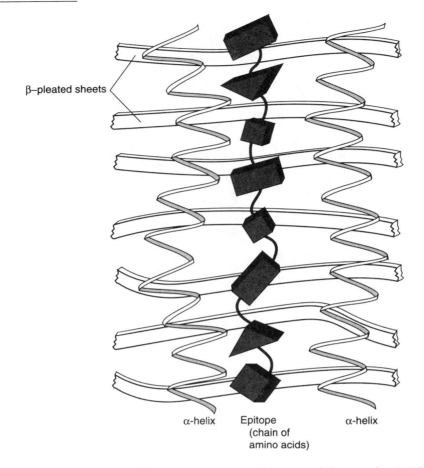

β–pleated sheets

α-helix   Epitope   α-helix
(chain of
amino acids)

FIGURE 5-5. Schematic representation of an epitope in a major histocompatibility complex (MHC) molecule. The essential features of the peptide-binding portion of the molecule are shown from the perspective of the T-cell receptor (TCR). The epitope is represented by a chain of amino acids that lies in the antigen-presenting cleft and is held in place by two coiled portions of the MHC molecule. The walls of the groove are formed by α_1 and α_2 domains of class I MHC molecules and by α_1 and β_1 domains of class II MHC molecules. The "floor" of the cleft is constructed of β-pleated sheets that comprise a portion of each domain.

    b. DAG activates **protein tyrosine kinase C. IP3 releases Ca^{2+}** from intracellular storage organelles, thus activating **calmodulin,** which in turn activates **protein tyrosine kinase A.**

    c. A **protein kinase cascade** occurs in the cytoplasm and activates specific transcription factors that translocate to the nucleus to activate genes for cytokine synthesis and cell division. The kinases become activated by dephosphorylation possibly by phosphatase domains on CD45.

    d. Protein kinases A and C are involved in the **expression of nuclear-binding proteins** that regulate several genes involved in cell proliferation and differentiation.

        (1) Nuclear factor of activated T cells (NFAT) is expressed after T-cell activation and binds to an enhancer sequence upstream from the **IL-2 gene.**

        (2) A second protein, **NFκB** (so designated because it was originally described as a transcription factor that bound to the enhancer for the κ chain), upregulates the **IL-2 receptor gene.**

        (3) Products of **proto-oncogenes** also are detected in high levels in activated T cells.

(a) The **c-*myc*** gene product is seen only transiently in normal cells; the translocation of the region of chromosome 8 that encodes this protein to chromosome 2, 14, or 22 at positions close to immunoglobulin chain loci is routinely found in **Burkitt's lymphoma cells.** The malignancy is linked to infection by the Epstein-Barr virus (EBV), an agent known to activate B lymphocytes.

(b) The **c-*fos*** gene product associates with, and activates, another nuclear-binding protein that upregulates the **IL-2 gene.**

(c) The **c-*jun*** gene product forms a heterodimer with the c-*fos* protein and diffuses into the nucleus, where it upregulates the **IL-2 receptor gene.**

V. GENERAL CHARACTERISTICS OF B CELLS.
In mammals, B cells originate from stem cells in the bone marrow. During maturation in the marrow, immunoglobulin gene rearrangements and the appearance of surface markers identify the stage of B-cell development. These markers and the B-cell products (immunoglobulins) identify B cells.

A. B-cell markers and development (Figure 5-6)

1. Surface markers

a. **The pro-B cell** expresses **CD45, CD19, and CD10** on its surface. **CD10** is found primarily on immature B cells and on malignant cells from some patients with **c**ommon **a**cute **l**ymphocytic leukemia; therefore, it is called the CALLA antigen.

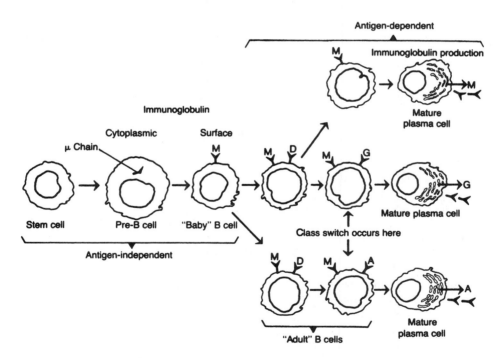

FIGURE 5-6. B-cell development. Gene rearrangements and RNA splicing occur during maturation and result in the production of a functional μ heavy (H) chain mRNA. The cell is now a pre-pre-B cell. The presence of the μ chain in the cytoplasm identifies the cell as a pre-B cell. Light (L) chain synthesis commences, and soon monomeric IgM appears in the B-cell membrane. It has now completed the antigen-independent phase of its development; further maturation is triggered by contact with specific antigen. Subsequent proliferation and differentiation with attendant class switching are influenced by cytokines secreted by helper T (Th) cells.

    b. The pre-B cell begins to synthesize mu heavy chain and eventually will express surface IgM (the immature B cell). Fully mature B cell, the next stage, synthesizes IgD as well, and this latter immunoglobulin predominates in the membrane.

2. Secreted products
    a. Immunoglobulins are the major secretory product of B cells.
    b. Some lymphokines secreted by T cells also are secreted by B cells (e.g., IL-1 and IL-6)

3. Development
    a. During the early maturation stages, the B cell undergoes several **immunoglobulin gene rearrangements** (see Chapter 3) that establish the B cell's **specificity for an antigen** before it travels to the secondary lymphoid organs.
    b. When the mature B cell moves to the blood and peripheral lymphoid tissues, it carries immunoglobulin on its surface and is ready to interact with antigen.
    c. Contact of an **epitope** with **immunoglobulin on the B-cell membrane** triggers cell division and the formation of plasma cells and memory B **cells.** This process is greatly enhanced by interleukins secreted by Th cells.
      (1) The **plasma cell** has abundant rough endoplasmic reticulum and actively secretes large amounts of antibody.
      (2) The **memory B cell** is a long-lived cell that is the progenitor responsible for rapid plasma cell proliferation in the anamnestic response.

B. | **Functions of B-cell markers**

1. Surface markers
    a. CD proteins. Both **CD19 and CD35 are receptors for C3b of the complement** system. The CD25 protein is an IL-2 receptor that is also found on activated T cells.
    b. Immunoglobulins M and D on B-cell surfaces function as antigen acceptors.
    c. The **B7 proteins** function as **adhesins,** enabling the antigen-presenting B cell to bind to T cells and stimulate T-cell proliferation.
    d. The **MHC class II** protein is an **antigen-presenting molecule** to one set of T cells: the CD4+ T cell.

2. Secreted molecules. The separate classes of immunoglobulins produced by B cells represent the major role of these cells in controlling the immune response. At different times, or from different B cells, different classes of antibodies are secreted, and each participates in the immune response in a slightly different way.

C. | **Chemistry of B-cell activation**

1. Adhesion of B7 on B cells with CD28 on T cells assists their cellular interaction.

2. The B-cell receptor (BCR) for antigen consists of the surface immunoglobulin and a heterodimer of the Igα and Igβ proteins. The cytoplasmic tails of the Igα and Igβ contain tyrosine kinase domains known as **immunoreceptor tyrosine-based activation motifs (ITAMs).** ITAM tyrosine residues become phosphorylated by enzymes (tyrosine protein kinases) of the Src family after **epitopes cross-link** surface IgM. This sends a signal for B-cell activation.

3. A second **tyrosine kinase, Syk,** participates in further phosphorylation, the hydrolysis of phosphatidyl-4,5-bisphosphate and activation of Ras.

4. The generation of active transcription factors that translocate to the nucleus to effect gene transcription are similar to those seen in T-cell activation. Tyrosine kinase and phosphatases are activated, phospholipase C is activated, PIP_2 is hydrolyzed to IP_3 and DAG. Calcium ions are mobilized and phosphokinase C and a calmodulin-dependent kinase are activated.

VI. | **EXPOSURE TO AN ANTIGENIC SUBSTANCE (see Figure 5-4)**

A. | An antigen injected into an animal is carried throughout the circulatory system, unfurls a complex series of events and eventually is deposited in lymphoid tissue.

1. **Deposition site**
   a. If the antigen is injected subcutaneously or intracutaneously, it is carried to the regional lymph node. This is followed by hyperplasia of the node.
   b. If the antigen is administered intravenously or intraperitoneally, it is then located primarily in the spleen. This organ becomes hyperplastic as a result of cellular infiltration and proliferation.

2. **Antigen processing and presentation** by the macrophage or other antigen-presenting cells (e.g., **Langerhans cells** of the skin, dendritic cells, and B lymphocytes) follows. B cells have limited antigen processing capability.

3. **Macrophages are activated by interaction with antigens and by cytokines** such as IFN-γ, granulocyte-macrophage colony-stimulating factor (GM-CSF), and TNF-α.

4. Activation results in an **increase** in the concentration of **class I and II MHC molecules** in the cell membrane. **Adhesion molecules** in the membrane also **increase** in number. Both of these events result in a higher degree of cellular interaction between antigen-presenting cells and B and T lymphocytes.

5. T-cell dependent antigens stimulate an immune response only when the epitope is presented to the T lymphocytes with a protein of the MHC. This is the basis of the term **MHC restriction** of the immune response.

6. T-cell independent antigens need not be processed and can directly stimulate antibody production by **B cells.** No anamnestic response occurs on secondary challenge with the same antigen (i.e., the antigens do not induce the development of memory cells), nor does class switching occur.

7. Besides presenting antigen to T and B cells, **macrophages release soluble mediators** such as IL-1, a monokine (i.e., a monocyte-derived mediator with hormone-like effects) that stimulates T cells to mature and to secrete lymphokines.

B. **Collaboration among cells** is required to induce a specific immune response.

1. **Humoral immunity.** Processed antigenic epitopes on the macrophage surface are presented toTh cells that recognize that epitope, as do B lymphocytes. The three cells—**Th cell, B cell,** and **macrophage**—interact, perhaps in a tricellular complex, and the B cell undergoes blastogenesis and differentiation (see Figure 5-4) under the influence of various cytokines (Figure 5-7; and see Table 5-2).

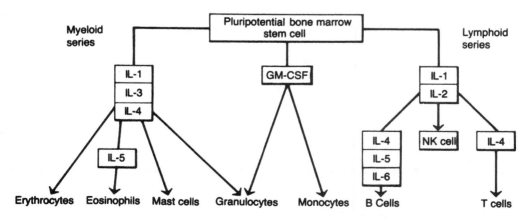

FIGURE 5-7. Cytokine regulation of the immune system. The major interleukins and their target cells are shown. Note the redundancy of stimuli and the multiplicity of targets for each lymphokine. Note also that more than one interleukin may have a similar effect. The interleukins (*IL-1* to *IL-6*) are lymphokines; granulocyte-macrophage colony-stimulating factor (*GM-CSF*) has multiple sources, including monocytes. *NK* cell = natural killer cell.

TABLE 5-2. Cytokines of Importance in Immune Response Induction*†

Cytokine	Sources	Targets	Effects
IL-1	Macrophages B cells NK cells	T cells B cells Macrophages	Lymphocyte activation Macrophage stimulation Pyrexia Acute-phase reaction‡ Increased cell adhesion
IL-2	T cells	B cells T cells NK cells Macrophages	Lymphocyte activation Macrophage activation Stimulation of lymphokine secretion
IL-3	T cells	Stem cells	Proliferation

IL-4	T cells	B cells
		Macrophages
			Lymphocyte proliferation
			Macrophage activation
			Influence on class switching:
			    Promotes IgG1 and IgE production
			    Decreases IgG2 and IgG3 production

IL-5	T cells	B cells Stem cells	Proliferation Differentiation Promotion to switch to IgA Eosinophilia
IL-6	Numerous	B cells Macrophages	Proliferation Stimulation of immunoglobulin secretion Acute-phase reaction‡
IL-7	Stromal cells	Pre-B cells T cells	Proliferation
IL-8	T cells Macrophages Vascular endothelium	Neutrophils T cells	Chemotaxis of leukocytes
IL-9	T cells	Th cells Mast cells	Proliferation
IL-10	T cells	T cells	Inhibition of lymphokine synthesis
IL-12	Antigen-presenting cells	T cells	Acts synergistically with IL-2 to stimulate proliferation and differentiation of cytotoxic lymphocytes (Tc, Tdth, and NK cells)
IL-13	Th cells	Macrophages	Downregulation
IL-16	T cells Eosinophils	CD4+ T cells	Chemotaxis Increases IL secretion
GM-CSF	T cells Monocytes	Stem cells Monocytes Granulocytes	Proliferation Differentiation
TNF-α	Macrophages T cells NK cells	B cells	Growth and differentiation Acute phase reaction
IFN-γ	T cells NK cells	Macrophages B cells	Differentiation

GM-CSF = granulocyte-macrophage colony-stimulating factor; IFN = interferon; IL = interleukin; NK cells = natural killer cells; Th cells = helper T cells; TNF = tumor necrosis factor.

*Lymphokines that are important in the expression of immunity are discussed in Chapter 7.

†Cytokines are soluble mediators with hormone-like actions. Cytokines produced by macrophages and other mononuclear phagocytes are called monokines; those produced by lymphocytes are called lymphokines.

‡Acute-phase reaction = increased concentration of certain serum proteins (C-reactive protein, amyloid A, haptoglobin, ceruloplasmin, and many complement components) in response to acute inflammation.

2. **Cell-mediated immunity.** This response is produced in a similar manner, except that the three interacting cells are the **Th cell, Tc cell precursor,** and **macrophage.**

3. The cytokines that regulate these interactions are effective only if the cells are very close together or perhaps even in direct contact. This cellular proximity is enhanced by the interaction of several **intercellular adhesion molecules** (see Figure 5-3).

C. Antibody synthesis

1. **Two signals** are needed for antibody synthesis to T-cell dependent antigens:
   a. An interaction between **antigen** and **monomeric IgM** on the B-cell surface
   b. **Communication between Th cells and B cells** mediated by lymphokines released from Th cells

2. Various **interleukins,** broadly referred to as **B-cell growth factors,** also affect B-cell proliferation and maturation.

VII. PHASES OF THE HUMORAL IMMUNE RESPONSE

A. Primary and secondary immune responses

1. **Characteristics** (Figure 5-8)
   a. **The primary immune response** occurs after the **first exposure to antigen** and produces a relatively **small amount of antibody.** The antibody level decreases over time in the absence of re-exposure to antigen.
   b. Subsequent exposure to even a small amount of antigen, however, evokes an **anamnestic response** (also called **booster response, memory response,** or **secondary immune response**).
      (1) The anamnestic response consists of a **rapid proliferation of plasma cells,** with the concomitant production of **large amounts of specific antibody.**
      (2) The anamnestic response occurs because a large population of **memory B and T cells** are recruited into the humoral immune system.

2. **Immunoglobulin class switching** (see Chapter 3). In the **primary immune response,** the immunoglobulin produced is mainly **IgM. Subsequent exposures** to antigen cause the response **to shift to IgG production** or some other Ig class.

B. Ontogeny of the immune response

1. **IgG** is the major fetal antibody, and it is **acquired from the mother** through the placenta almost exclusively during the last 8–10 weeks of gestation. Term newborns have adult levels of IgG, but infants born younger than 32 weeks' gestational age have very low levels of immunoglobulins. The development of full immunocompetence takes several years. Adult levels of antibodies are not reached until the teenage years.

FIGURE 5-8. Phases of the humoral immune response. The time between initial and subsequent exposure to a specific antigen must be sufficient for an adequate immune response to be mounted. *(A)* A primary immune response occurs upon initial exposure; if the time between initial and subsequent antigen exposure is short, only a low-grade immune response is mounted. *(B)* If sufficient time elapses between exposures, an anamnestic response occurs, in which there is a rapid proliferation of plasma cells and production of a large amount of antibody specific for the antigen.

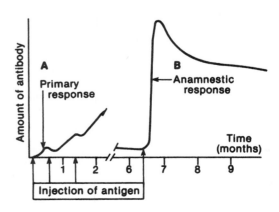

2. **IgM is the major antibody produced by a fetus.** IgM synthesis begins before birth. If the level of IgM is elevated at birth, an in utero infection may have occurred. Several months after birth, the maternal IgG is at a very low level, and the infant has not yet begun to synthesize large quantities of IgG. This is the most dangerous time for an infectious disease in infants.

VIII. REGULATION OF THE IMMUNE RESPONSE

A. **Suppression** can read to opportunistic infections but may be appropriate in the following circumstances:

1. **Allergic conditions** involving either immediate or delayed hypersensitivities

2. **Autoimmune disease,** in which the body destroys its own tissues through immune mechanisms

3. **Transplantation to prolong graft survival**

B. **Enhancement** of the immune response is advantageous in the management of immunodeficient patients (see XI).

C. **Responsiveness** is the key to immune regulation.

1. **Unresponsiveness**
   a. **Definition.** Unresponsiveness is the absence of an immune response to a substance that would be immunogenic under ordinary conditions. **Anergy** is a term used for this lack of response.
   b. **Classification. Two** broad **categories** of unresponsiveness exist: immunosuppression and immunotolerance. The difference between them is primarily quantitative.
      (1) **Immunosuppression** refers to a general or broad reduction in the host's immune responsiveness. This may be caused by:
         (a) A **congenital defect** in cells of the immune system
         (b) An **acquired condition** such as infection with HIV, malignancy, malnutrition, or cytotoxic medication
      (2) **Immunotolerance** is the absence of an immune response to a **specific** antigenic stimulus.

D. **Natural processes** control the immune response.

1. **Major histocompatibility complex (MHC) restriction** is a self-imposed regulatory mechanism.

2. The **idiotypic network** has been proposed as a negative regulatory system.
   a. **Anti-idiotypic antibodies are** antibodies to the epitope-binding region of the original antibody.
   b. These anti-idiotypic antibodies can **down-regulate the immune response.**
      (1) They do so by mimicking the original epitope and binding with epitope-specific immunoglobulins or T-cell receptors on immunocommitted lymphocytes.
      (2) Because this binding on T cells takes place in the absence of class II MHC molecules, it interferes with effective epitope triggering of lymphocyte proliferation and maturation.
      (3) Anti-idiotypic antibodies could also react with antibody-forming cells and sensitize them to complement or NK cell-dependent destruction.

3. Considerable evidence suggests that the immune system is under **neuroendocrine control.**
   a. The **sympathetic nervous system** interacts with the immune system.
      (1) **Lymphocytes and macrophages** have membrane receptors for neurotransmitters such as acetylcholine, norepinephrine, and endorphins, and lymphocytes secrete endorphin-like compounds.

(2) Brain neurons in the hypothalamus have membrane receptors for interleukins, interferons, histamine, serotonin, and prostaglandins, which are mediators of inflammation.

(3) Stress usually produces immunosuppressive effects in the body by causing release of corticosteroids.

b. The **endocrine glands** appear to be involved in these regulatory networks as well.

    (1) Lymphocytes and macrophages have receptors for adrenocorticotropic hormone (ACTH), corticosteroids, insulin, growth hormone, prolactin, estradiol, and testosterone.

    (2) Lymphocytes secrete ACTH.

IX. IMMUNOSUPPRESSION

A. Physical means of immunosuppression

1. Surgically removing central (primary) lymphoid organs is immunosuppressive but only if the organs are removed in the perinatal period.

    a. If the **bursa of Fabricius,** the **thymus,** or both, are surgically removed **in the neonatal period, immunologic competence** does not develop in the corresponding lymphoid cell line.

    b. If these tissues are surgically removed after immunologic development, immune competence is affected very little.

2. Surgical excision of the **peripheral lymphoid tissues (lymph nodes** and **lymphoid cells) has little effect** because these tissues are too diffuse to be totally removed. Removal of the **spleen** does not grossly impair antibody production but does make the person **susceptible to bacterial infections,** particularly septicemias caused by encapsulated pathogens.

3. Ionizing radiation damages the lymphoid organs and bone marrow.

    a. Radiation damages DNA by impairing cell division needed for **clonal expansion** and expression of the immune response. Irradiation suppresses the **inductive phase of the primary immune response,** but the **secondary immune response** is less affected because mature cells are not dependent on DNA synthesis.

    b. Shielding the lymphoid organs from whole-body irradiation protects against damage to their immune capacity.

B. Chemical and biologic means of immunosuppression

1. General considerations. All chemical and biologic immunosuppressive agents are **more effective in preventing a primary immune response** than they are in preventing a secondary immune response or in interrupting an ongoing response. Therefore, the immunosuppressive agent should be given just before or at the same time as the antigen.

2. Types of immunosuppressive agents and their actions

    a. Lympholytic agents

        (1) Action. Lympholytic agents are able to lyse lymphocytes in vivo.

        (2) The **two** major **types** of lympholytic immunosuppressants are **ionizing radiation** and **antibodies** (i.e., antilymphocyte serum or antithymocyte serum). These agents are used to minimize renal and heart transplant rejection, both of which are based on cell-mediated activities.

        (3) Corticosteroids (e.g., cortisone) are both **immunosuppressive and anti-inflammatory.** They are lympholytic in laboratory animals but not in humans. Cortisone has as many as 12 or more different actions that influence the immune response. These include influencing cell motility, destabilizing macrophage lysosomes, decreasing the binding of immune complexes to phagocytic cell receptors, depressing antigen processing and IL-1 production, and interfering with the release of IL-2 and TNF from macrophages.

    b. Lymphocytotoxic agents
      (1) Action. These agents **interfere with DNA, RNA, and protein synthesis.**
      (2) Major lymphocytotoxic agents include:
        (a) Antimetabolites of DNA bases (e.g., azathiaprine, a purine analogue) and folic acid antagonists (e.g., methotrexate) interfere with DNA synthesis.
        (b) Alkylating agents, such as cyclophosphamide, interfere with cell division by altering guanine so that DNA base-pairing errors occur, and they also can cross-link DNA strands.
        (c) Cyclosporine, a peptide of fungal origin, is particularly effective in suppressing graft rejection. It penetrates T cells in the G_0 or G_1 phase and exerts its immunologic effects by **blocking transcription** of the genes for interleukins 2, 3, and 4 and IFN-γ. It binds to cyclophilin and this complex binds to and inactivates the serine/threonine phosphatase **calcineurin.**
        (d) FK506, or tacrolinus, is another immunosuppressive polypeptide that inhibits signal transduction from the T-cell receptor, thus inhibiting lymphokine synthesis.
        (e) Rapamycin is a macrolide antibiotic that interferes with the intracellular signalling pathways of the IL-2 receptor.
    c. Antibodies can be used to inhibit immune responses in four ways.
      (1) Antibodies that react with T cells (i.e., **antithymocyte globulin** or **serum**) will, in the presence of complement, lyse the cells.
      (2) If exposure to a specific antigen follows injection of a preformed antibody, the immune response in the host is blocked.
        (a) This is the principle used in the development of **Rh$_o$(D) immunoglobulin (RhoGAM)** to combat Rh incompatibility (i.e., erythroblastosis fetalis, a hemolytic disease of the newborn).
        (b) Injection of **anti-Rh$_o$(D)** into the mother facilitates clearance of the fetal Rh+ cells from the body, thus aborting an immune response.
      (3) The **anti-idiotypic network** was described briefly in Chapter 3 III B 2. (see also VIII D 2).
        (a) An anti-idiotypic antibody against IgM on the B-cell surface or against the TCR on the T-cell surface blocks binding of antigen to these cells and causes their activation.
        (b) In addition, anti-idiotypic antibodies can destroy B and T cells directly by sensitizing the cells to complement-mediated damage or antibody-dependent cell-mediated toxicity (ADCC).
      (4) Monoclonal antibodies directed against CD antigens (e.g., CD3) on lymphocyte membranes may be immunosuppressive via complement-mediated cytolysis.

C. **Immunosuppression associated with diseases and other conditions.** In certain genetic conditions (see Chapter 9), there is a loss or defect in the immune apparatus itself. This also may occur as a side effect of an infectious disease or malignancy.

    1. Congenital immunodeficiencies
      a. In **Bruton's hypogammaglobulinemia,** B-cell immunity fails to develop and scant amounts of antibodies are formed, resulting in repeated bacterial infections unless treated with infusions of pooled immunoglobulin.
      b. In **DiGeorge syndrome,** T-cell immunity is deficient because the third and fourth pharyngeal pouches, the origin of the thymus, fail to develop during embryogenesis, and the individuals are subject to recurrent fungal and viral diseases.
      c. In **chronic granulomatous disease** phagocytes are unable to kill ingested microorganisms because of an inability to form toxic oxygen metabolites, thereby permitting recurrent or chronic bacterial infections.

    2. Malignancies. Particularly when lymphoid tissues are involved (e.g., lymphomas, Hodgkin's disease, leukemias), normal lymphocyte functions may be "crowded out" from bone marrow and peripheral lymphoid tissues by the excessive and uncontrolled growth of the malignant cells.

3. **Infections**
   a. **HIV infection** causes a profound immunosuppression. The virus attacks CD4+ cells and renders patients susceptible to numerous opportunistic infections and certain types of tumors, particularly Kaposi's sarcoma.
   b. **Viral infections** (e.g., measles, mumps, herpes) also may have a negative effect on macrophage functions and cell-mediated responses.
   c. Specific T-cell anergy is seen in **lepromatous leprosy** and in the terminal stages of **tuberculosis.**

4. **Malnutrition.** Adequate nutrition is essential for proper functioning of the immune system.
   a. Cell-mediated immunity appears to be the most sensitive to nutritional deprivation, but humoral immunity, complement, and phagocytic functions also are affected.
   b. Nutrient deficiencies that adversely affect immune functions include those involving proteins, vitamins (particularly those involved in DNA and protein synthesis) and minerals, especially zinc or iron, which can cause decreases in T-cell functions and in the microbicidal activity of phagocytes.

5. **Chemicals. Alcohol** adversely affects both innate and acquired immunity and is reflected in a high incidence of opportunistic infections in alcoholics. Alcohol adversely affects chemotaxis and the ciliary action in airways, which facilitates lung clearance. Alcohol also depresses acquired cell-mediated immunity.

X. TOLERANCE

A. **Definition.** Tolerance is the absence of specific immune responses in an otherwise fully immunocompetent person.

1. **Types.** This type of unresponsiveness can be either naturally acquired (**autotolerance**) or specifically induced (**acquired or immune tolerance**).

2. **Clinical importance.** Tolerance is of importance in clinical medicine in several ways.
   a. Failure of autotolerance may result in **autoimmune diseases.**
   b. Specifically induced tolerance could represent an avenue for the therapy of **autoimmune diseases, allergic conditions,** and **allograft rejection.**

B. **Autotolerance and acquired tolerance**

1. **Autotolerance (neonatal, natural,** or **self-tolerance)**
   a. **Definition.** Autotolerance is tolerance to one's own antigens. This is acquired early in life, probably in utero, as the result of negative selection of T cells in the thymus.
   b. **Clonal deletion theory.** Clones of autoreactive cells may develop steadily throughout life. These **forbidden clones** are deleted by encounters with the overwhelming concentration of self-antigens present in the body. Th cells are apparently more susceptible to this than B cells.

2. **Acquired (immune) tolerance**
   a. **Simulation.** Autotolerance can be simulated by experimentally induced tolerance called acquired or immune tolerance.
      (1) Unresponsiveness to a specific antigen can be induced by the injection of the antigen into a fetal animal, which mimics the autoantigen exposure that induces autotolerance.
      (2) Because the animal's immune system regards the injected antigen as a self-antigen, it does not produce an immune response to that antigen when it is encountered later in life. This tolerance will fade over time unless re-exposure to the antigen occurs.
   b. **Induction** of acquired tolerance in adult animals usually requires excessive amounts of antigen. Tolerance involves each epitope of the antigen, now referred to as a

tolerogen. Tolerance is not simply in vivo neutralization or absorption of the antibody; it is the specific absence of antibody formation induced by the tolerogen.

C. **Characteristics of immune tolerance**

1. Tolerance is a **specific cellular defect** that is probably due to the loss of functional or immunologically reactive T and B lymphocytes.
   a. The **role of the T cell** has been extensively investigated in mice. In mice, Th-cell tolerance occurs 1 day after the tolerogen is administered and lasts 120–150 days. In contrast, it takes 5–7 days for the B cell to be deleted or inactivated, and this tolerance lasts for only 50 days or so.
   b. Induction of Th-cell tolerance requires 1000 times less antigen than that required to induce B-cell tolerance.

2. Tolerance is **epitope specific:** the unresponsiveness is to all or only some of the epitopes of a particular antigen.

3. In **immune deviation (split tolerance),** either the humoral- or cell-mediated response is disrupted but not both.

4. **Cross-reacting antigens** can break tolerance to some epitopes if the cross-reacting antigen contains one or more new epitopes plus the cross-reactive (shared) epitope(s) to which the animal is unresponsive.

5. Several **factors influence the induction of tolerance.**
   a. Because tolerance involves deletion of specifically reactive cells, it is easier to induce if there are fewer cells to be deleted. Thus, immune tolerance of either T cells or B cells is easiest to induce in the **prenatal** or the **neonatal animal.**
   b. The **simpler the antigen, the better a tolerogen it is.** A more complex antigen is less effective at inducing tolerance because tolerance to numerous epitopes is more difficult to achieve than to the smaller number in simple antigens.

D. **Induction of immune tolerance**

1. **Methods of inducing immune tolerance in adult animals**
   a. Adult animals often are immunosuppressed by the injection of cyclosporine or another suitable immunosuppressant before they receive antigen.
   b. Alternatively, they can be injected with a tolerogenic form of antigen. For example, a saline solution of human gamma globulin, which contains aggregated globulins, is normally immunogenic in a nonhuman species, but nonaggregated forms of the antigen are tolerogenic.
   c. The antigen can be **complexed with a toxic compound,** such as ricin, or **labeled with a radioactive isotope,** such as iodine-125, to deliver a lethal hit to B and T cells bearing membrane receptors for the antigen.
   d. **Anti-idiotypic cytotoxic antibody** can be injected to eliminate a specific clone of B cells.

2. **Two theories concerning induction of tolerance**
   a. One theory states that the immunocyte is rendered tolerant by an **antigen blockade** at the membrane. When the antigen receptor reacts with its homologous epitope, the receptor is fixed (or frozen) so that no messages for antibody production can get into the cell or the cell may be killed.
   b. The alternative theory suggests that the tolerogen induces apoptotic events during maturation of T cells in the thymus.

XI. **IMMUNOPOTENTIATION**

A. **Overview.** The immune response can be **enhanced** by increasing the rate at which the response occurs, elevating its magnitude, or increasing the duration of the response.

1. In some instances, cell-mediated responses can be enhanced with no change in the humoral response, as in the use of certain mycobacterial cell-wall components.

2. Representative immunostimulants are listed in Table 5-3.

B. **Adjuvants**

1. **Definition.** Adjuvants are nonspecific potentiators of the immune response.

2. **Mechanisms of potentiation.** Adjuvants enhance immune responses by several mechanisms:

   a. Increasing phagocytosis by insolubilizing the antigen and increasing its apparent size, a feature that improves macrophage processing of the antigen.

   b. Prolonging the period of exposure to the antigen by forming semi-soluble depots of the antigen, which dissolve over time. Aluminum hydroxide, alum, and other **precipitants** or **adsorbents** are examples.

   c. Amplifying the proliferation of immunologically committed lymphocytes by enhancing lymphokine activity

3. **Examples of adjuvants**

   a. **Freund's adjuvant** is a classic adjuvant used in experimental animals.

      (1) **Incomplete Freund's adjuvant (IFA)** is a water-in-oil emulsion with antigen in the water phase. IFA increases the humoral immune response approximately 100-fold and prolongs the phase of active immunoglobulin synthesis by months.

      (2) **Complete Freund's adjuvant (CFA)** is IFA with the addition of mycobacteria or their cell wall components, which does not alter the antibody response but adds a cell-mediated response.

   b. **Bacille Calmette-Guérin (BCG),** an attenuated mycobacterium used as a vaccine against tuberculosis, activates macrophages and enhances NK cell activity. The **adjuvant activity** resides in its cell wall glycolipids (e.g., wax D). A synthetic **muramyl dipeptide,** N-acetylmuramyl-L-alanyl-D-isoglutamine, has similar properties.

   c. **Mitogenic substances,** such as **endotoxin** and some plant lectins [e.g., **phytohemagglutinin (PHA)**], produce an immunostimulatory effect by increasing the clonal expansion of B cells and T cells.

TABLE 5-3. Classification of Immunopotentiator Compounds

Compound	Class	Mechanism of Action
Freund's adjuvant, water-in-oil emulsion	Depot	Delays release of antigen; prolongs lymphoid tissue exposure to antigen
Calcium alginate	Precipitants	Same as above
Alum, aluminum hydroxide, bentonite, polyacrylamide, methylated bovine serum albumin	Adsorbents	Same as above
Foreign bodies	Irritants	Induces chronic inflammatory response, which increases antigen exposure to macrophages and B and T cells
Lipopolysaccharide (endotoxin) of gram-negative bacteria, phytohemagglutinin, concanavalin A	Mitogens	Increases clonal expansion of B and T cells during an immune response
Interleukins 1, 2, and 3; macrophage-activating factor; interferons	Lymphokines	Enhances proliferation or differentiation of lymphoid cells; activates macrophages
Polyadenylate-polyuridylate nucleotides	Synthetic	Stimulates antigen processing and T helper cell activity

C. Immunorestoration

1. **Lymphokines,** such as interleukins 1, 2, and 3, and IFN-γ, have been used therapeutically to stimulate sluggish immune responses. These agents are available as recombinant, genetically engineered molecules and are used to proliferate, differentiate, and activate lymphocytes and macrophages (see Table 5-3).

2. **Transplantation** of functional immunoreactive cells or their precursors into an individual with an immune deficiency is a successful restorative process if the recipient has the necessary tissues in which the immature cells can mature (see Chapter 9).

Vignette Revisited

Normal recovery from a viral disease such as measles suggests an intact T-cell immunity. This is supported by the fact that the child has recently experienced poison ivy, an allergic condition that is also due to cell-mediated immunity. Although the history is lacking in this regard, the child should also be able to handle fungal infections, such as candidiasis, well.

The white blood cell count is elevated and shows an increased percentage of neutrophils. This is a normal occurrence in acute infections. All other values are within normal limits for a child of this age.

The extreme hypogammaglobulinemia suggests a B-cell deficiency, because these cells are the precursors to the plasma cells that actually synthesize immunoglobulins. Patients with B-cell immunodeficiencies are particularly susceptible to bacterial infections, particularly of the skin and the respiratory system. The decrease in lymphocytes in the peripheral blood could also be associated with this type of disease, although the majority of lymphocytes in the blood are of the T-cell lineage. If secondary lymphoid organs (e.g., the spleen, Peyer's patches) were examined, an absence of plasma cells would be noted. Germinal centers would be missing as well. In fact, lymphoid tissues in general would be hypoplastic.

There are two therapeutic measures that would be appropriate for this patient. The prophylactic administration of pooled gamma globulin would passively confer resistance to many bacterial pathogens. This would need to be administered every 4–6 weeks because the half-life of IgG is approximately 3 weeks in humans. The child also should be started on antibiotics at the earliest sign of a pulmonary infection. Because staphylococci are a common problem, it would be a good idea to use an antibiotic such as oxacillin, methicillin, or cefoxitin, which are resistant to penicillinase. These penicillin-type drugs are also effective against other gram-positive cocci, such as the pneumococcus, which cause significant disease in this immunodeficient population. For a detailed discussion of immunodeficiency diseases, see Chapter 9.

1. The rapid rise, elevated level, and prolonged production of antibody that follows a second exposure to antigen is known as the

(A) delayed hypersensitivity reaction
(B) autoimmune response
(C) anamnestic response
(D) conditioned response
(E) thymus-independent response

2. The mammalian counterpart of the avian bursa of Fabricius is the

(A) spleen
(B) gut-associated lymphoid tissue (GALT)
(C) thymus
(D) bone marrow
(E) liver

3. One of the characteristics of the secondary immune response is that it

(A) is mainly IgM antibody
(B) requires only a low dose of immunogen for induction
(C) has low-affinity antibodies
(D) has a short duration of antibody synthesis
(E) has a slow rate of antibody synthesis

4. The monokine (macrophage-derived cytokine) that is intimately involved in the immune response is

(A) interleukin-1 (IL-1)
(B) IL-2
(C) IL-3
(D) macrophage-activating factor (MAF)
(E) migration-inhibiting factor (MIF)

5. The antigens in thymus-dependent humoral immune responses show which of the following properties? They

(A) induce primarily an IgM response
(B) are mainly carbohydrate in nature
(C) induce an active anamnestic response on booster injection
(D) are exemplified by the polymerized protein flagellin
(E) are not very common

6. Class I major histocompatibility complex (MHC) molecules are involved in MHC restriction of

(A) cytotoxic T (Tc)-cell interaction with virus particles
(B) Tc-cell interaction with virally infected host cells
(C) helper T (Th)-cell interaction with antigen-presenting cells
(D) Th-cell interaction with B cells
(E) B-cell interaction with antigen-presenting cells

7. The injection of large doses of protein results in immune tolerance that is due to

(A) removal of antibody by excess antigen
(B) catabolism of antibody as rapidly as it is formed
(C) production of a nonreacting antibody
(D) suppression of B cells, T cells, or both
(E) induction of cytotoxic anti-idiotype antibodies

8. The immunosuppressive effect of cortisone is attributed to its ability to

(A) produce lymphopenia
(B) destroy immunoglobulins
(C) block DNA synthesis
(D) stabilize lysosomal membranes
(E) cross-link DNA strands

9. Which of the following adjuvants activates macrophages and natural killer (NK) cells?

(A) Incomplete Freund's adjuvant (IFA)
(B) Endotoxin
(C) *Bordetella pertussis*
(D) Bacille Calmette-Guérin (BCG)
(E) Alum

10. Which of the following is a serious complication associated with the use of immunosuppressive agents?

(A) Increased incidence of autoimmune diseases
(B) Increased susceptibility to opportunistic infections
(C) Loss of tuberculin sensitivity in patients with tuberculosis
(D) Hair loss
(E) Decreased complement levels

11. Which of the following immunosuppressive agents is lympholytic in humans?

(A) Cortisone
(B) Actinomycin D
(C) Ionizing radiation
(D) Cyclosporine
(E) Methotrexate

ANSWERS AND EXPLANATIONS

1. The answer is C [VII A 1 b]. Immunologic memory (anamnesis) is an important characteristic of the immune response. It allows booster shots 7–10 years after a primary immunization. More importantly, the rapid rise in antibody levels after reexposure to a particular infectious agent is responsible for long-lasting "convalescent" immunity.

2. The answer is D [III C 2]. In birds, the bursa of Fabricius is the organ responsible for the maturation of the B-cell component of the immune system. Although gut-associated lymphoid tissue (GALT) was once considered to be the likeliest mammalian counterpart of this avian organ, the bone marrow is now believed to be the site where mammalian B cells mature. The thymus is the organ (in birds as well as in mammals) that is responsible for the maturation and differentiation of T cells. Splenectomy decreases the antibody content of serum transiently, but it does not cause permanent immunosuppression. This procedure is used in the treatment of people with idiopathic thrombocytopenic purpura (ITP) and a few other immunologic diseases. Removal of the spleen renders a person susceptible to bacterial sepsis; *Streptococcus pneumoniae* infection is a common cause.

3. The answer is B [VII A 1,2]. The secondary immune response, also referred to as the booster or anamnestic response, is triggered by relatively low doses of immunogen. The secondary immune response is mainly IgG antibody, and the antibodies produced have a high affinity for the antigen. Another feature of the secondary immune response is a rapid rate of production of antibody, usually accompanied by an antibody level that exceeds the previous, or primary, immune response.

4. The answer is A [II B 2 a; Table 5-2]. Interleukin-1 (IL-1) is a product that the macrophage secretes during antigen processing. IL-1 reacts with the helper T (Th) cell, inducing it to produce IL-2. IL-2 in turn acts on other Th cells and causes them to proliferate and elaborate IL-3 and a host of other interleukins that cause the proliferation of many cells. Among these are B cells, which would be the most important in the context of the humoral immune response. IL-1 is also known as endogenous pyrogen.

5. The answer is C [VI A 5,6]. Thymus-dependent humoral immune responses do show a vigorous anamnestic response. Most humoral responses are thymus dependent in that antibody synthesis requires the action of helper T (Th) cells, and these cells in turn require an intact thymus. In contrast, antigens that are independent of thymic influence are characterized by the presence of repeating epitopes, as are seen in carbohydrates and polymerized proteins such as flagellin. These antigens induce IgM only and fail to induce immunologic memory; an anamnestic response is not shown.

6. The answer is B [IV D 2]. Class I major histocompatibility complex (MHC) restriction requires that the T cell interact only with viral antigens present in membranes that bear the class I antigen of the host. The CD8 molecule interacts with the class I molecule at the same time that the T-cell receptor (TCR) is interacting with the viral capsid protein, thus ensuring successful delivery of the cell's toxic molecules. If these cells could be triggered to release lymphotoxins and other substances by chance interaction with naked viral particles or proteins, the effectiveness of this protective response would be greatly diminished. The T cells would then be prematurely releasing cytoplasmic contents anywhere in the body rather than at the actual site of viral replication. Class II MHC restriction is involved in T- and B-cell interactions with antigen-presenting cells.

7. The answer is D [X B 2 b, D 2 b] Large doses of antigen induce immune tolerance by eliminating helper T (Th) cells and specifically reactive B cells. In most experimental systems, circulating antibody would not be present before tolerogen administration. In fact, free antibody can interfere with induction of tolerance. Cytotoxic anti-idiotype antibodies can induce immune tolerance, but their production would not be induced by the injection of antigen.

8. The answer is A [IX B 2 a (3)]. Cortisone produces lymphopenia, either by direct lympholytic action, as seen in rodents, or by altering the tissue distribution of these cells, as seen in humans. T cells are more sensitive than B cells to this effect of corticosteroids. These drugs also have an anti-inflammatory action and interfere with the formation of phagolysosomes.

9. The answer is D [XI B 3]. Bacille Calmette Guérin (BCG) is an attenuated strain of tubercle bacilli that potentiate the action of (activates) both macrophages and natural killer (NK) cells. *Bordetella pertussis* has an adjuvant action that induces the production of IgE antibodies in experimental animals. Freund's adjuvants [either complete (CFA) or incomplete (IFA)] are water-and-oil emulsions in which the antigen is emulsified in the oil phase. CFA has mycobacteria or mycobacterial cell products incorporated into the emulsion. CFA and IFA are used in experimental situations, but are not used in humans because they cause granuloma formation. They function, as does alum, by being irritants, causing an inflammatory response at the site of adjuvant deposition, and by serving as depots from which antigen is slowly released to the antibody-forming system of the body.

10. The answer is B [VIII A]. Drug-induced immunodeficiency commonly increases the incidence of infections, particularly by opportunistic pathogens. The frequency of cancer also is higher in people receiving immunosuppressive therapy. Tuberculin sensitivity probably would not be affected because immunosuppression is not very effective against established responses. Hair loss is a common complication of cancer chemotherapy, but the dosages of immunosuppressive drugs used in the control of autoimmune diseases, graft rejection episodes, and so forth usually are not high enough to manifest this unpleasant side effect.

11. The answer is C [IX B 2 a]. In humans, lysis of lymphoid cells can be caused by ionizing radiation and by specific antibodies to appropriate cell membrane markers. Cortisone causes lympholysis in some animal species but not in humans. Here its action is directed more to changing the traffic patterns of the cells. Azathiaprine, cyclosporine, and methotrexate interfere with DNA replication or function and hence cause immunosuppression.

Chapter 6

Laboratory Methods

Vignette

The patient is a 1-day-old neonate born in the 34th week of gestation. Labor and delivery were uncomplicated, and the child's Apgar scores were within normal limits. The infant appeared slightly anemic at birth but rapidly developed severe hyperbilirubinemia during the first day of life. The pediatrician feared a possible hemolytic disease of the newborn and ordered a direct Coombs' tests on the cord blood. The test was positive. Blood group and Rh typing revealed that the mother was group O, Rh-positive and the baby was group A, Rh-negative. An exchange transfusion was performed, and the child was monitored for increases in bilirubinemia over the next week. The infant was sent home on the sixth day of life.

1. What are the causes of hemolytic disease of the newborn?
2. What is the Apgar test?
3. What is the Coombs' test?
4. What should the parents be told about future pregnancies?

I. **IN VITRO ANTIGEN–ANTIBODY REACTIONS** (i.e., serologic reactions) provide methods for the diagnosis of disease and for the identification and quantitation of antigens and antibodies.

A. The **titer,** or level, of antibody in a serum often is expressed as the greatest dilution of antibody that gives a positive reaction with antigen. Such titers can be of diagnostic and prognostic importance (e.g., a fourfold rise in antibody titer for a pathogenic bacterium between the acute and convalescent serum samples can be diagnostic for a specific disease).

B. **Antigen–antibody interactions are affected by various environmental factors.** The antigen–antibody complex is not bound firmly together and may dissociate spontaneously unless pH, salt concentration, and temperature are properly adjusted. The major forces that hold antigen–antibody complexes together are their ionic attractions.

C. **Avidity** refers to the firmness with which an antibody binds to an antigen. **Affinity** is another term used to indicate the strength of an antigen–antibody reaction. The **physical state of the antigen** is responsible for the naming of antibodies and serologic reactions exemplified by the following terms.

1. **Agglutinins** are antibodies that clump or aggregate cellular antigens.

2. **Lysins** are antibodies that cause dissolution of cell membranes. **Hemolysins** lyse erythrocytes with the help of complement proteins.

3. **Precipitins** are antibodies that form insoluble complexes with soluble antigens.

II. **PROCEDURES INVOLVING DIRECT DEMONSTRATION AND OBSERVATION OF REACTIONS.** The relative sensitivity of serologic tests for antigens and antibodies are presented in Table 6-1.

TABLE 6-1. Relative Sensitivity of Tests Measuring Antibody and Antigen

Test	Sensitivity
Precipitation	Low
Immunoelectrophoresis	Low
Double diffusion in agar gel	Low
Complement fixation	Intermediate
Radial immunodiffusion	Imtermediate
Bacterial agglutination	Intermediate
Hemolysis	Intermediate
Passive hemagglutination	Intermediate
Hemagglutination inhibition	Intermediate
Antitoxin neutralization	Intermediate
Radioimmunoassay (RIA)	High
Enzyme-linked immunosorbent assay (ELISA)	High
Virus neutralization	High

A. **Agglutination reactions** detect and quantitate agglutinins and identify cellular antigens. When the cells interact with the antibody, clumps aggregate into masses visible to the naked eye. When antibodies combine with bacteria in vivo, **opsonization** occurs.

 1. Agglutination occurs because antibodies are at least **bivalent** (i.e., have at least two combining sites).

 2. Two sites on the antibody and multiple sites on the antigen result in **antigen–antibody lattice formation** that can build up into large complexes (Figure 6-1).

B. **In the presence of complement, an antigen–antibody reaction on a cell membrane may result in membrane damage that leads to cell lysis.** This phenomenon is important in the host's defense against microbial infections. **Hemolysis** is the lysis of red blood cells, **bacteriolysis** is the lysis of bacteria, and **cytolysis** is a more general term referring to the lysis of any cell.

C. **Fluid precipitation** occurs when the antigen is soluble.

 1. **Immunodiffusion** is a term used to describe a method of performing precipitation tests in gels. If an antigen–antibody reaction takes place in a **semisolid medium** (e.g., agar), bands of

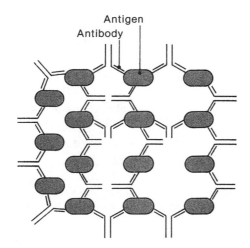

FIGURE 6-1. Lattice structure composed of antigen and antibody.

precipitate form as the reactants diffuse toward each other from separate wells in the agar. An example of this is the **double immunodiffusion** method called the Ouchterlony technique (Figure 6-2). The advantage of the procedure is that **antigenic relationships can be detected by the precipitation pattern.** The three basic patterns are illustrated in Figure 6-3.
   a. In **reactions of identity,** if the two antigens are identical, the two precipitin bands merge into a **solid chevron.**
   b. In **reactions of nonidentity,** where the two antigens are completely different, the lines of precipitate **cross.**
   c. The **reaction of partial identity** is indicated by **spur formation,** indicating that one of the antigens is cross-reactive with (but not identical to) the other. The spur occurs because one of the antibodies does not react with the cross-reacting antigen but migrates past that antigen until it reaches the antigen that has an epitope for which the antibody has specificity.

2. **Quantitative radial immunodiffusion** is a variation of immunodiffusion that can be used to quantitate antigens, such as human serum immunoglobulins.
   a. In this test, the desired quantity of an antiserum (e.g., antibody to human IgG) is incorporated into the agar. A serum source containing an unknown concentration of IgG is placed in wells in the agar.
   b. As the serum sample diffuses through the agar and encounters the antibody, a concentric ring, or halo of precipitate, forms. **The diameter of the halo of precipitate directly correlates with the concentration of IgG in the sample.** The level of IgG in the sample can be determined by referring to a standard curve based on halo diameters of known concentrations of IgG.

3. **Immunoelectrophoresis** was developed because the double immunodiffusion technique could not always resolve highly complex mixtures of antigens with similar diffusion rates.

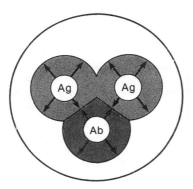

FIGURE 6-2. Diffusion of reactants in double immunodiffusion. *Ag* = antigen; *Ab* = antibody.

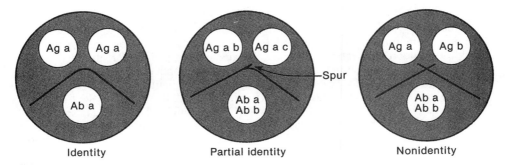

FIGURE 6-3. Types of patterns seen in immunodiffusion. *Ag* = antigen; *Ab* = antibody. The spur in Figure 6-3 contains *antibody B* only; *antibody A* reacted with *epitope A* on *antigen AC.*

    a. In this procedure, the antigen mixture (placed in a well in agar) is subjected to electrophoresis.

    b. Under these conditions, the individual antigenic components migrate through the agar at variable rates. If antibody is then placed in a well situated parallel to the path of migration, the reactants diffuse toward one another and form separate arcs of precipitate for each antigenic component.

4. Counterimmunoelectrophoresis (CIE) is another variant of the precipitation procedure. This technique is a double diffusion method (both antigen and antibody migrate from separate wells toward each other) under the influence of an electric current. Precipitation occurs where the reactants meet.

D. **If a serum contains an antitoxin (i.e., an antibody to a toxin), that antibody will neutralize the toxin** if the reactants are mixed in the proper proportions. A similar test is done to measure neutralizing antibodies to viruses.

E. **Flocculation** is another form of antigen–antibody reaction that occurs if the antigen is neither cellular nor soluble, but is an **insoluble particulate.** The Venereal Disease Research Laboratory (VDRL) test is such a test used for the diagnosis of syphilis. The antigen is a soluble cardiolipin coated onto the surface of cholesterol particles that aggregate in the presence of an antibody (the syphilitic reagin) in the serum of patients with syphilis. The test may be performed on a glass slide or on commercially available cards as the **rapid plasma reagin (RPR) test.**

III. **COMPLEX SEROLOGIC PROCEDURES.** Antigen–antibody reactions in which the visible manifestation requires the participation of accessory factors, indicator systems, and specialized equipment can be measured by several techniques.

A. **Complement,** a protein constituent of normal blood serum, is consumed (i.e., fixed) during the interaction of antigens and antibodies and will not be available to lyse hemolysin-coated RBGs. This phenomenon forms the basis for the **complement fixation test,** which is a sensitive test that can be used to detect and quantitate antigens and antibodies.

B. **Fluorescent dyes** (e.g., fluorescein isothiocyanate) can be conjugated to antibody molecules to allow visualization of the molecules under ultraviolet light and fluorescence microscopy. Such labeled antibody may then be used to identify antigens by either the direct or indirect technique.

1. Direct immunofluorescence uses antibody that is labeled with a fluorescent dye. This is allowed to react with an unknown tissue or organism that may contain the antigen for which the antibody is specific. If the antibody reacts with antigen, it is seen as a green stain on the specimen under ultraviolet light. This method also has been adapted to the identification of viruses by either light or electron microscopic techniques. In one variation, horseradish peroxidase is conjugated to the antibody. After the enzyme–antibody complex has reacted with the antigen, a substrate for the enzyme is added. Bound antibody is detected by the presence of visible colored precipitate created by the enzyme at the site of antibody binding. The immunoperoxidase test is an example of an enzyme-linked immune assay (EIA).

2. Indirect immunofluorescence procedures use a fluorescent antibody directed against antibody (e.g., fluorescent rabbit antiserum to human gamma globulin). In this technique, an antibody (the human gamma globulin) also serves as an antigen; it is the meat in an immunologic sandwich. In the serodiagnosis of syphilis by the **fluorescent treponemal antibody absorption (FTA-ABS) test,** *T. pallidum* fixed to a slide is flooded with the patient's serum. Antibodies to the spirochete in the patient's serum bind to the organisms. The slide is then overlain with fluorescein-tagged antibody to human gamma globulin, and the *T. pallidum* spirochetes will fluoresce when the slide is viewed under an ultraviolet microscope.

C. **Hemagglutination inhibition test.** Hemagglutination is the agglutination of red blood cells by antibodies (i.e., hemagglutinins), certain virus particles (e.g., influenza and mumps viruses), or other substances. Although viral hemagglutination is a nonimmunologic phenomenon, it forms the basis for the hemagglutination inhibition test, which is extremely valuable as a viral diagnostic test. To examine the serum of a patient suspected of having **influenza,** the patient's serum is mixed with known influenza virus and red blood cells. If antibody is present, hemagglutination normally caused by the virus will be inhibited because the antibody will bind to the virus and block its contact with the erythrocytes. This is an example of a **virus neutralization test**.

D. **Passive agglutination** is the result of converting a precipitation reaction to one that agglutinates antigen. Latex particles coated with a soluble antigen and then exposed to specific antibody become agglutinated. This is the basis for latex agglutination tests to identify antigens of pathogenic bacteria and to detect rheumatoid factor in serum.

E. **Coombs' (antiglobulin) test.** In certain instances, nonagglutinating antibodies are unable to form visible aggregates when subjected to precipitation or agglutination procedures. To demonstrate the presence of such antibodies, the Coombs' (antiglobulin) test may be used. The Coombs' test involves adding an antibody directed against gamma globulin to provide a bridge between two cells or particles coated with the primary antibody. The test may be performed in two ways, as illustrated by the two methods to detect nonagglutinating anti-red cell antibodies.

1. **The direct Coombs' test** is used to detect cell-bound antibody. The red blood cells are washed free of serum and unbound antibody, and the antiglobulin reagent is added directly to the cell suspension. The direct Coombs' test is of value in the detection of antibodies to red blood cells associated with syndromes such as hemolytic diease of the newborn (i.e., erythroblastosis fetalis) and autoimmune hemolytic disease. Some antibodies associated with these diseases have the ability to attach to, but not agglutinate, the target red blood cell. The absorbed antibody (i.e., gamma globulin) can be detected, however, by the use of an antibody (i.e., Coombs' serum) to human gamma globulin.

2. **The indirect Coombs' test** is used to detect the presence of nonagglutinating anti-erythrocyte antibodies in a person's serum that might complicate a blood transfusion. The serum suspected to contain such an antibody is incubated with donor red blood cells, the cells are washed, and the antiglobulin reagent is added. At this point, if antibody is adsorbed to the red blood cells, the cell will be agglutinated. The indirect Coombs' test also is of value in detecting antibody in the serum of a pregnant woman that might be directed at the Rh antigen of her fetus and thus be at risk for erythroblastosis fetalis.

F. **Radioimmunoassay (RIA)** is an extremely sensitive method (to the picogram level) that can be used for the quantitation of any substance that can be labeled with a radioactive isotope (e.g., iodine-125).

1. **Liquid-phase RIA** depends on the competition between labeled (known) and unlabeled (unknown) antigen for the same antibody. This requires separation of the antigen–antibody complex from free antigen or antibody, measurement of the amount of radiolabel in the complex, and comparison of this measurement to the amount of label attached to the antibody in the absence of any competing antigen.

2. **Solid-phase RIA** involves adsorption or covalent linkage of antibody to a solid matrix. Unlabeled antigen is then added, followed by labeled antigen. Determination of bound versus free labeled antigen is then made, and the amount of antigen in the unknown sample is calculated by referring to a standard curve.

3. **Applications.** RIA is useful in the quantitation of a **wide range** of biologic substances that function as antigens or haptens, including a number of hormones (e.g., insulin, growth hormone), serum proteins (e.g., IgE), metabolites (e.g., cyclic AMP, folic acid), drugs (e.g., digoxin, digitoxin), and microbial capsules and other products such as hepatitis B surface antigen (HBsAg).

G. **Enzyme-linked immunosorbent assay (ELISA)** has virtually the same sensitivity as RIA. The ELISA is both highly sensitive (> 99%) and specific (> 99%). The only difference in the two tests is that an enzyme replaces the radioisotope in ELISA tests. ELISA tests are developed by adding a substrate to the enzyme and measuring the amount of enzyme product formed. As with RIA, ELISA may be used to measure either antigen or antibody by either direct or indirect methods.

IV. ASSAYS OF IMMUNE COMPETENCE often require evaluating phagocytic cells, B cells, and T cells.

A. **Analysis of phagocytic cells** may require one of three different assays.

1. **Assays for metabolism and generation of toxic molecules** determine whether phagocytic cells are generating toxic metabolites of oxygen needed to kill microorganisms. The **nitroblue tetrazolium (NBT) test** determines this by using the dye as the terminal receptor of the electron transport system instead of oxygen. This test may be conducted on both resting phagocytes and those stimulated to engage in phagocytosis.

2. **Assay for phagocytosis and killing of microorganisms.** Some phagocytic disorders are defects in either ingestion or killing, even if normal NBT values exist.
   a. **Phagocytosis.** Cells can be incubated with bacteria or other engulfable materials (e.g., latex, polystyrene particles) for 1–3 hours and then examined for uptake of the foreign bodies.
   b. **Microbicidal activity.** Intracellular killing by phagocytic cells can be measured by direct plate counting of the number of microorganisms that survive incubation with phagocytes compared to the number of bacteria in control tubes not containing phagocytes.

3. **Assays for chemotaxis** are available to test the ability of neutrophils to move in a directed migratory pattern toward a chemotactic stimulus such as endotoxin or the complement-split product, C5a.

B. **Analysis of B and pre-B cells.** In all evaluations of immunity, it is important to establish both the number of immune cells that are present and whether these cells are functional.

1. **Membrane marker assays** are used to enumerate B cells. For B cells, the **marker** can be a surface immunoglobulin molecule or a cluster of differentiation (CD) molecule such as CD19 or CD20; all these molecules are integral membrane components. ELISA or RIA-labeled antibodies are used for this.

2. **Enumeration of pre-B cells.** The pre-B cells have μ heavy (H) chains in their cytoplasm but none on their cell membrane. Antibody does not normally enter viable B cells, so the cells are first treated to make them permeable. Rhodamine (red)-labeled anti-human μ serum is added to label any μ chains in the cytoplasm. Pre-B cells show **red fluorescence in the cytoplasm but not on the cell surface.**

3. **Evaluation of B-cell function**
   a. The quantitation of **serum immunoglobulin levels** is accomplished by radial immunodiffusion.
   b. Some patients have normal serum immunoglobulin levels but lack specific antibodies. In this case, it must be determined whether the patient has antibodies that should have been induced by exposure to antigens used in previous immunizations. **This is determined by agglutination, precipitation, or other tests.**
   c. If the patient has not been immunized, vaccination followed by evaluation of the immune response is necessary. An attenuated vaccine should never be given to an immunodeficient person.
   d. **Isohemagglutinin levels.** People in blood groups A, B, or O should have anti-B, anti-A, or anti-A and anti-B antibodies, respectively, in their serum by the age of 2 years. If these antibodies are absent, a defect in B-cell function is indicated.

C. **Analysis of T cells and their subsets**

1. **Enumeration of T-cell subsets**
   a. **Fluorescent monoclonal antibodies** to specific T-cell surface markers (CD4 or CD8) can be used to enumerate individual T-cell subsets (Table 6-2).

b. The **fluorescence-activated cell sorter (FACS)** uses flow cytometry techniques to analyze and separate cells according to their fluorescence and light-scattering properties. This technique relies on an instrument that can detect the staining of T cells and direct them into collecting vessels specific for their T-cell type based on their different fluorescence.

2. **Evaluation of T-cell function**

a. **Delayed-type hypersensitivity skin tests** determine the T-cell response to past encounters with antigens. The patient is subjected to a battery of intradermal skin tests intended to evoke a response to one or more antigens. Possible antigens include mumps virus, candidin (a yeast antigen to which most humans have been exposed), purified protein derivative (PPD) skin test reagents for *Mycobacterium tuberculosis* infection), and diphtheria toxoid.

b. **Lymphocyte proliferation assays**. These assays test T-cell function by determining the amount of radioactive tritium incorporated into the DNA of a cell exposed to a mitogen, such as phytohemagglutinin, in the presence of tritiated thymidine.

c. **Mixed lymphocyte culture** (see Chapter 10 I C 3 c) or **mixed lymphocyte reaction (MLR)**. This test is especially useful in determining if a recipient has cells that will attack those in a proposed graft. Lymphocytes of the donor and recipient are mixed in culture. If the recipient cells react to antigens on the donor cells, the recipient cells will begin to enlarge and replicate. This is a positive MLR response.

d. **Cell-mediated cytotoxicity assays** are essentially the same as mixed lymphocyte assays, except tumor cells often are used as the target rather than lymphocytes.

V. IDENTIFICATION OF IMMEDIATE (TYPE I) HYPERSENSITIVITY REACTIONS DUE TO IgE

A. **General considerations.** A **thorough patient history** is extremely valuable for the identification of allergies.

B. **In vivo tests.** A series of potential allergens are administered via a **scratch test** or intradermally, and the injection sites are examined within 15–20 for minutes the appearance of the **wheal (edema)-and-flare (erythema) reaction.**

C. **In vitro IgE assays.** Either total IgE or specific IgE levels may be measured.

1. **Radioimmunosorbent test (RIST)** is the technique used to measure **total IgE concentration.** In this case, the IgE serves as antigen and is detected and quantitated by an indirect ELISA or RIA test.

2. **Radioallergosorbent test (RAST)** is the technique used to measure the amount of IgE spe-

TABLE 6-2. Immunologic Specificity of Selected Anti-T-Cell Serums

Antibody Against	Cells Detected	Normal Blood Values (%)
CD2*	T cells and natural killer (NK) cells	85 +
CD3[†]	T cells	75
CD4	Helper and dth T cells	50
CD8	Suppressor and cytotoxic T cells	25

*CD = cluster of differentiation molecules, which are membrane components of various cells of the body that aid in identification of cellular function.

[†]Called the pan-T reagent because it reacts with all peripheral blood cells; CD3 antigen is complexed with the T-cell antigen receptor in the T-cell membrane.

cific for a known allergen. In this instance, the allergen on a solid phase is incubated with the IgE source and, subsequently, the amount of IgE bound is measured by the ELISA or RIA method with an enzyme or isotope-labeled reagent anti-IgE.

VI. PRODUCTION AND USE OF MONOCLONAL ANTIBODIES

A. Present and potential uses of monoclonal antibodies

1. Monoclonal antibodies are extremely valuable in **laboratory procedures** because they are easily purified and react with a single epitope of an antigen.

2. A potential **long-range benefit** of monoclonal antibodies is as **therapeutic agents.** Monoclonal antibodies are being used in the **treatment of cancer,** primarily as carriers of anticancer agents such as radioisotopes or cytotoxic agents. In addition, monoclonal antibodies may represent an alternative source of immunogens as **anti-idiotypic vaccines.**

B. Production of monoclonal antibodies by the murine hybridoma technique. Hybridomas are artificially created cells that produce pure or monoclonal antibodies.

1. A mouse is injected with antigen, and plasma cells from its spleen are fused with cancerous mouse cells (i.e., plasmacytoma or myeloma cells).
   a. The cells are cultured at high dilutions to allow only one fused cell per culture well.
   b. Only hybrid (fused) cells replicate because plasma cells are fully differentiated cells (which do not multiply), and the plasmacytoma cells used are deficient in hypoxanthine–guanine phosphoribosyltransferase (HGPRT), which makes them susceptible to metabolic poisoning by appropriate chemical alterations of the medium.

2. Each **hybrid cell** formed by this technique has two important properties:
   a. It produces a single molecular form of antibody dictated by its spleen cell parent.
   b. It continually grows and divides, like its plasmacytoma cell parent.

3. The clone of hybrid cells that produces the desired antibody is identified and is then grown as a continuous cell line, from which large amounts of the homogeneous or monoclonal antibody can be harvested.

Vignette Revisited

1. Hemolytic disease of the new born (HDNB) occurs when the mother has made antibodies of the IgG class that are reactive with the infant's red blood cells (RBCs). The most serious disease is erythroblastosis fetalis, wherein the Rh-negative mother makes antibodies against the Rh antigen found on the RBCs of the baby. In some instances the mother will have IgG antibodies against the A and/or B blood group antigens. These isoagglutinins are usually of the IgM class and do not cross the placenta but occasionally transfusions of other unique antigenic experiences will induce an IgG response.
2. The Apgar score reflects respiratory and neurologic functions at birth. The tests are done at 1 and 5 minutes of age and would be expected to be normal in this infant.
3. The Coombs' test detects human gamma globulin on RBCs. The direct test looks at the infant's RBCs to see if they have antibodies on their surface. If they do, the Coombs' reagent (goat anti-human gamma globulin) will cause the cells to agglutinate. In the indirect test the presence of antibodies reactive with human RBCs can be detected. The serum of the infant in our case would probably contain antibodies reactive with blood group A erythrocytes. The exchange transfusion with compatible blood will remove these excess antibodies as well as the sensitized RBCs and bilirubin (a breakdown product of hemoglobin which signals hemolysis in vivo).
4. The parents should be warned that the disease may recur in future infants and will most likely be more severe with each pregnancy. If the father is heterozygous for the blood group A gene (i.e., A/O) then half of the children would be expected to be blood group O and Would not be in any danger.

1. Which one of the following is included in the indicator system of a complement fixation test?

(A) Specific antibody and complement
(B) Specific antigen and complement
(C) Red blood cells and hemolysin
(D) The patient's heat-inactivated serum
(E) Guinea pig serum

2. Which of the following procedures gives the most sensitive measure of antibody?

(A) Precipitation
(B) Agglutination
(C) Radial immunodiffusion
(D) Radioimmunoassay (RIA)
(E) Immunoelectrophoresis

3. In enumerating immune cells, the important marker in the cytoplasm of the pre-B cell is immunoglobulin heavy (H) chain

(A) α
(B) δ
(C) ε
(D) γ
(E) μ

4. In the direct immunofluorescence identification of a specific infectious agent (e.g., *Treponema pallidum* or *Streptococcus pyogenes*), fluorescein may be conjugated to

(A) the microorganism
(B) sheep red blood cells (SRBCs)
(C) antibody specific to human gamma globulin
(D) antibody specific to the microorganism
(E) antibody specific to complement

5. The radioimmunosorbent test (RIST) is a technique used to measure

(A) cellular antigens
(B) both antigen and antibody activity
(C) allergens in food
(D) specific IgE levels
(E) total IgE concentration

6. A 65-year-old woman has had previous immunizations against influenza, as recommended by her HMO. She wishes to know if she is still immune to influenza. The physician explains that the influenza virus is recognized to alter its antigenicity frequently and that antibodies to only a limited number of influenza type A strains can be measured. The best test for this purpose is

(A) the radioallergosorbent test
(B) an immunodiffusion test
(C) a hemagglutination inhibition test
(D) a Coombs' test
(E) a precipitation test

7. A professor gives a student a preparation of a fluid protein antigen and asks the student to arrange a sensitive serologic test to determine the presence of an antibody to this antigen. Of the following procedures, which would be the most sensitive and suitable test?

(A) Passive hemagglutination
(B) Radioallergosorbent test
(C) Counterimmunoelectrophoresis
(D) Ouchterlony double diffusion test
(E) Fluid precipitation test

8. The immunology laboratory has not received the reagents needed to perform the radioimmunosorbent test (RIST) and the radioallergosorbent test (RAST) usually ordered by the allergy unit of the dermatology department. The attending physician in dermatology should advise the residents to substitute which one of the following for the RAST test?

(A) Mixed lymphocyte reaction tests
(B) Raji cell tests
(C) Complement fixation tests
(D) Scratch tests
(E) Ouchterlony tests with patient sera and anti-IgE

ANSWERS AND EXPLANATIONS

1. The answer is C [III A 2 b]. The indicator system in a complement fixation test consists of sheep red blood cells (SRBCs) plus antibody (hemolysin) specific for SRBCs. Complement fixation requires both a test system and an indicator system. The test system contains antibody, antigen, and a source of complement (e.g., guinea pig serum). To ascertain that the complement in the test system has been fixed (i.e., consumed), it is necessary to add a second set of reagents, the indicator system, which must react to the presence of active complement in a visible way. When complement has not been fixed, the SRBCs will be lysed if they are first sensitized to complement lysis by anti-SRBC antibody, such as hemolysin.

2. The answer is D [III F, G; Table 6-1]. Radioimmunoassay (RIA) and enzyme-linked immunosorbent assay (ELISA) are the most sensitive of the methods available for the detection of antigens and antibodies. Precipitation is among the least sensitive tests, followed by (in order of increasing sensitivity) immunoelectrophoresis, radial immunodiffusion, and bacterial agglutination.

3. The answer is E [IV B 2]. The pre-B cell has μ heavy (H) chains in its cytoplasm but not IgM in its membrane. Pre-B cells are enumerated by incubating a suspension of viable cells with fluorescein-labeled anti–human μ chain antiserum. At this point, the antibody is unable to enter the cell cytoplasm. After the cells are washed and fixed on a slide, the membrane is permeable, and rhodamine (red)-labeled anti–human μ chain serum is added to label any μ chain in the cytoplasm.

4. The answer is D [III B 1]. During direct immunofluorescence, the fluorescein is conjugated directly onto the antibody that will react with the specific pathogen. Fluorescein-tagged anti–human gamma globulin is used in indirect tests. Some procedures use two labeled antibodies—one fluorescein conjugated and a second labeled with rhodamine, which fluoresces red. Thus, different cellular structures or organisms can be visualized at the same time.

5. The answer is E [V C 1]. The radioimmunosorbent test (RIST) is used to measure to-tal IgE concentration, and is useful in identifying people at risk for immediate hypersensitivity (type I) reactions. Specific IgE levels are measured by the radioallergosorbent test (RAST), in which particular allergens are complexed to insoluble carrier materials. These tests permit measurement of picogram quantities or less of immunogenic or haptenic substances. Both antigen and antibody activity can be measured by the enzyme-linked immunosorbent assay (ELISA). Cellular antigens are identified by means of agglutination reactions. Allergens in foods could be quantitated by a radioimmunoassay (RIA) procedure if the capture molecule was an allergen-specific antibody; however, RIST "captures" serum IgE.

6. The answer is C [III C]. The influenza virus is one of the viruses that binds to erythrocytes and agglutinates them. Consequently, antibodies bound to the virus block viral attachment to these red cells and result in a hemagglutination inhibition (HAI) reaction. If serum of the patient incubated with the viral strains available produces an HAI reaction, the breadth of the patient's antibodies to these strains of the virus can be elucidated.

7. The answer is A [III D, Table 6-1]. All forms of precipitation assays are relatively insensitive. The radioallergosorbent test (RAST) is designed to measure IgE specific for an antigen but could be modified for use in this instance, except that it requires considerable skill to perform the test and uses radioisotopes in its original form. Thus, passive hemagglutination is the best answer.

8. The answer is D [V C 2]. The radioallergosorbent test (RAST) test is a sensitive test to measure the presence of serum IgE antibody that is specific for a certain allergen. None of the suggested answers will give the exact amount of IgE in the patient's serum that will react with certain allergens. However, simple skin tests (e.g., the scratch test) determine very economically if the patient has IgE specific for the different allergens selected. The size of these positive scratch tests may indicate the relative amount of IgE to the different allergens. On this basis, scratch tests are a good substitute for the RAST test.

Chapter 7

Immunologic Mechanisms of Tissue Damage

Vignette

A group of Girl Scouts were on a weekend trip to Big Bend National Park. Deb and Dana, who also came along on the trip last year, wandered through the woods to a small meadow to look for wildflowers. As they were gathering flowers, they were both stung several times by bees. As they ran back to the campsite, Dana started wheezing and became extremely short of breath. She felt her chest begin to tighten, and she quickly broke out in a diffuse, pruritic rash over her entire body.

Dana was rushed to the hospital where she was stabilized and admitted for observation. The next day, Deb developed severely pruritic, erythematous papules on her lower legs and hands. These were treated with a topical ointment, and she was advised not to scratch the lesions and to avoid rubbing her eyes.

1. What is the most likely cause of Dana's symptoms?
2. Why did Deb not become ill? Is she likely to get sick later?
3. How should Dana be treated?
4. What is the cause of Deb's itching episode?
5. How should Deb be further treated?
6. Why should she not scratch the lesions?

I. INTRODUCTION. Although the immune system generally is protective, the same immunologic mechanisms that defend the host may at times result in severe damage to tissues and occasionally may cause death.

A. Hypersensitivity reactions (allergies). This term refers to damaging immunologic reactions that result from the in vivo interaction of an antigen and the immune response the individual makes to that antigen (usually called an **allergen** in this context). The person's first contact with the allergen induces an immune response. Subsequent exposure produces a reaction that leads to tissue damage. These reactions are called **hypersensitivity reactions** because they are exaggerated responses (or sensitivities) to materials that are usually innocuous when first encountered.

B. Classification. Gell and Coombs have classified hypersensitivity reactions into four major types.

1. **Type I**—immediate hypersensitivity reactions

2. **Type II**—cytotoxic reactions

3. **Type III**—immune complex-mediated reactions

4. **Type IV**—cell-mediated reactions

II. IMMEDIATE HYPERSENSITIVITY (TYPE I) REACTIONS

A. Definition. Immediate hypersensitivity reactions are initiated by antigens reacting with cell-bound immunoglobulin E (IgE) antibody. This type of hypersensitivity may be manifested in many ways, depending on the target organ or tissue, and may range from life-threatening anaphylactic reactions to lesser annoyances, such as hay fever.

B. | **Pathogenic mechanisms**

    1. Immediate hypersensitivity reactions involve the release of pharmacologically active mediators from mast cells or basophils. This release is triggered by the cross-linking of cell-bound IgE molecules by antigens (Figure 7-1).

    2. Allergens
        a. Strictly speaking, allergens are antigens that induce the production of specific IgE antibodies in humans. By extension, the term "allergen" is also used at times to refer to antigens that produce other types of hypersensitivity reactions.
        b. Allergens include such diverse substances as:
            (1) Plant pollens (e.g., ragweed) and mold spores (e.g., *Alternaria, Aspergillus*)
            (2) House dust (e.g., excreta of house dust mites)
            (3) Animal hair, dander, and feathers
            (4) Foods (e.g., milk, gluten, wheat, eggs, fish, peanuts, chocolate)
            (5) Animal antiserums and hormones
            (6) Insect venoms (e.g., bee, wasp)
            (7) Drugs and chemicals (e.g., antibiotics, antiseptics, anesthetics, vitamins)

    3. IgE (reaginic antibody). The **primary antibody** responsible for immediate hypersensitivity reactions in humans is **IgE.**
        a. IgE antibodies are **homocytotropic.** This means they have a high affinity for mast cells and basophils, both of which have a receptor for the epsilon heavy chain (FcεR) in their membranes.
        b. IgE is produced by **plasma cells** in the mucosa of the **respiratory and gastrointestinal tracts.**
        c. IgE in the gut **may protect against intestinal parasites.**
        d. Regulation of IgE production appears to be under the control of helper T (Th) cells and the lymphokines they produce. Th2 cells produce interleukin-4 (IL-4), which induces class switching from immunoglobulin M (IgM) to IgE.

    4. Mediators of atopic disease
        a. Release of mediators
            (1) Background. If the initial exposure to an allergen has resulted in the production of specific IgE and its ultimate fixation to mast cells and basophils, subsequent exposure to the allergen will trigger an antigen—antibody reaction on the cell mem-

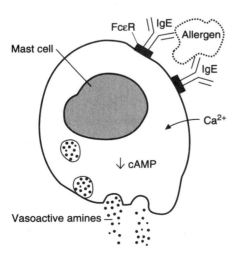

FIGURE 7-1. The mechanism of allergic injury in atopic disease (type I reaction). The allergen cross-links two immunoglobulin E (*IgE*) molecules that are anchored in the membrane of the *mast cell.* This causes an influx of Ca^{2+} and a decrease in the level of intracellular cyclic adenosine monophosphate (*cAMP*). Degranulation occurs, and *vasoactive amines* are released into the extracellular environment. *Fc*εR = receptor for Fc of IgE.

brane. A critical step is the bridging of adjacent membrane-bound IgE molecules by the allergen. This initiates degranulation and release of mediators stored in mast cells and basophils; it also induces synthesis of other vasoactive compounds.

    (2) Sequence of mediator release. Mediator release requires energy and occurs in the following sequence:

        (a) An **influx of calcium** into the mast cell occurs.

        (b) A cytoplasmic **phosphodiesterase** is activated.

        (c) Intracellular cyclic adenosine 3,5-monophosphate **(cAMP) levels fall.**

        (d) Mediator-rich **cytoplasmic granules migrate** to the cell surface.

        (e) Exocytosis occurs, and the granule contents are released to the exterior of the cell.

  b. Sources of mediators. Some mediators (i.e., those derived from mast cells and basophils) (Table 7-1) are stored within the cell in a **preformed** state. Others are **synthesized** on allergen contact.

TABLE 7-1. Mast Cell and Basophil Mediators of Atopic Disease

Mediators	Effects	Comments
Preformed mediators		
Histamine	Smooth muscle contraction (e.g., bronchospasm) Increased capillary permeability Increased mucus secretions Increased airway resistance Chemokinesis	Probably the most important mediator in anaphylaxis
ECF-A	Chemotaxis of eosinophils that control allergic reactions by releasing arylsulfatase B (inactivates SRS-A) and histaminase (inactivates histamine)	
Synthesized mediators		
PAF	Platelet aggregation and release of vasoactive amines Increased vascular permeability Smooth muscle contraction Bronchoconstriction Neutrophil chemotaxis	An acetyl glyceryl ether phosphoryl choline; inactivated by phospholipases
SRS-A leukotrienes LTC4, LTD4, LTE4	Smooth muscle contraction Increased capillary permeability Mucus secretion in airways	Lipoxygenase metabolite of arachidonic acid; probably a major factor in asthmatic bronchospasm
LTB4	Chemotaxis	
Prostaglandins PGE$_1$, PGE$_2$	Strong bronchodilation Strong vasodilation	Cyclooxygenase metabolites of arachidonic acid

ECF-A = eosinophil chemotactic factor of anaphylaxis; *LT* = leukotrienes; *PAF* = platelet-activating factor; *PG* = prostaglandin; *SRS-A* = slow-reacting substance of anaphylaxis.

(1) **Preformed mediators** are important in the early events of a type I reaction. They include **histamine** and **eosinophil chemotactic factor of anaphylaxis (ECF-A)**

(2) **Synthesized mediators**

    (a) **Platelet-activating factor (PAF)** is generated from a stored precursor.

    (b) Other synthesized mediators are **arachidonic acid derivatives (e.g., the leukotriene slow-reacting substances of anaphylaxis [SRS-A]).**

        (i) After degranulation, changes in the cell membrane allow phospholipase A_2 to break down membrane lipids producing arachidonic acid.

        (ii) Arachidonic acid is subsequently degraded, via lipoxygenase or cyclooxygenase pathways, to leukotrienes or prostaglandin and thromboxane mediators, respectively.

    (c) **Bradykinin,** a nonapeptide derived from serum α_2-macroglobulin through the action of kallikrein enzyme**,** causes smooth muscle contraction and increases vascular permeability in a slow, prolonged manner. It also increases mucus secretion and activates **phospholipase A_2** to augment arachidonic acid production.

  c. **Fate of mediators.** These substances are rapidly degraded in the body by various enzymes (e.g., histaminase and aryl sulfatase).

5. Genetic factors appear to play a role in **atopic allergies.**

  a. Hay fever, asthma, and food allergies, for example, show a **familial tendency;** there is a strong probability (about 75%) that children of two atopic parents also will be atopic.

  b. Population studies suggest that total IgE levels are regulated by a single gene that is not linked to the major histocompatibility complex (MHC).

  c. Specific IgE responses to ragweed and ryegrass allergens have a **linkage** with particular **human leukocyte antigens (HLA-DR2 and -DR3).**

C. **Clinical features**

1. **Tests for identifying specific allergens** are described in Chapter 6.

  a. In vivo **skin tests** to identify the **range of allergen sensitivities** are the most common tests**.**

  b. **Radioimmunoassays** are also used to **quantitate IgE levels in serum.**

2. **Symptoms and signs** of immediate hypersensitivity reactions begin very shortly (10–20 minutes) after allergen exposure and vary greatly in severity and character depending on the target organ or tissue and on whether the condition is anaphylactic or atopic.

  a. **Anaphylaxis** is an immediate hypersensitivity response elicited in an otherwise healthy host that has been appropriately sensitized.

    (1) The response may be either **systemic (anaphylactic shock)** or **local,** but in all species it is characterized primarily by smooth muscle contraction and increased capillary permeability.

    (2) The primary **target organ,** or **shock organ,** varies from species to species. Examples of primary target organs include the lung in guinea pigs and humans, the heart in rabbits, and the liver in dogs. These differences are related to the mast cell content of the tissues.

    (3) The immediate hypersensitivity response in the guinea pig has a classic presentation of **itching, sneezing, urination, defecation,** and **convulsions.** Death occurs within minutes because of severe bronchoconstriction, smooth muscle contraction, and trapping of air in the lungs (these symptoms may also be seen in humans as well).

  b. **Atopy** is an immediate hypersensitivity response that occurs only in genetically predisposed hosts on sensitization to specific allergens.

    (1) As in anaphylactic reactions, the response in atopic reactions is characterized by **smooth muscle contraction** and **increased capillary permeability** with **resultant local edema. Mucus secretion** adds to the **airway obstruction.**

    (2) Specific types of atopic reactions include **bronchial asthma, allergic rhinitis (hay fever), urticaria (hives), angioedema,** and **atopic dermatitis (eczema).**

3. **Incidence of disease** (Table 7-2)
    a. **Anaphylactic shock** of sufficient severity to require hospitalization occurs in approximately **20,000 people each year** in the United States, causing 200–400 deaths. Over 25% of the adult population were recently reported to have **anti-insect venom IgE,** suggesting that sting anaphylaxis should be considered in cases of unexpected death, particularly in summer.
    b. **Atopic reactions** are much more common.
       (1) Approximately **5% of the population of the United States have asthma,** and more than 5000 people die of this condition yearly. Asthma is slightly more common in boys than in girls (3:2).
       (2) About 10% of the population of the United States suffer from hay fever.
       (3) Atopic dermatitis affects only 1%–2% of the population.

D. **Therapeutic measures for hypersensitivity reactions (Table 7-3)**

1. **Avoidance of the responsible allergens (environmental control).** Environmental control is the most effective way to manage allergic disease. This can be accomplished easily with food allergies; however, it may be difficult with inhalant allergens.

2. **Hyposensitization** involves injecting the patient, over time, with gradually increasing doses of the responsible allergen. This stimulates the production of immunoglobulin G

TABLE 7-2. Impact of Selected Allergic Conditions on the Population of the United States

Allergic Condition	Estimated Number Affected (millions)
Chronic sinusitis	35
Allergic rhinitis	20
Asthma	14
Contact dermatitis and eczema	6

TABLE 7-3. Possible Methods of Therapy of Atopic Diseases

- Avoidance of allergen
- Hyposensitization—IgG blocking antibody
- Desensitization—saturate or exhaust IgE
- Drugs
    - Block mediator release*
        Cromolyn sodium—blocks Ca^{++} influx
        Theophylline—$\downarrow$ phosphodiesterase
        Epinephrine—$\uparrow$ adenylate cyclase
    - Block mediator effect
        Antihistamine
        Epinephrine—relax smooth muscle
        Cortisone inhibits mediator synthesis and phospholipase A_2; also
            inhibits chemotaxis

*The goal of therapy is to prevent degraulation by maintaining homeostatic cAMP level in the cell.

Ca^{++} = calcium ions; $cAMP$ = cyclic adenosine monophosphate; $\uparrow$ = acativate; $\downarrow$ = block

(IgG)-blocking antibody, which reacts with the offending allergen and prevents its combining with IgE on the mast cell membrane.

3. **Desensitization** is a transient ablation of the sensitivity to the allergen. It is induced by multiple minute injections of the allergen given over a period of a few hours. The patient is usually treated with anti-histaminic drugs and corticosteroids prior to desensitization therapy. The allergen injections cause all of the mast cells and basophils bearing the homologous IgE to degranulate. Sensitivity will return once new mast cells and basophils become coated the IgE, a process that will take a few weeks. In the intervening time the individual will be non-responsive to that particular allergen. This process is sometimes done to allow the administration of life saving drugs (e.g., antibiotics) to allergic individuals.

4. **Drug treatment** involves the administration of agents designed to reverse various allergic mechanisms (see Table 7–3). This may be achieved in several ways:
    a. **Mediators can be blocked from binding to target tissue** (e.g., by using antihistaminics such as diphenhydramine).
    b. **Granules** or **cell membranes and vascular endothelium** (e.g., with corticosteroids) can be **stabilized.**
    c. **Mediator release can be blocked** in one of three ways:
        (1) **Inhibiting calcium influx** (e.g., by using cromolyn sodium)
        (2) **Stimulating adenylate cyclase,** the enzyme that converts adenosine triphosphate (ATP) to cAMP (e.g., by using isoproterenol or β-adrenergic agents such as epinephrine)
        (3) **Preserving the necessary levels of cAMP** by **inhibiting phosphodiesterase,** an enzyme that converts cAMP to AMP (e.g., by using theophylline or other methyl xanthines)
    d. Synthesis of the slow reactive substances of anaphylaxis can be interfered with by blocking production of arachidonic acid.
        (1) Cortisone induces proteins (e.g., macrocortin) in the cytoplasm of mast cells that alter arachidonic acid metabolism.
        (2) **Macrocortin** and other cortisone-induced proteins block phospholipase A_2, thus inhibiting the breakdown of cell membrane lipids into arachidonic acid.

III. CYTOTOXIC (TYPE II) REACTIONS

A. **Definition.** Cytotoxic reactions are initiated by antibody—either IgG or IgM—reacting with cell-bound antigen.

B. **Pathogenic mechanisms** (Figure 7-2)

1. Cytotoxic reactions primarily involve one of two pathogenic mechanisms for sensitization of the cell:
    a. The **combination of IgG or IgM antibodies with epitopes** on cell surface or tissue

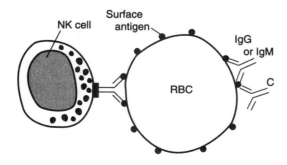

FIGURE 7-2. The mechanism of cytotoxic antibody action (type II reaction). Immunoglobulin G (*IgG*) or M (*IgM*) reacts with an antigen on a red blood cell (*RBC*) membrane and activates the complement cascade (*C*); this results in opsonization or cell membrane perturbation and lysis (as shown in Figure 4–3). IgG and IgM may sensitize the cell to cytotoxic attack by natural killer (*NK*) cells.

    b. The **adsorption of antigens** or **haptens to tissues** or **to the cell membrane,** with **subsequent attachment of antibodies** to the adsorbed antigens

2. Either of these sensitization mechanisms may lead to one of the following destructive processes:

    a. Lysis or inactivation of target cells by activation of **complement**

    b. **Phagocytosis** of target cells, with or without complement participation

    c. Lysis or inactivation of target cells by **antibody-dependent cell-mediated cytolysis (ADCC)** through the **action of natural killer (NK) cells**

C. **Clinical features.** Cytotoxic reactions can be grouped according to the nature of the target cell or the tissue damage that occurs in the reaction.

1. **Red blood cell lysis** is the most important clinical phenomenon associated with cytotoxic reactions.

    a. **Mechanisms of red blood cell lysis. Immunologically mediated transfusion reactions** may occur by two different mechanisms.

        (1) Rapid **intravascular hemolysis** of transfused red blood cells is usually associated with **ABO system incompatibility.** The ABO blood group system consists of genetically determined antigens on the red blood cell surface.

        (2) **Phagocytosis and destruction** of red blood cells, primarily by the reticuloendothelial system (RES), is almost invariably associated with Rh incompatibility. The Rh antigen most commonly involved is $Rh_o(D)$.

        (3) **Clinical consequences**

            (a) Symptoms of transfusion reactions include fever, back pain, chills, malaise, hypotension, nausea, and vomiting.

            (b) Acute renal failure is a serious complication of transfusion reactions and is highly correlated with the severity of the lower back pain.

        (4) **Prevention of transfusion reactions** includes careful blood typing and cross-matching to avoid incompatibility.

    b. **Hemolytic disease of the newborn**

        (1) **Etiology and pathogenesis**

            (a) Hemolytic disease of the newborn occurs because **the mother has made IgG antibodies against antigens on the infant's red blood cells (RBCs).** The antigenic stimulus may have been a previous transfusion, a graft, or an earlier pregnancy. The major blood group antigens A and B may be involved, as may Rh antigens, and minor blood group antigens like M and N.

            (b) **Erythroblastosis fetalis** occurs when an Rh-negative mother gives birth to an Rh-positive infant. Most often $Rh_o(D)$ is involved.

               (i) The major risk of sensitization occurs during delivery, when large amounts of cord blood enter the mother's circulation.

               (ii) Sensitization may occur during pregnancy if fetal blood leaks into the maternal circulation. A small amount of transplacental blood leakage is normal.

            (c) After sensitization, IgG antibodies to the $Rh_o(D)$ antigen are produced. These antibodies may cross the placenta and destroy fetal cells. The first child usually is not affected, but the chance of sensitization increases with subsequent pregnancies.

        (2) **Symptoms.** Anemia and jaundice usually develop in affected infants during the first 24 hours of life. Hepatosplenomegaly and bilirubin encephalopathy also occur.

        (3) **Management.** In severe cases, infants require **exchange transfusion,** a procedure in which the infant's blood is removed and replaced with a neutral blood for which the baby has no antibodies.

            (a) Amniocentesis and spectrophotometric examination of the amniotic fluid for bilirubin is the best way to determine the status of fetal erythrocytes.

            (b) An **indirect Coombs' test can be done with the mother's serum** before the baby is born and a **direct Coombs' can be done on the infant's RBCs** to determine sensitization (see Chapter 6 for a discussion of these tests).

(4) **Prevention.** Hemolytic disease of the newborn is best avoided by **preventing maternal sensitization to fetal Rh antigens** or by **inhibiting the production of antibodies** to those antigens.

(a) Administering **anti-Rh$_0$ IgG antibodies (RhoGAM)** to an Rh-negative mother within 72 hours after delivery of an Rh-positive infant prevents sensitization, probably via rapid destruction and clearance of Rh-positive cells from the circulation.

(b) The anti-Rh$_0$ IgG is a blocking agent; it does not induce immune tolerance to the Rh$_0$(D) antigen. Therefore, it must be given **after each pregnancy.**

(c) In the past, approximately 10% of Rh-negative women who gave birth to Rh-positive infants became sensitized even after RhoGAM injection, probably as a result of placental leakage during pregnancy. Current obstetric practice recommends injection of RhoGAM at 26 weeks' gestational age and again at parturition; this has virtually eliminated earlier treatment failures.

c. **Autoimmune hemolytic disease.** Warm-antibody hemolytic anemia, cold-antibody hemolytic anemia, and paroxysmal cold hemoglobinuria are discussed in Chapter 8.

2. **White blood cell lysis**

a. **Granulocytopenia.** Cytotoxic reactions involving antibodies to neutrophils or to drugs adsorbed to neutrophil surfaces can result in granulocytopenia and a consequent phagocytic defect, which leads to an increased susceptibility to infection.

b. **Idiopathic thrombocytopenic purpura (ITP)** is characterized by the presence of platelet-specific IgG antibodies, which can lead to various bleeding disorders.

c. **Systemic lupus erythematosus (SLE)**

(1) This autoimmune disease can be considered a mixed disease—that is, it involves both type II and type III hypersensitivity reactions.

(2) In patients with SLE, several types of antibodies are present in the serum, including antinuclear antibodies, antibodies to membrane and cytoplasmic components, and antibodies cytotoxic to blood cells (lymphocytes, red blood cells, platelets).

D. | **Therapeutic measures.** Therapy for cytotoxic reactions involves treatment of the underlying cause as well as the manifestations of the reaction. Examples include:

1. **Suppression of the immune response** by means of corticosteroids, with or without cytotoxic immunosuppressive drugs (e.g., cyclophosphamide and methotrexate), or by splenectomy

2. **Removal of the offending antibodies** via exchange transfusion (in the case of hemolytic disease of the newborn) or plasmapheresis (in the case of Goodpasture's syndrome)

3. **Withholding the offending drug** (in the case of a drug-induced syndrome such as ITP or drug-induced hemolytic disease)

IV. IMMUNE COMPLEX-MEDIATED (TYPE III) REACTIONS

A. | **Definition.** Immune complex-mediated reactions are initiated by antigen—antibody (i.e., immune) complexes that are formed in the blood vessels and are then deposited in tissues.

1. **Immune complex disorders** are characterized by the presence of such complexes on vascular and glomerular basement membranes.

2. **Symptoms** depend on the location of the immune complex deposition, and can include arthritis, nephritis, vasculitis, or skin lesions.

B. | **Pathogenic mechanisms.** Pathogenesis involves an interplay of antigen, antibody, complement, and neutrophils (Figure 7-3).

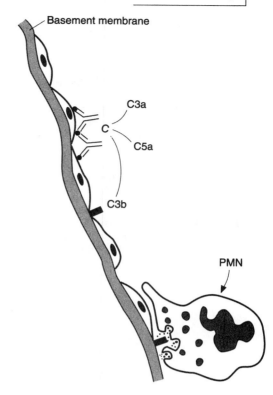

FIGURE 7-3. The mechanism of tissue damage caused by immune complexes (type III reaction). Immune complexes of antigen and either immunoglobulin G (*IgG*) or M (*IgM*) are deposited on *basement membranes.* Complement (*C*) is activated, and polymorphonuclear neutrophils (*PMNs*), which have receptors for C3b, move into the area in response to the *C5a* chemotaxin. In the process of attempting to engulf the immune complexes, these phagocytic cells degranulate and release proteolytic enzymes and other toxic molecules that injure tissues in the area.

1. The first step is the intravascular formation of **soluble immune complexes,** which generally occurs when there is **excess antigen.**
   a. **Antigens.** Virtually any antigen that induces a detectable antibody response is suitable; autoantigens are commonly involved. **Microbial antigens** (e.g., *Streptococcus pyogenes, Mycobacterium leprae, Treponema pallidum, Plasmodium* and *Trypanosoma* species), can also induce significant immune complex-caused tissue damage, as can **viruses** such as Epstein-Barr, hepatitis B, and hemorrhagic dengue.
   b. The **antibodies** involved are IgG and IgM, both of which are capable of activating complement.

2. Only **small immune complexes** cause damage because, being very small, these immune complexes escape phagocytosis. They penetrate the endothelium of blood vessel walls (probably with the aid of vasoactive amines released from platelets and basophils) and are deposited on the vascular basement membrane.

3. **Complement** is activated, and C3a and C5a are released.
   a. These anaphylatoxins **increase the permeability of the vascular endothelium.** They react with receptors on mast cells and basophils, causing the release of vasoactive amines. This increases vascular permeability.
   b. C5a is also chemotactic for neutrophils, which then infiltrate the area and release lysosomal enzymes and toxic oxygen metabolites that destroy the basement membrane, thus altering the structural integrity and function of the tissue (e.g., the glomerular basement membrane of the kidney).

4. **Platelets** also interact with immune complexes through membrane-bound Fc receptors. This leads to platelet aggregation and microthrombus formation.
   a. Platelets **release vasoactive amines and tissue cell growth factors.**
   b. These growth factors may be responsible for the cellular proliferation found in certain immune complex diseases such as rheumatoid arthritis and lupus nephritis.

5. **Large immune complexes** are destroyed by phagocytosis. The complexes are first bound to red blood cells through CRI complement receptors in the cell membrane. The red cells circulate to the liver where the immune complexes are removed by the RES.

C. **Clinical features.** The following are classic examples of type III reactions mediated by immune complex deposition in tissues.

1. **Arthus reaction.** This necrotic dermal reaction is considered to be a **local immune complex-deposition phenomenon.** It was observed first in rabbits, but similar reactions are observed in other animals, including humans.
   a. Animals are immunized with antigen.
   b. On subsequent exposure, foci of erythema, edema, and necrosis occur at the injection site. Microscopic examination of tissue reveals an accumulation of neutrophils plus a vasculitis related to destruction of the basement membrane of blood vessel walls.

2. **Serum sickness.** This syndrome follows the injection of foreign serum into humans. It is considered to be a **systemic immune complex-deposition phenomenon.** Serum sickness was first seen after the administration of horse antitoxin in humans.(Figure 7-4).

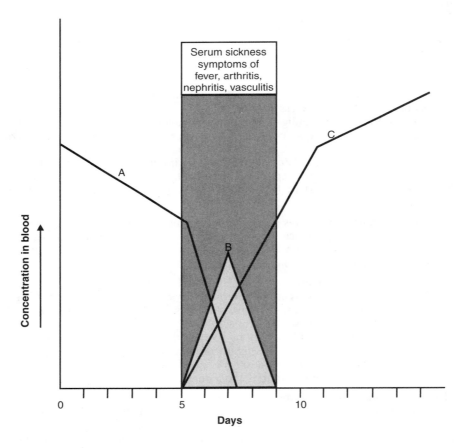

FIGURE 7-4. Horse antitoxin injected at Day 0. A=horse antitoxin; B=immune complexes; C=antibodies against horse serum proteins.

a. **Clinical observation.** The primary damage observed in serum sickness, as in the **Arthus reaction,** appears to be a vasculitis associated with destruction of vascular basement membrane.

b. **Symptoms.** The syndrome is characterized by fever, rash, splenomegaly, lymphadenopathy, arthritis, and glomerulonephritis.

   (1) The hallmark of immune complex glomerulonephritis is **granular ("lumpy-bumpy") appearance of the immune complexes on the basement membrane** as detected by direct immunofluorescence using tagged antibody specific for immunoglobulin or complement.

   (2) This technique can differentiate immune complex glomerulonephritis from that caused by autoantibodies to the glomerular basement membrane, in which a smooth, linear pattern of immunoglobulin deposition is observed.

3. **Poststreptococcal glomerulonephritis.** The immune complex glomerulonephritis that can follow a streptococcal pharyngitis is characterized by proteinuria and hematuria with red blood cell casts in the urine.

   a. Antibody, complement, and bacterial antigens are present in the renal vasculature.

   b. Poststreptococcal glomerulonephritis, like serum sickness glomerulonephritis, has a "lumpy-bumpy" appearance under immunofluorescence.

4. **Autoimmune disease.** Endogenous antigen—antibody—complement complexes are involved in the pathogenesis of certain autoimmune diseases, such as rheumatoid arthritis and SLE.

5. **Hypersensitivity pneumonitis.** Both type III and type IV hypersensitivity reactions appear to play a role in this interstitial lung disease (see V C 3).

D. **Therapeutic measures.** Treatment for immune complex-mediated reactions includes:

1. **Reduction of inflammation** by means of aspirin, antihistamines, non-steroidal anti-inflammatory agents, and corticosteroids

2. **Suppression of the immune response** by means of corticosteroids and cytotoxic immunosuppressive drugs (e.g., cyclophosphamide, methotrexate)

3. **Removal of offending complexes** via plasmapheresis

V. CELL-MEDIATED REACTIONS (TYPE IV): DELAYED HYPERSENSITIVITY AND CELL-MEDIATED CYTOTOXICITY

A. **Overview.** Cell-mediated immune reactions do not involve antibody and complement; instead, they are dependent on functioning T cells (Figure 7-5).

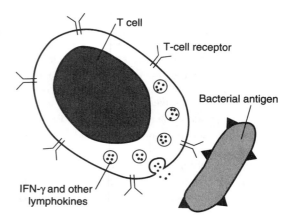

FIGURE 7-5. The mechanism of injury in cell-mediated immune responses (type IV reaction). *T cells* interact via their *T-cell receptor* with a homologous antigen in the antigen-binding groove of a class I major histocompatibility complex (MHC) molecule (see Figure 5-5). This interaction perturbs the T-cell receptor and the CD3 molecules; it initiates a series of reactions that culminate in the release of gamma interferon (*IFN-γ*) and other lymphokines by the T cell (see text for details).

1. There are **two kinds** of cell-mediated immunity: **delayed-type hypersensitivity** (Gell and Coombs type IV reactivity) and **cytotoxic T (Tc) cell responses.** Each response is initiated by a different type of sensitized (antigen-reactive) T cell.
   a. The **effector cells** that are responsible for **delayed-type hypersensitivity reactions (Tdth cells)** recruit other cells (e.g., macrophages) that actually do most of the tissue damage.
   b. The **effector cells** that are responsible for **cell-mediated cytotoxic reactions (Tc cells)** are themselves cytotoxic due to the release of cytotoxic lymphokines.

2. **Cell-mediated reactions differ from antibody-mediated reactions.**
   a. Delayed hypersensitivity reactions and cell-mediated cytotoxic reactions are **delayed in time,** in contrast to antibody-mediated immune reactions, which may occur minutes after antigen exposure as in anaphylaxis.
      (1) **Delayed hypersensitivity reactions** usually peak 24–48 hours after exposure and manifest as inflammation at the site of antigen exposure.
      (2) **Tc cell reactions** have a similar manifestation and time course.
   b. Antibody-mediated and cell-mediated hypersensitivities also differ in the **nature of their inflammatory process.**
      (1) **Antibody-mediated reactions** have more edema and erythema (wheal and flare).
      (2) **Cell-mediated immune reactions** are characterized by significant mononuclear cell infiltration with resultant induration.

B. **Pathogenic mechanisms**

1. **Effector cells**
   a. **Two types of effector T cells** can be identified.
      (1) **Tdth cells**
         (a) Tdth cells recognize foreign antigens, primarily those of intracellular pathogens.
         (b) They confer resistance by secreting IFN-γ and other lymphokines, thereby activating macrophages to cytotoxic activity and enhancing other T-and B-cell responses.
      (2) **Tc cells,** often called **cytolytic T lymphocytes (CTLs)**
         (a) Tc cells recognize foreign antigens on most cells of the body.
         (b) They confer resistance in two ways:
            (i) Secretion of IFN-γ, which induces other cells to produce antiviral proteins. IFN-γ is a major lymphokine that is important in expression of cell-mediated immunity. Its biologic effects are summarized in Table 7-4.
            (ii) Direct destruction of target cells (e.g., grafted tissue, tumors, and virus-infected cells) by release of perforin, proteases, nucleases, and tumor necrosis factor with subsequent target cell destruction. (see Table 1–9).
   b. **Tc cells** are **directly cytotoxic, whereas Tdth cells act** primarily **through recruitment of other cells.**

TABLE 7-4. Major Biologic Activities of Interferon Gamma (IFN-γ)

Inhibiting viral replication by interfering with viral protein synthesis
Inducing the expression of class II major histocompatibility complex (MHC) molecules on tissue cells, allowing these cells to become active in antigen presentation
Increasing the expression of Fc receptors on macrophages
Activating neutrophils and macrophages to heightened microbicidal and tumoricidal activity
Inhibiting cell growth (e.g., Th2 cells)
Enhancing the activity of natural killer (NK) cells

c. Tdth cells can be distinguished serologically from Tc cells by their **cluster of differen-tiation (CD)** surface antigens.
  (1) Tdth cells are CD4$^+$ (i.e., they carry the CD4 surface antigen).
  (2) Tc cells are CD8$^+$.

2. **Induction of reactions.** Cell-mediated reactions are induced by the uptake and process-ing of antigen and the activation of T cells.
  a. There are several **different types of antigen-processing cells.**
    (1) **Macrophages.** Antigen-processing cells for B cells and for CD8$^+$ cells are usually macrophages. Macrophages, however, do not normally have much class II anti-gen in their membranes.
    (2) **Langerhans cells.** Hence, a delayed-type hypersensitivity reaction is probably ini-tiated by the interaction of Tdth CD4$^+$ cells with epitope—class II MHC com-plexes on dendritic cells, which express high concentrations of class II molecules.
  b. Antigen-processing cells and T cells can interact, but only if the two participants are **MHC-identical.**
    (1) CD4$^+$ cells recognize antigen in conjunction with class II MHC molecules (e.g., HLA-DR).
    (2) CD8$^+$ cells recognize antigen in conjunction with class I MHC molecules (HLA-A, -B, and -C).
  c. Under the influence of antigen and MHC gene products, antigen-reactive (sensitized) Tdth and Tc cells are produced.
  d. Role of **interleukins**
    (1) The Th population of CD4$^+$ cells aids in the development of CD4+ dth cells and CD8$^+$ cytotoxic cells by releasing **lymphokines (interleukins)** that augment prolif-erative and maturational signals generated by antigen contact.
    (2) Interleukin IL-12, produced by antigen processing cells such as the Langerhans cells of the skin, is a particularly important lymphokine that acts synergistically with IL-2 to enhance proliferation and maturation of Tdth and Tc cells of the cell-mediated immune responses.

3. **Expression of delayed hypersensitivity** (see Figure 7-5)
  a. On interaction with homologous epitope (probably presented on the surface of den-dritic cells), the Tdth subpopulation of CD4$^+$ cells responds by secreting lymphokines such as IFN-γ.
  b. The lymphokines in turn activate nearby lymphocytes and macrophages and induce the immigration of more cells into the area. It is not known how many biochemically distinct lymphokines exist; however, the following are among those generally recog-nized as **mediators of delayed hypersensitivity.**
    (1) **Migration-inhibiting factor** inhibits migration of macrophages.
    (2) **Macrophage-activating factors** such as IFN-γ, granulocyte-macrophage colony-stimulating factor, and tumor necrosis factor α (TNF-α) enhance the microbicidal and cytolytic activity of macrophages. IFN-γ has numerous other functions (see Table 7-4).
    (3) **Leukocyte-inhibiting factor** inhibits random migration of neutrophils.
    (4) **Macrophage-chemotactic factor [interleukin-8 (IL-8)]** stimulates infiltration of neutrophils and T cells.
    (5) **Interleukin-2 (IL-2),** a mitogenic factor, stimulates the growth of activated T cells. It also activates cytotoxic lymphocytes and macrophages.
    (6) **TNF-β (lymphotoxin)** has the ability to kill certain tumor cells.
  c. **Activated macrophages** secrete a variety of biologically active compounds that cause inflammation and destroy bacteria, tumors, and other cells considered foreign by the immune apparatus. These compounds include:
    (1) **Cytokines**
      (a) Interleukins 1, 6, 8, and 12
      (b) TNF-α
    (2) **Reactive oxygen metabolites** such as superoxide anion, hydroxyl radical, and hy-drogen peroxide

        (3) Proteases and other lysosomal enzymes
- **d.** An **amplification loop** is activated.
  - **(1)** The IFN-γ secreted by activated Tdth cells stimulates macrophages to express MHC class II proteins in their membranes.
  - **(2)** The interferon-activated macrophages can now present epitopes to Tdth cells, with the resultant release of more IFN-γ and more efficient antigen presentation.
- **4. Expression of Tc cell cytotoxicity**
  - **a.** Tc cells destroy only those target cells that they recognize as antigenically foreign.
    - **(1)** When a Tc cell encounters a cell, it explores the other cell's surface for an epitope that its T-cell receptor can recognize.
    - **(2)** If recognition occurs, the Tc cell releases cytotoxic proteins from its intracytoplasmic granules (see Table 1–9).
  - **b.** The effector molecules released by Tc cells are more cytotoxic than those of Tdth cells, and commonly lead directly to cell death.
    - **(1)** The most important of the Tc cell's cytotoxic proteins is **perforin,** which resembles the complement component C9, both in terms of function and amino acid sequence.
      - **(a)** Like C9, perforin inserts itself into target cell membranes, and polymerizes, forming transmembrane channels that allow the influx and exit of water, ions, and low molecular-weight metabolites. The perforin-induced channels cause the target cell to lose electrolytes, absorb water, swell, and burst.
      - **(b)** Perforin is a highly hydrophobic molecule that integrates very rapidly into the lipid membrane of target cells. Hence, its diffusion is limited and lysis of non-target cells is minimal.
      - **(c)** Tc cells have a membrane proteoglycan (a chondroitin sulfate called **protectin**) that interacts with perforin molecules to prevent their polymerization, thus protecting the Tc cells from perforin damage.
    - **(2) Other molecules** released from these intracytoplasmic granules include serine proteases, nucleases, and molecules that resemble TNF.
    - **(3)** An endogenous endonuclease is activated by the interaction of a Fas ligand in the membrane of the cytotoxic cell with the Fas protein in the target cell membrane. This initiates the process of apoptosis **(programmed cell death).**
  - **c.** After the Tc cell initiates lysis of the target cell, it searches for another "victim."

C. **Clinical features**

- **1. Role of T-cell-mediated immunity in disease**
  - **a. Delayed hypersensitivity and Tc cell reactions can be protective** as well as damaging. They provide resistance to:
    - **(1)** Chronic intracellular bacterial infections (e.g., tuberculosis)
    - **(2)** Fungal and viral infections
    - **(3)** Tumors (cytotoxic antibody is also sometimes involved)
  - **b. Tc cells** play a role in the **rejection of grafted tissues and organs.** Humoral immunity also may be involved in allograft rejection.
  - **c. Sensitized T lymphocytes** provide the basic **mechanism of tissue injury** in the following diseases:
    - **(1) Contact dermatitis,** which is a delayed hypersensitivity reaction that occurs in response to exposure of the skin to certain allergens (e.g., urushiol allergen of poison ivy and poison sumac)
    - **(2)** Some **autoimmune diseases,** in which Tc cells play a major role in pathogenesis (e.g., Guillain-Barré syndrome)
- **2.** The **tuberculin skin test reaction** is the classic example of delayed hypersensitivity.
  - **a.** A small amount of antigen—usually purified protein derivative (PPD) of the tuberculosis bacillus is injected intradermally into a sensitized person.
  - **b.** The reaction appears slowly, about 12–24 hours after the injection, and reaches maximal reactivity 24–48 hours later.

(1) Initially, there is erythema and a neutrophil infiltrate.

(2) Later, a mononuclear cell (lymphocyte and macrophage) infiltrate causes induration in the region of the injection.

3. **Hypersensitivity pneumonitis (extrinsic allergic alveolitis).** These terms refer to the parenchymal reaction that develops in the lung on repeated inhalation of particulate allergens.

   a. **Pathogenesis**

      (1) Patients often have antibodies to the offending substances, with deposition of antigen-antibody complexes in target (lung) tissue during the early phase of the disease.

      (2) Evidence indicates that **delayed hypersensitivity (type IV) reactions** play a major role in the pathogenesis of hypersensitivity pneumonitis.

   b. **Symptoms.** Fever, chills, chest pain, cough, and dyspnea occur 4–8 hours after exposure. In severe, chronic cases, irreversible lung damage (fibrosis) may occur.

D. Therapeutic measures

1. **Avoidance of allergens** is the first line of therapy.

2. **Reduction of inflammation** is achieved with aspirin and other nonsteroidal anti-inflammatory agents (NSAIDs).

3. **Immunosuppression** (See also Chapter 5). Agents that suppress cell-mediated immunity include

   a. **Corticosteroids,** which are both immunosuppressive and anti-inflammatory

   b. **Antibodies** (e.g., anti-lymphocyte serum and anti-thymocyte serum)

   c. **Cytotoxic immunosuppressive drugs** (e.g., azathioprine, cyclosporine, and cyclophosphamide).

Vignette Revisited

1. Dana had an anaphylactic reaction and could have easily slipped into anaphylactic shock. The vasoactive compounds released from her mast cells and basophils caused local edema in the bronchioles, mucus secretion, and smooth muscle contractions, all of which narrowed the airway.

2. Deb may have never been stung by bees before this incident and therefore, may have never been sensitized to their venom. The initial exposure is the basis for the later allergic (or, in Dana's case, anaphylactic) reaction. Deb may become ill from a subsequent bee sting if she made an IgE response to the venom following this exposure.

3. Epinephrine should be given immediately on recognition of the anaphylactic reaction. Once this is accomplished, care is focused on ensuring that the patient has a patent airway and is ventilating adequately. Steroids may help to reduce inflammation over the ensuing hours and days, but they are of no use in the initial management.

4. Deb most likely has poison ivy or poison sumac. At some point in her life, she came in contact with and was sensitized to an allergenic resin of the plant which contains complex catechols and is known as urushiol. These compounds bind to proteins in the skin and become immunogenic. A second exposure triggers an allergic contact dermatitis, which occurs because the sensitized Tdth lymphocytes release lymphokines when they encounter the urushiol—protein conjugate in the dermal layers.

5. Deb should be treated with oral antihistamines and calamine lotion. The use of topical antihistamine lotions should be discouraged because they may actually make symptoms worse and lead to secondary problems in some patients. In younger children, the lesions may need to be bandaged to prevent scratching, because this could lead to spreading of the reaction and secondary infection of open sores. Topical antibiotics can be used if infection is suspected.

6. Deb is advised not to scratch because she can transfer the allergen to her fingers and the reaction will "spread" via this form of autoinoculation. If the allergen is transferred to her eyes, the reaction is uncomfortable and difficult to treat.

STUDY QUESTIONS

Questions 1–2

1. A 26-year-old male patient has a severe allergy to mold spores. Avoidance is not a practical solution because of the ubiquity of the fungus, and hyposensitization is recommended. This form of immunotherapy for atopic allergies induces formation of which of the following blocking antibodies?

(A) IgA
(B) IgD
(C) IgE
(D) IgG
(E) IgM

2. Three weeks after a severe case of pharyngitis, this patient begins to have protein and blood in his urine. A diagnosis of post-streptococcal glomerulonephritis is made. The pathogenesis of immune complex disorders such as this involves an interplay of antigen, antibody, neutrophils, and which of the following complement-derived factors?

(A) C1s
(B) C1a4b
(C) C3b inactivator
(D) C3 activator
(E) C5a

3. The patient is a 25-year-old female with a rash over the bridge of her nose. She complains of low grade fever and joint pain. There is protein and erythrocytes in her urine. A diagnosis of systemic lupus erythematosus is made. The pathogenic requirements for this type of immune complex-induced glomerulonephritis include

(A) red blood cell and complement interaction
(B) lymphocytes
(C) neutrophils
(D) kidney-derived antigen
(E) large aggregated immune complexes

4. The neonate is lethargic and jaundiced. Laboratory studies reveal profound anemia and elevated bilirubin levels in the blood. A direct Coombs' test is positive; the child is blood group O. The mother is blood group A, Rh negative, but was not injected with RhoGAM after an elective abortion when she was 16 years of age. The most likely cause of this child's disease is

(A) ABO blood group incompatibility
(B) congenital syphilis
(C) sickle cell disease
(D) minor blood group incompatibility
(E) erythoblastosis fetalis

5. The mother of an undersized 10-month-old child comes to her pediatrician for help. The child is colicky and does not eat well. Chronic diarrhea has also been a problem. Skin testing of the infant reveals an allergy to milk proteins. The immunologic basis of this disease is most likely

(A) IgA
(B) IgG
(C) IgE
(D) Tdth cells
(E) Tc cells

6. Atopic allergies such as asthma and hay fever affect over 25 million individuals in the United States. What is the most effective method of treating these allergies?

(A) Hyposensitization
(B) Environmental control
(C) Administration of modified allergens
(D) Administration of antihistamines
(E) Administration of corticosteroids

7. Mediators of immediate hypersensitivity (type I) reactions are either preformed and stored in host cells or are newly formed from precursor constituents. Which one of the following is a preformed mediator of type I reactions?

(A) Platelet-activating factor (PAF)
(B) Anaphylatoxin I
(C) Slow-reacting substance of anaphylaxis (SRS-A)
(D) Histamine
(E) Leukotriene LTC4

8. A patient has a history of stillbirths. Fearing hemolytic disease of the newborn in the infant she is currently carrying, amniocentesis is performed. Spectrophotometric examination reveals hemoglobin breakdown products in the amniotic fluid. Erythrocyte injury in cytotoxic (type II) hypersensitivity reactions is initiated by which of the following pathogenic mechanisms?

(A) Antibody interfering with the functioning of biologically active substances
(B) Antigen reacting with cell-bound antibody
(C) Antibody reacting with cell-bound antigen
(D) Formation of antigen-antibody complexes
(E) Sensitized T cells reacting with specific antigens

9. A 9-year-old grade school boy is seen by the school nurse. He complains of hives that began to develop shortly after lunch. She is familiar with the child's allergic history and suspects that some food product has triggered this episode. This patient's allergic urticaria is best described as being a manifestation of

(A) an IgE-mediated disorder
(B) delayed hypersensitivity
(C) cytotoxic IgG antibodies
(D) cytotoxic T (Tc) cells
(E) an immune complex-mediated disorder

1. The answer is D [II D 2]. Immunotherapy for atopy involves the deliberate injection of the offending allergen, beginning at a low dosage and increasing to a maintenance dosage (i.e., the highest dose the patient can tolerate). The procedure stimulates production of IgG-blocking antibody, which binds the allergen and forms complexes that are removed by the reticuloendothelial system (RES), thus preventing the allergen from reaching and combining with the IgE on basophils and mast cells. The IgA level will be unaffected; however, the amount of allergen-specific IgE will decrease during the course of the allergen injections. T cells are not involved in atopic allergies.

2. The answer is E [IV B 3]. In immune complex disorders, antigen-antibody (immune) complexes are formed either locally or in the circulation and are deposited on the vascular or glomerular basement membrane. This causes inflammation by the following sequence of events: The antigen-antibody complexes, once deposited, fix complement component C1q, thus activating the classic complement pathway. C5a is generated, which is chemotactic for neutrophils; neutrophils then infiltrate the area and release lysosomal enzymes and toxic oxygen metabolites that destroy the surrounding tissue. None of the other complement proteins listed (C1s, C1a4b, C3b inactivator, and C3 activator) are chemotactic.

3. The answer is C [IV B]. The pathogenetic requirements for immune complex-induced glomerulonephritis include neutrophils and complement, as well as antibody and antigen (any of several antigens may be involved; they need not be derived from the kidney). The small size of the immune complex is critical to its pathogenicity; complexes that are small are not cleared from the circulation readily and are deposited on blood vessel walls. Such immune complexes form in a region of antigen excess and are soluble, escape phagocytosis, penetrate the vascular endothelium, and lodge on the basement membrane. Activation of complement attracts neutrophils, which release lysosomal enzymes that destroy basement membrane. Studies have shown that in humans, red blood cells participate in clearing immune complexes from the circulation. Complexes that have been coated with C3b attach to C3b receptors on red blood cells, are transported to the liver and spleen, and then are removed from the red blood cells by phagocytes.

4. The answer is E [III C 1 b]. Erythroblastosis fetalis is a very serious form of hemolytic disease of the newborn which occurs when an Rh-negative mother gives birth to an Rh-positive infant, the Rh antigen having been acquired from an Rh-positive father. The most commonly involved antigen is $Rh_o(D)$. For this condition to occur, the mother must be sensitized to blood group antigens of the infant's blood; sensitization usually occurs during a previous delivery or an abortion. After sensitization, IgG antibodies to the acquired antigen are produced, which may cross the placenta and destroy fetal cells. This is not an ABO blood group incompatibility as the infant is blood group O. It could be a minor blood group incompatibility but that would be much less common than an Rh (antigen D) mismatch with resultant erythroblastosis.

5. The answer is C [II A, B 2 b (4)]. Food allergy is an immediate, or type I, (IgE-mediated) hypersensitivity reaction. Immediate hypersensitivity reactions are initiated by antigens reacting with cell-bound IgE antibody. The reaction may manifest in many ways, ranging from life-threatening systemic anaphylaxis to the lesser annoyance of atopic allergies, such as food allergies, allergic rhinitis (hay fever), and urticaria (hives).

6. The answer is B [II D 1]. The most effective method of managing atopic allergies is through environmental control (i.e., avoidance of the specific allergen or allergens responsible for the allergic reaction). Atopic allergies are immediate hypersensitivity reactions that occur only in genetically predisposed hosts on sensitization to specific allergens. Other forms of management of atopic allergies include immunotherapy, which can be accomplished through hyposensitization or administration of modified allergens, and drug treatment (e.g., with antihistamines, corticosteroids, or epinephrine).

7. The answer is D [II B 4 b; Table 7-1]. Immediate hypersensitivity (type I) reactions involve the release of pharmacologically active substances (mediators) from mast cells or basophils, a mechanism that is triggered by antigens reacting with cell-bound IgE. Some type I mediators are stored within the mast cells and basophils in a preformed state; others are newly synthesized on initiation of the immediate hypersensitivity response. Preformed mediators include histamine (probably the most important), and eosinophil chemotactic factor of anaphylaxis (ECF-A). Mediators that are synthesized and released after the antigen-antibody reaction include slow-reacting substances of anaphylaxis (leukotrienes), platelet-activating factor (PAF), and prostaglandins. The anaphylatoxins are products of the complement cascade (C3a and C5a that are able to induce mast cell degranulation by reacting with specific receptors in the cell membrane.

8. The answer is C [III A, B 1]. The same immunologic mechanisms that defend the host may at times cause severe damage to tissues. These damaging immunologic reactions (also called hypersensitivity reactions) have been classified into four types according to the

mechanism of tissue injury. Cytotoxic (type II) hypersensitivity reactions are initiated by antibody—usually IgG or IgM—reacting with cell-bound antigen. Immediate hypersensitivity (type I) reactions are initiated by antigen reacting with cell-bound antibody—usually IgE. Immune complex-mediated (type III) reactions are initiated by antigen-antibody complexes that form locally or are deposited from the circulation. Delayed hypersensitivity (cell-mediated; type IV) reactions are initiated by sensitized (antigen-reactive) T cells reacting with specific antigens. A fifth mechanism of tissue injury exists, in which antibody interferes with the functioning of biologically active substances (e.g., clotting factors, insulin); this has sometimes been referred to as a type V reaction, but is more commonly called type II.

9. The answer is A [II A, B 1, 3]. Allergic urticaria (hives) is one of the milder manifestations of immediate hypersensitivity—specifically, atopic allergy. A more serious, sometimes life-threatening form of immediate hypersensitivity is systemic anaphylaxis. Although other immunoglobulin classes have been implicated in immediate hypersensitivity reactions, the primary antibody responsible for such reactivity in humans is IgE.

Chapter 8

Autoimmune Diseases

Vignette

A 54-year-old white man had been in good health until approximately 2 weeks before hospital admission, when, after receiving an influenza vaccination, he developed generalized fatigue and malaise. When his condition persisted for almost 1 week, he became concerned that it was more than just a reaction to the vaccine. Four days before admission he developed a severe, diffuse headache with accompanying muscle and bone pain. Forty-eight hours before admission, the patient noticed marked bilateral weakness in his extremities. On the day of admission, the patient had been unable to get out of bed and was brought to the hospital by ambulance.

The physical examination revealed a well-nourished, well-developed man in mild respiratory distress with rapid, shallow breathing. He was alert and oriented to person, place, time, and circumstance. His blood pressure was 160/120, his pulse was 115 beats/min, and his respirations were 28/min. His cardiac, pulmonary, and abdominal examinations all were unremarkable. During the neurologic examination, the patient demonstrated bilateral extremity weakness. Deep tendon reflexes were absent. The cranial nerves were intact. A computed tomography scan of the brain revealed no gross structural abnormalities. A lumbar puncture was performed. Opening pressure was 120 mm H_2O (normal is 50–200 mm H_2O) and the fluid was clear. White blood cells were 5/mm^3; red blood cells were absent; protein was 60 mg/dl (normal is 10–45 mg/dl); and glucose was 60 mg/dl (normal is 40–80 mg/dl).

During the next 2 days, the patient's vital signs fluctuated erratically, and his pulmonary capacity decreased from 3600 to 1000 ml. Arterial blood gases at this time were: PaO_2 70 mm Hg (normal is 80–100 mm Hg); $PaCO_2$ 48 mm Hg (normal is 35–45 mm Hg); HCO_3^-, 15 mEq/L; and pH, 7.38. A tracheostomy was performed, and the patient was placed on a ventilator.

Over the next 4 weeks, the patient's condition continued to deteriorate. The paralysis became nearly complete, and he developed pneumococcal pneumonia, which was treated successfully with penicillin. Seven weeks after admission, the patient began to regain neurologic function. His strength slowly returned, and his pulmonary mechanics improved. He was removed from the ventilator on his sixty-third day in the hospital. The patient was discharged 2 weeks later and began an active physical therapy program. The patient's recovery was complete, and 4 months after his initial illness he was able to return to work full time.

1. Based on the history, the physical examination, and the cerebrospinal fluid studies, what is the diagnosis?
2. What is the treatment for this disease?
3. Is there any significance between the influenza vaccine and the onset of symptoms?

I. GENERAL CONSIDERATIONS

A. **Definition.** Autoimmune responses are immune responses of an individual to antigens present in the individual's own tissue. These disorders are characterized by chronicity and usually are nonreversible (i.e., patients never fully recover and must learn to "live with their disease").

B. | **Incidence**

1. Autoimmune diseases affect more than 20 million Americans.

2. **Factors that affect incidence** include:
   a. **Sex.** Autoimmune diseases tend to occur at **higher frequencies in women than in men** (Table 8-1).
   b. **Age.** The frequency of autoimmune diseases **increases with age.** Very few autoimmune diseases occur in children and adolescents (juvenile diabetes is an exception); most of these disorders first appear in the 20-to 40-year age-group.

C. | **Etiology**

1. A defect in the mechanisms underlying self-recognition (autotolerance, self-tolerance) can result in autoimmune disease.

2. Autoimmune responses can be mediated by humoral factors (circulating antibodies, immune complexes) or cellular factors [delayed hypersensitivity, cytotoxic T (Tc) cell-mediated immunities.
   a. Most autoimmune diseases have associated **autoantibodies.**
      (1) These antibodies are believed to be etiologically involved in autoimmune diseases and to cause the resultant damage; namely, Gell and Coombs types II and III hypersensitivity reactions.
      (2) The autoantibodies, however, may merely reflect the damage done to an organ. As such, they are of diagnostic but not etiologic interest.
   b. Some of the autoimmune diseases that involve nervous tissue (the encephalomyelitides and Guillain-Barré syndrome) are thought to result from Gell and Coombs type IV hypersensitivity reactions. Guillain-Barré syndrome also may have an antibody component.
   c. Some autoimmune diseases (Hashimoto's thyroiditis, diabetes mellitus) are "mixed"—that is, they have both an antibody and a T-cell component.

3. **Possible mechanisms.** The basic process most likely involves recruitment of a helper/inducer T cell that cooperates with preexisting autoreactive B cells or Tc-cell precursors to induce a self-destructive immune response. The immunologic imbalance may arise from one or more of the following:
   a. **An excess of self-reactive helper T (Th)-cell activity**
      (1) The Th-cell hyperactivity may be induced by:

TABLE 8-1. Sex Ratio and Incidence of Certain Autoimmune Diseases

Disease	Female-Male Ratio	Estimated Incidence*
Rheumatoid arthritis	3:1	1000
Insulin-dependent diabetes mellitus	1:1	300
Systemic lupus erythematosus (SLE)	4:1	100
Multiple sclerosis	3:1	100
Polymyositis-dermatomyositis	2:1	0.5–1
Ankylosing spondylitis	1:9	0.5–1

*Per 100,000 United States population.

   (a) Altered forms of self-antigen
   (b) Antigens that cross-react with self-antigens as a result of epitope similarity
   (c) **Molecular mimicry,** in which self-antigens and foreign materials such as viruses or bacteria share identical epitopes
   (2) Altered forms of cross-reacting antigens may be produced by coupling of a virus, chemical, or drug (e.g., hydralazine) to self-antigen.
b. **A bypass of the requisite self-reactive Th-cell activity**
   (1) Such a bypass may occur via polyclonal B-cell activation by materials such as bacterial lipopolysaccharide or Epstein-Barr virus.
   (2) Modified chemical–host or viral–host antigens could recruit a cross-reactive Th cell and elicit autoantibody production.
c. **A release of sequestered antigen** (e.g., from the lens of the eye or from sperm)
   (1) Sequestered antigens are not ordinarily available for recognition by the immune system.
   (2) Release may be the result of trauma or infection.

4. Genetic predisposition. Genetic factors clearly play a role in autoimmune disease.
   a. The observed familial incidence is believed to be largely genetic rather than environmental.
   b. This association is thought to relate to those major histocompatibility complex (MHC) genes that code for the class II antigens that are important in the presentation of antigens during the induction of an immune response.
      (1) Most autoimmune diseases appear to be associated with class II MHC molecules [also called human leukocyte antigens (HLAs)] DR2, DR3, DR4, and DR5 (Table 8-2).
      (2) Over 90% of patients with ankylosing spondylitis have the HLA-B27 antigen, compared to only 8% of the normal population.

5. Drugs. Certain drugs are known to precipitate autoimmune episodes. For example, systemic lupus erythematosus (SLE) may follow administration of procainamide or hydralazine. Most of these diseases disappear when the drug is withheld.

D. **Clinical categories**

   1. Autoimmune diseases have been divided into two clinical types, **organ-specific** and **systemic,** based on the distribution of lesions (Table 8-3).

TABLE 8-2 Association Between HLA-DR Alleles and Selected Autoimmune Diseases

Disease	HLA Antigen	Relative Risk*
Multiple sclerosis	DR3	4.0
Systemic lupus erythematosus (SLE)	DR2	3.0
	DR3	3.0
Myasthenia gravis	DR3	3.0
Rheumatoid arthritis	DR4	6.0
Hashimoto's thyroiditis	DR5	3.0
Insulin-dependant diabetes mellitus	DR3/DR4 heterozygote	2.0–5.0

*Increase in risk for white individuals who bear the antigen as opposed to those who do not (e.g., a DR2-positive person is four times more likely to have multiple sclerosis than someone who is DR2-negative).

TABLE 8-3. Tissue Distribution and Presumed Immune Mediation in Representative Autoimmune Diseases

Disease	Presumed Mediation	Tissue Involvement
Systemic		
Rheumatoid arthritis	H	Joints and vascular bed
Systemic lupus erythematosus (SLE)	H	Kidney, skin, central nervous system, cardiovascular system
Organ- or tissue-specific		
Sjögren's syndrome	H	Lacrimal and salivary glands
Acute disseminated encephalomyelitis	T	Nervous system
Guillain-Barré syndrome	T	Nervous system
Multiple sclerosis	T	Nervous system
Myasthenia gravis	H	Nervous system
Hashimoto's thyroiditis	H,T	Thyroid
Graves'disease	H	Thyroid
Diabetes mellitus	H,T	Pancreas
Goodpasture's syndrome	H	Lung and kidney
Pernicious anemia	H	Stomach
Autoimmune hemolytic diseases	H	Red blood cells
Idiopathic thrombocytopenic purpura (ITP)	H	Platelets
Pemphigus	H	Skin
Dermatomyositis	H,T	Skin and muscle

H = humoral (circulating antibodies, immune complexes); T = T-cell mediated.

2. Systemic autoimmune diseases are sometimes called **collagen-vascular diseases,** indicating the widespread distribution of lesions in connective tissues and the vascular system.

E. Diagnosis

1. **General signs** of autoimmune disease that may have diagnostic value include:
   a. Elevated serum gamma globulin levels
   b. Presence of autoantibodies
   c. Depressed levels of serum complement
   d. Immune complexes in serum
   e. Lesions detected on biopsy (e.g., glomerular lesions) resulting from deposition of immune complexes

2. **Diagnostic tests** are designed to detect antibodies specific to the particular antigen involved in the autoimmune disease (Table 8-4). Certain facts should be noted.
   a. Patients may have more than one autoantibody and, in fact, may suffer from **multiple autoimmune diseases.**
      (1) Approximately 10% of patients with autoimmune thyroiditis also suffer from pernicious anemia, and 30% have antibodies to gastric parietal cells. Fully 50% of people with pernicious anemia have antibodies reactive with thyroid antigens.
      (2) Nearly 50% of patients with sicca complex [see II C] suffer from rheumatoid arthritis or other autoimmune arthritic diseases. This syndrome is called Sjögren's syndrome.
      (3) Patients with SLE may have 10 to 15 autoantibodies of differing specificities.
   b. **Multiple antibodies.** Although SLE is associated primarily with antinuclear antibodies, and rheumatoid arthritis primarily with rheumatoid factor, both types of antibodies may be found in both diseases (Table 8-5).
   c. **Autoantibodies are not unique to autoimmune disease.** Antinuclear antibodies may

TABLE 8-4. Representative Examples of Organ-Specific Antigens

Disease	Antigen
Addison's disease	Microsomal proteins of adrenal cells
Acute disseminated encephalomyelitis	Basic protein of myelin
Diabetes mellitus	Islet cell antigens Insulin
Goodpasture's syndrome	Type IV collagen of basement membranes
Grave's disease	Thyroid-stimulating hormone receptors
Hashimoto's thyroiditis	Thyroglobulin
Myasthenia gravis	Acetylcholine receptors
Pernicious anemia	Gastric parietal cell antigens Intrinsic factor
Sjögren's syndrome	Salivary gland duct epithelial cells

TABLE 8-5. Incidence of Antinuclear Antibodies and Rheumatoid Factor in Various Autoimmune Diseases

Disease	Incidence	
	Antinuclear Antibodies	Rheumatoid Factor
Systemic lupus erythematosus (SLE)	90%+	20%
Rheumatoid arthritis	20%	90%+
Sjögren's syndrome	70%	75%

be found in tuberculosis, histoplasmosis, and malignant lymphoma and other neoplasia.

F. Treatment

1. **Metabolic control** may be effective in certain organ-specific diseases.
   a. In thyrotoxicosis (Graves' disease), antithyroid drugs (e.g., propylthiouracil, methimazole) may be prescribed. Surgical or radionuclide (iodine-131; ^{131}I) ablation of the gland also is effective. These patients must go on l-thyroxine maintenance therapy.
   b. Vitamin B_{12} is given to patients with pernicious anemia.

2. Aspirin, **nonsteroidal anti-inflammatory drugs, steroidal anti-inflammatory drugs** (e.g., cortisone, which also may be immunosuppressive), and **immunosuppressive cytotoxic drugs** (e.g., cyclophosphamide, azathioprine) are useful in treating disease symptoms. The latter agents are used only in advanced disease.

3. **Anticholinesterase drugs** and **thymectomy** are of value in myasthenia gravis.

4. Plasmapheresis, or plasma exchange therapy, appears to be useful in the treatment of certain diseases (e.g., Guillain-Barré disease, SLE, Goodpasture's syndrome).
  a. The removal of the offending antibodies and immune complexes is beneficial.
  b. The plasma that is removed is replaced with normal serum albumin or fresh frozen plasma.

5. Splenectomy is of value in hemolytic diseases and idiopathic thrombocytopenic purpura (ITP).

II. REPRESENTATIVE AUTOIMMUNE DISEASES

A. **Rheumatoid arthritis** is a chronic, inflammatory joint disease with systemic involvement. It primarily affects women and is associated with HLA-DR4, which may confer genetic susceptibility.

1. Clinicopathologic features
  a. An **unknown etiologic agent** initiates a nonspecific immune response. An inflammatory joint lesion that begins in the synovial membrane can become proliferative, destroy adjacent cartilage and bone, and result in joint deformity.
  b. **General symptoms** include weight loss, arthritis, malaise, fever, fatigue, and weakness.

2. Immunologic findings
  a. **Rheumatoid factor.** A hallmark of rheumatoid arthritis is the presence of rheumatoid factor, an anti-IgG immunoglobulin (classically IgM, but also IgG and IgA) that is produced by B cells and plasma cells in the synovial membrane. IgM and IgG rheumatoid factors are the primary components of immunoglobulin production in the rheumatoid synovial membrane.
    (1) Most patients (90%) with established rheumatoid arthritis have rheumatoid factor in their serum. In these patients, the disease is generally more severe than in patients without rheumatoid factor.
    (2) Rheumatoid factor has antibody specificity for the heavy chain (γ chain) of IgG. Apparently, an unglycolsylated IgG is produced by some plasma cells; this is the nonself immunogen that triggers the autoimmune response.
  b. **Immune complexes.** The synovial fluid of patients with rheumatoid arthritis contains immune complexes consisting of rheumatoid factor, IgG, and complement. These complexes can trigger an immunologic reaction in two ways.
    (1) **Immune complex activation of complement**
      (a) Rheumatoid factor combines with IgG away from its antibody-combining site, which leaves the IgG molecule free to combine with its homologous antigen or with more antibodies to form large complexes.
      (b) These aggregates can become large enough to activate both the classic and alternative complement pathways, with production of neutrophil chemotactic factor (C5a).
    (2) **Phagocytic cell participation.** The inflammatory response is amplified as immune aggregates of IgG and rheumatoid factor are phagocytized by macrophages, which release cytokines, and by neutrophils, which release digestive enzymes and toxic oxygen metabolites.
  c. **Antinuclear antibodies.** These also are present in some patients with rheumatoid arthritis (see Table 8-5).

B. **SLE** is a chronic, inflammatory, systemic (multiorgan) disorder that predominantly affects young women of childbearing age. At least 5000 Americans die of SLE each year, but most cases are controlled by medical treatment. Death usually results from renal failure or from infection brought on by immunosuppressive therapy.

1. **Clinicopathologic features**
   a. **General symptoms** include malaise, fever, lethargy, and weight loss. Multiple tissues are involved, including the skin, mucosa, kidney, brain, and cardiovascular system.
      (1) The most characteristic feature is the **butterfly rash,** an erythematous rash that occurs over the nose and cheeks. Other skin lesions (e.g., discoid, psoriasiform, maculopapular, bullous) also have been described.
      (2) **Renal involvement** occurs in 50% of patients with SLE. Diffuse proliferative glomerulonephritis and membranous glomerulonephritis are common.
      (3) **Central nervous system manifestations** appear in 50% of patients and include depression, psychoses, seizures, and sensorimotor neuropathies.
   b. **Mixed connective tissue disease,** or overlap syndrome, occurs primarily in female patients who have features of rheumatoid arthritis, SLE, polymyositis–dermatomyositis, or scleroderma.
   c. **Drug-induced SLE** occurs as a complication of treatment with hydralazine, a vasodilator used in the treatment of hypertension; procainamide, an antiarrhythmic drug; and, to a lesser degree, other drugs such as isoniazid.
      (1) Onset of the disease is abrupt following exposure to the drug.
      (2) The serum contains antinuclear [but not anti–double-stranded DNA (dsDNA)] antibodies.
      (3) The symptoms are similar to those of SLE (see II B 1 a); however, they are usually milder and the patient has a complete return to normalcy following cessation of drug administration.
   d. SLE may **first appear during pregnancy** or may have an **increase in symptoms during pregnancy.**
      (1) Abortion, stillbirths, intrauterine growth retardation, and preterm delivery occur frequently in women who are later diagnosed with SLE.
      (2) Infants born of mothers with active SLE have increased mortality due to hypertension, nephritis, hemolytic anemia, leukopenia, and thrombocytopenia. The serum of the infant has various IgG autoantibodies (e.g., antinuclear antibodies) that have been acquired from the mother.
      (3) The lupus anticoagulant, present in 10% to 15% of women, reacts with cell membrane phospholipids, and its presence is correlated with increased morbidity in children born of patients with SLE. This antibody causes vascular thromboses in the placenta and maternal organs and is thought to be responsible for congenital heart block in the infant. It will cause a false positive RPR (see Chapter 6 II E).

2. **Immunologic findings**
   a. **Lupus erythematosus (LE) cell phenomenon.** The discovery of this phenomenon led to the current understanding of the immunologic basis of SLE.
      (1) When peripheral blood from a patient is incubated at 37°C for 30 to 60 minutes, the lymphocytes swell and extrude their nuclear material.
      (2) This nuclear material is opsonized by anti-DNA antibody and complement and is then phagocytized by neutrophils, which in this situation are called LE cells.
   b. **Antinuclear antibodies.** The detection of antinuclear antibodies by indirect immunofluorescence is of diagnostic importance in SLE. Three primary types of antibodies (either IgG or IgM) to DNA can be detected:
      (1) Antibodies to single-stranded DNA (ssDNA)
      (2) Antibodies to dsDNA [most closely associated with active SLE and the glomerulonephritis triggered by the deposition of immune complexes (consisting of DNA, antibody, and complement) on the basement membrane of blood vessels of renal glomeruli]
      (3) Antibodies that react with both ssDNA and dsDNA
   c. **Other autoantibodies**
      (1) Some patients with SLE also form antibodies against RNA, red blood cells, platelets, mitochondria, ribosomes, lysosomes, thromboplastin, or thrombin.
      (2) Some patients (30%) demonstrate a positive test for rheumatoid factor.

    d. Genetic aspects. Autoantibody formation is in part genetically determined. There is an increased incidence of SLE in individuals of HLA-DR2 and DR3 haplotypes.

    e. T-cell changes. The number of T cells decreases; thus, the ability to develop delayed hypersensitivity is impaired. Antibodies cytotoxic for T cells correlate with this T-cell deficiency.

    f. Animal studies. These studies have shown that estrogens enhance anti-DNA antibody formation and increase the severity of renal disease in genetically susceptible mice (e.g., the NZB/NZW hybrids), whereas androgens have the opposite effect. These findings suggest that hormones may be involved in the predominance of SLE in women.

C. **Sicca complex** is a chronic, inflammatory disease that affects the exocrine glands. The primary targets appear to be the lacrimal and salivary gland duct epithelium. Most patients are women.

    1. Clinicopathologic features

      a. The disease is characterized by dry eyes (keratoconjunctivitis sicca) and dry mouth (xerostomia). Dryness of the nose, larynx, and bronchi also is seen. Little moisture is evident in the vaginal mucosa.

      b. Sjögren's syndrome usually is sicca complex associated with another connective tissue disease such as rheumatoid arthritis or SLE.

    2. Immunologic findings. Numerous features suggest an immunologic etiology.

      a. Patients demonstrate hypergammaglobulinemia, which suggests excessive B-cell activity, and have several types of autoantibodies, such as rheumatoid factor, antinuclear antibodies, and antibodies to salivary duct epithelium.

      b. The salivary and lacrimal glands of affected people are infiltrated with plasma cells, B cells, and T cells. Some patients show quantitative and qualitative T-cell suppression in peripheral blood.

D. **Encephalomyelitis**

    1. Acute disseminated encephalomyelitis may occur after vaccination (e.g., rabies immunization) or viral infection (e.g., measles, influenza).

      a. Clinicopathologic features

        (1) Symptoms include headache, backache, stiff neck, nausea, low-grade fever, malaise, and weakness or paralysis of the extremities. Vaccination with attenuated viruses (e.g., measles, rubella) may produce symptoms such as elevated body temperature, convulsions, drowsiness that may progress to a comatose state, and paralysis of the extremities (particularly the legs).

        (2) Pathologic examination reveals perivascular accumulation of macrophages, lymphocytes, and some neutrophils throughout the gray or white matter of the brain with variable demyelination.

        (3) Although survivors of the acute stages of disease usually experience no permanent neurologic sequelae, mental retardation, epileptic seizures, or even death can result.

      b. Immunologic findings. These suggest that the disease represents a cell-mediated allergic response to **myelin basic protein,** similar to that seen in experimental allergic encephalomyelitis. Antibodies to myelin basic protein do not appear to be involved in the disease process, although they are useful diagnostically.

    2. Experimental allergic encephalomyelitis is the experimental model for acute disseminated encephalomyelitis in humans. This disease can be induced in animals by the injection of either homologous or heterologous brain or spinal cord extracts emulsified in complete Freund's adjuvant. (See Table 5–3).

      a. Clinicopathologic features

        (1) Two to three weeks after sensitization, animals begin to lose weight and then develop impaired righting reflex, ataxia, flaccid paralysis of the hind legs, urinary incontinence, and fecal impaction. Although most animals ultimately die, some recover completely.

(2) Histologic lesions consist of demyelination and perivascular accumulation of lymphocytes, mononuclear cells, and plasma cells throughout the brain and spinal cord.

b. Immunologic findings

(1) The encephalitogenic factor appears to be certain polypeptide sequences of myelin basic protein.

(2) Although both B cells and T cells respond to basic protein, T cells evidently are responsible for lesions (demyelination).

(a) Animals demonstrate classic cutaneous delayed hypersensitivity to basic protein, and lymphoid cells can passively transfer the disease.

(b) Antibodies to basic protein are formed, but they correlate poorly with disease and cannot passively transfer it.

E. **Guillain-Barré syndrome (acute idiopathic polyneuritis)** occurs after an infectious disease (e.g., measles, influenza, hepatitis) or after vaccination (e.g., influenza), and it affects all age-groups. This self-limiting, paralytic syndrome occurs rarely (1 per 100,000 vaccinees), but is associated with a 5% mortality rate.

1. Clinicopathologic features

a. Symptoms include progressive weakness, first of the lower extremities, and then of the upper extremities and respiratory muscles; this weakness can lead to paralysis. Deep tendon reflexes are absent. In most patients, normal function returns in 6 to 10 months.

b. Examination of peripheral nerve tissue reveals a perivascular mononuclear cell infiltrate and demyelination.

2. Immunologic findings

a. Experimental disease, induced by injections of nervous tissue in complete Freund's adjuvant, appears to be T-cell mediated, as evidenced by sensitivity of lymphocytes to nerve extracts and passive transfer of disease with sensitized cells.

b. Several of the immunologic features in the experimental animal model characterize Guillain-Barré syndrome in **humans.** Lymphocytes are sensitive to peripheral nerve extracts, lymphokines are produced, and antinerve antibodies are present.

F. **Multiple sclerosis** is a relapsing neuromuscular disease with periods of exacerbation and remission. It is more common in females (6:1 ratio), and the incidence in the United States is 0.1%.

1. Clinicopathologic features

a. Symptoms include motor weakness, ataxia, impaired vision, urinary bladder dysfunction, paresthesias, and mental aberrations.

b. Inflammatory lesions (sclerotic plaques), consisting of mononuclear cell infiltrates and demyelination, are confined to the myelin in the central nervous system (CNS).

2. Immunologic findings

a. The cause of multiple sclerosis remains unknown, but the clustering of cases suggests an infectious agent. The antigen appears to be a myelin structural protein.

(1) Epidemiologic studies indicate that a virus may play a role. Molecular mimicry between a virus and a myelin protein could trigger a T-cell response. (see I C 3 a(I)(C)).

(2) Patients with this condition tend to have elevated levels of antibodies to measles virus in their serum and spinal fluid. Measles antigens have also been detected in CNS tissues.

b. Similar associations with measles infection and nervous system disease are found in another condition of suspected autoimmune etiology, **subacute sclerosing panencephalitis.**

G. **Myasthenia gravis** is a chronic disease resulting from faulty neuromuscular transmission.

1. **Clinicopathologic features**
   a. The disease is characterized by muscle weakness and fatigue, particularly of the ocular, pharyngeal, facial, laryngeal, and skeletal muscles.
   b. Muscle weakness and neuromuscular dysfunction result from blockade and depletion of acetylcholine receptors at the myoneural junction (Figure 8-1).

2. **Immunologic findings.** Approximately 60% to 80% of patients have an enlarged thymus, and 80% to 90% have antibodies against the acetylcholine receptor. Apparently, this antibody binds to acetylcholine receptors at the myoneural junction, causing endocytosis of the receptors.

H. **Chronic thyroiditis (Hashimoto's thyroiditis)** is a thyroid disease that mainly affects women between 30 and 50 years of age.

1. **Clinicopathologic features**
   a. The thyroid gland may be enlarged (goiter) and firm or hard. Histologic examination reveals a lymphocyte and plasma cell infiltrate, disappearance of colloid, and varying amounts of fibrosis.
   b. As the disease progresses, signs of hypothyroidism (e.g., low values of circulating thyroid hormones, decreased thyroidal uptake of radioiodine) may be seen.

2. **Immunologic findings**
   a. Antibody to thyroglobulin are detected by enzyme-linked immunosorbent assay and radioimmunoassay.
   b. Antibody to thyroid microsomal antigen can also be detected.

I. **Graves' disease (thyrotoxicosis, hyperthyroidism)** results from the overproduction of thyroid hormone (thyroxine).

1. **Clinicopathologic features.** Patients exhibit fatigue, nervousness, increased sweating, palpitations, weight loss, and heat intolerance.

2. **Immunologic findings**
   a. An increase in the number of peripheral B cells correlates with the severity of the disease.
   b. Current evidence suggests that patients produce several antibodies to thyrotropin receptors (Figure 8-2).

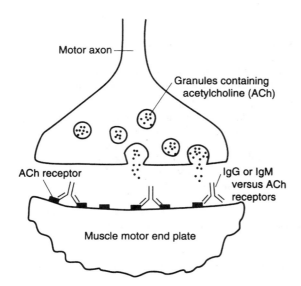

Motor axon

Granules containing acetylcholine (ACh)

ACh receptor

IgG or IgM versus ACh receptors

Muscle motor end plate

FIGURE 8-1. Mechanism of action of Gell and Coombs type II cytotoxic antibodies in myasthenia gravis. Immunoglobulin G (*IgG*) or M (*IgM*) antibodies react with acetylcholine (*ACh*) receptors and prevent binding of ACh, thus inhibiting muscle contractions.

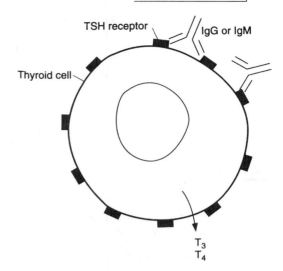

FIGURE 8-2. Mechanism of action of Gell and Coombs type II cytotoxic antibodies in Graves' disease. Immunoglobulin G (*IgG*) or M (*IgM*) antibodies against the thyroid-stimulating hormone (*TSH*) receptor on thyroid cells mimic the hormone and cause the thyroid cell to secrete triiodothyronine (T_3) and thyroxine (T_4).

    (1) One type of antibody blocks the binding of thyroid-stimulating hormone (TSH) to thyroid epithelial cells.

    (2) A second antithyroid antibody causes thyroid cells to proliferate.

    (3) A third type, referred to as **thyroid-stimulating antibody,** reacts with TSH receptors on the thyroid cell membrane and mimics the action of the pituitary hormone thyrotropin. The result of this interaction is overproduction of thyroid hormones and hyperthyroidism.

  c. Because thyroid-stimulating antibodies are IgG, they can cross the placenta and cause hyperthyroidism in the newborn. The condition resolves spontaneously as the maternal IgG is catabolized by the infant over a period of several weeks.

  d. Increased frequencies of HLA-Bw35 and HLA-DR3 have been found.

J. **Type 1 diabetes mellitus [insulin-dependent diabetes mellitus (IDDM), juvenile diabetes]** results from immunologic destruction of the insulin-producing beta cells of the islets of Langerhans in the pancreas. This disease affects approximately 1 of every 500 people in the United States. Its onset peaks between the ages of 10 and 15 years.

  1. Clinicopathologic features

    a. An **inability to synthesize insulin** makes the patient susceptible to wide fluctuations in blood glucose levels. Acute manifestations of insulin insufficiency include ketoacidosis, polyuria, polydipsia, and polyphagia.

    b. Chronic hyperglycemia and associated abnormal metabolic events lead to cardiovascular disease, neuropathies, kidney problems, and cataracts.

    c. **Treatment.** Patients with IDDM are refractory to dietary control and require daily insulin injections. Immunosuppression with cyclosporine has produced some beneficial results.

    d. **Insulin-resistant diabetes** is a similar clinical entity in which the patient does not respond to insulin injections because he has antibodies that react with the **insulin receptor** on cells of the body and block hormone action in this manner.

  2. Immunologic findings

    a. **Affected people produce antibodies to insulin and to membrane and cytoplasmic constituents of beta cells.**

      (1) Anti-islet cell antibodies are observed in most patients (> 90%) with juvenile diabetes.

      (2) Anti-insulin antibodies are produced by most patients with diabetes on insulin therapy. These are most likely induced by the hormone injections; however, these same antibodies may be seen in patients with IDDM at the time of diagnosis (i.e., before any insulin therapy).

    b. Cytotoxicity of T cells for islet cells also has been reported. The islets are infiltrated with B and T cells and are eventually destroyed.

    c. The onset of IDDM is often preceded by a **viral infection;** mumps, cytomegalovirus, influenza, rubella, and coxsackievirus have been implicated.

        (1) Mumps and coxsackievirus can destroy islet cells *in vitro.* A B4 coxsackievirus, isolated from the pancreas of a diabetic child, has produced a similar disease in experimental animals.

        (2) IDDM develops in 15% of children with congenital rubella.

K. **Goodpasture's syndrome** is a rare, progressive disease of the lungs and kidneys. This disorder occurs in all age-groups, but unlike most other autoimmune diseases, it mainly affects young men. The prognosis is poor.

    1. Clinicopathologic features

        a. Classic **symptoms** include pulmonary hemorrhage, hemoptysis, hematuria, and glomerulonephritis.

        b. Pulmonary infiltrates may show on radiographs.

    2. Immunologic findings

        a. Immunofluorescence reveals linear deposits of immunoglobulin (usually IgG) and complement on alveolar and glomerular basement membranes. The IgG appears to represent an antibody specific for type IV collagen shared by these kidney and lung membranes.

        b. Some cases have characteristics suggestive of an immune complex phenomenon.

L. **Pernicious anemia** results from defective red blood cell maturation caused by faulty absorption of vitamin B_{12}. Normally, dietary vitamin B_{12} is transported across the small intestine into the body as a complex with intrinsic factor, which is synthesized by parietal cells in the gastric mucosa. In patients with pernicious anemia, this process is blocked.

    1. Clinicopathologic features

        a. The hallmark of the disease is the progressive destruction of gastric glands and the associated loss of parietal cells. The consequent lack of intrinsic factor leads to failure of vitamin B_{12} absorption.

        b. Mononuclear leukocytes and neutrophils infiltrate the gastric mucosa. Defective red blood cell maturation leads to megaloblastic anemia with attendant weakness, loss of appetite, fatigue, pallor, and weight loss.

        c. Neurologic damage can occur as a result of vitamin B_{12} deficiency and may be irreversible. Patients also may show an increased incidence of stomach cancer.

    2. Immunologic findings. Patients produce antibodies (mainly IgG) to **three different gastric parietal cell antigens,** all of which are cell-specific. In addition, antibody to **intrinsic factor** is produced.

        a. Antibody to intrinsic factor may block the attachment of vitamin B_{12} to intrinsic factor or may bind to intrinsic factor or the intrinsic factor–B_{12} complex.

        b. Some patients also show cell-mediated immunity to intrinsic factor and parietal cell antigens.

M. **Autoimmune hemolytic diseases.** These include warm-antibody hemolytic anemia (the most common type of autoimmune hemolytic disease), cold-antibody hemolytic anemia, and paroxysmal cold hemoglobinuria.

    1. Clinicopathologic features. Classic symptoms include fatigue, fever, jaundice, and splenomegaly relating to the presence of antibodies directed against self red blood cell antigens and the resultant anemia. Splenectomy prolongs RBC life in vivo.

    2. Immunologic findings

        a. Warm-antibody hemolytic anemia

            (1) "Warm" antibodies show optimum reactivity at 37°C. They are primarily IgG, are poor at complement fixing, and can be detected on the red blood cell surface by the antiglobulin (Coombs') test. Warm antibodies are directed primarily against Rh determinants.

   (2) Various patterns of red blood cell coating can be detected in different patients. Cells can be coated with IgG alone, IgG plus complement, or complement alone. Antibody-coated red blood cells appear to be opsonized for phagocytosis primarily in the spleen.

b. Cold-antibody hemolytic anemia. Hemolysis is usually mild and the symptoms are confined to cold, exposed extremities.

   (1) "Cold" antibodies show optimum reactivity at 4°C. They are primarily of the IgM class, fix complement, and agglutinate red blood cells directly, without the requirement for Coombs' antiglobulin.

   (2) The IgM is specific against red blood cell antigen I.

   (3) Cold agglutinins also may be detected secondary to infections (e.g., mycoplasmal pneumonia).

c. Paroxysmal cold hemoglobinuria. This rare syndrome is associated with Donath-Landsteiner antibody, a cold antibody of the IgG class directed against red blood cell antigen P.

   (1) The antibody is biphasic in that it sensitizes cells in the cold, usually below 15°C, and then hemolyzes them when the temperature is elevated to 37°C.

   (2) Patients demonstrate symptoms (e.g., fever, pain in the extremities, jaundice, hemoglobinuria) after exposure to cold.

N. **ITP,** which may be either acute or chronic, results from antibody-mediated platelet destruction. In children, this disease is sometimes preceded by a viral infection.

1. Clinicopathologic features

   a. Patients demonstrate bleeding problems in the gums, gastrointestinal and genitourinary tracts.

   b. Platelet counts are profoundly suppressed. Splenectomy is beneficial.

2. Immunologic findings

   a. IgG antibodies specific for platelets can be demonstrated. Antibody-coated platelets are sequestered and destroyed by macrophages of the spleen and liver primarily.

   b. Thrombocytopenia sometimes may be drug-induced.

   (1) Causative drugs include sulfonamides, antihistamines, quinidine, and quinine.

   (2) Drug–antibody complexes are adsorbed onto the platelet surface, resulting in complement activation.

   (3) Treatment consists of withholding the drug.

O. **Bullous (vesicular) diseases** are chronic dermatologic problems that result when destruction of intercellular bridges (**desmosomes**) interferes with cohesion of the epidermis. This process leads to the formation of blisters (bullae).

1. Clinicopathologic features

   a. Pemphigus vulgaris, an erosive disease of the skin and mucous membranes, is characterized by intraepidermal blisters.

   b. Bullous pemphigoid, a bullous disease of the skin and mucosa, is usually seen in middle-aged and older people. The blisters form beneath the epidermis at the dermal–epidermal junction.

2. Immunologic findings

   a. Pemphigus vulgaris skin lesions show antibody (mainly IgG) deposition and complement components in squamous intercellular spaces when examined by immunofluorescence.

   b. Bullous pemphigoid lesions demonstrate deposition of antibody and complement along skin basement membrane. Circulating antibasement membrane antibodies also can be detected.

P. **Polymyositis-dermatomyositis** is an acute or chronic inflammatory disease of the muscles (polymyositis) and frequently also involving the skin (dermatomyositis).

1. **Clinicopathologic features.** Patients demonstrate weakness of striated muscle, with some muscle pain and tenderness, and a characteristic skin rash.

2. **Immunologic findings**
   a. Hypergammaglobulinemia is common, along with deposition of immunoglobulin and complement in the vessel walls of the skin and muscle.
   b. Studies showing cellular passive transfer and lymphokine release by T cells indicate that cellular immunity also may play a role in pathogenesis.

Q. **Scleroderma** is a slowly progressive, chronic, disabling disease characterized by abnormally increased collagen deposition in the skin and occasionally in the internal organs. This disorder commonly begins in the third or fourth decade of life and affects women twice as often as men.

1. **Clinicopathologic features**
   a. **Raynaud's phenomenon** (i.e., intermittent bilateral attacks of ischemia of the fingers or toes, or sometimes the ears or nose, marked by severe pallor and accompanied by paresthesia and pain) frequently is the first symptom noted. Skin involvement may be limited to the hands, forearms, feet, or face.
   b. The unique pentad of symptoms, the so-called **CREST syndrome** (**c**alcinosis, **R**aynaud's phenomenon, **e**sophageal dysmotility, **s**clerodactyly, **t**elangiectases) may remain stable for years.
   c. Progressive systemic sclerosis usually begins with polyarthritis, but symptoms vary depending on the organs involved in the abnormal collagen deposition.

2. **Immunologic findings**
   a. Patients with CREST syndrome have antibodies of diagnostic importance that react with **centromeres**.
   b. Antinuclear antibodies having reactivity with nucleolar antigens are commonly found.

R. **Rheumatic fever** is a nonsuppurative sequela of group A streptococcal disease, usually pharyngitis, which manifests 2 to 4 weeks after the acute infection. Disease severity abates with time, but recurrences occur with each subsequent *Streptococcus pyogenes* infection.

1. **Clinicopathologic features**
   a. The three major clinical features of rheumatic fever include:
      (1) Arthritis (most common manifestation)
      (2) Carditis
      (3) Chorea (uncontrollable, irregular movement of the muscles of the face, arms, and legs)
   b. Cutaneous symptoms include a transient, painless rash and subcutaneous nodules. These symptoms usually develop in patients that exhibit some of the major clinical features and are seldom seen alone.

2. **Immunologic findings**
   a. The patients make a cross-reacting antibody in response to the M protein of the infecting organism. This streptococcal antigen shares an epitope with human heart myocardial tissues, and the autoantibody attacks the heart (e.g., tissues, valves).
   b. Biopsy of heart valves reveals plasma cell infiltration and deposition of antibodies and complement proteins in the tissues.

S. **Postpericardiotomy syndrome** and **postmyocardial infarction syndrome** (Dressler's disease) is a transient, acute inflammatory disease that may follow damage to cardiac tissues (e.g., open heart surgery, myocardial infarction).

1. **Clinicopathologic features.** It usually manifests as a pericarditis, with or without pleural effusion, pulmonary infiltrates, and transient arthritis which develops 2–3 weeks after pericardial damage. It usually responds well to nonsteroidal anti-inflammatory drug (NSAID) therapy.

2. Immunologic findings
   a. Antibodies and complement proteins are detected in myocardial tissues
   b. Increased concentration of antobodies against coxsackie and other viruses suggest the disease may follow reactivation of a latent viral infection.

Vignette Revisited

1. Based on the history, the physical examination, and cerebrospinal fluid studies, this patient has acute idiopathic polyneuropathy, or Guillain-Barré syndrome. This disease is an acute or subacute polyneuropathy that can follow infective illness, surgical procedures, or inoculations. The mechanism of action is unknown, but it is thought to have an immunologic basis. There is no specific test to diagnose this disease, although patients may have antibodies reactive with peripheral nervous tissue and their T cells respond to these same antigens.

   The chief complaint in Guillain-Barré syndrome is frequently symmetrical weakness, with weakness being greater in proximal limbs than in distal limbs. Criteria required for diagnosis are progressive weakness of more than one limb, progression for up to 4 weeks, symmetrical deficits, mild sensory involvement, absence of fever, autonomic dysfunction, and increased cerebrospinal fluid protein 1 week after the onset of symptoms.

2. Initial treatment of Guillain-Barré syndrome consists of supporting the patient's vital signs and pulmonary function. Tachycardia and fluctuating blood pressure may require pharmacologic intervention. Decreased pulmonary function due to respiratory muscle paralysis may require ventilator support. Plasmapheresis may reduce the time required for recovery and decrease the likelihood of residual neurologic deficits. Corticosteroids were prescribed in the past, but recent studies have shown that they may adversely affect the outcome and prolong the recovery time.

3. Viral infections and vaccinations have been associated with Guillain-Barré syndrome, but no direct link has been found.

STUDY QUESTIONS

1. A patient who has suffered from severe, disabling arthritis for several years presents with the joints in his hands distorted due to the severity of the inflammation. The spinal column has become involved and the patient has a stooped appearance due to the involvement of the thoracic vertebrae. The patient is diagnosed with rheumatoid arthritis. Upon further examination, which of the following signs would be absent in this patient?

(A) Lesions detected on biopsy
(B) Immune complexes in serum
(C) Depressed levels of serum complement
(D) T cells reactive with autoantigens
(E) Hypergammaglobulinemia

2. A 27-year-old skier is in training for the next winter Olympics. He has recently been running a low-grade fever and is fatigued beyond what would be expected from his workouts. His coach sent him to the infirmary because his skin and sclera were yellow. Physical examination reveals a jaundiced, well-developed man with splenomegaly. Laboratory results of interest include marked hemoglobinuria and a serum that apparently reacts with antigen P–positive human erythrocytes in the refrigerator but does not cause lysis until the temperature of the reaction mixture is raised to 37°C. The antibody detected is characteristic of

(A) warm-antibody hemolytic anemia
(B) cold-antibody hemolytic anemia
(C) paroxysmal cold hemoglobinuria
(D) idiopathic thrombocytopenic purpura (ITP)
(E) pernicious anemia

3. Autoimmune diseases may be organ-specific or they may have multiple target tissues. The latter are sometimes called collagen-vascular diseases or connective tissue diseases. Which of the following autoimmune diseases is systemic?

(A) Thyroiditis
(B) Systemic lupus erythematosus (SLE)
(C) Pernicious anemia
(D) Multiple sclerosis
(E) Myasthenia gravis

4. Louis Pasteur developed a vaccine for rabies. The immunizing antigen was spinal cord tissues from a rabbit infected with the rabies virus. Side effects of the immunization included headache, nausea, stiff neck, malaise, paralysis of the extremities, and occasionally coma. Subsequent laboratory studies have shown that a T-cell response to myelin basic protein appears to be responsible for the pathogenesis of this condition, which is

(A) Guillain-Barré syndrome
(B) Graves' disease
(C) acute disseminated encephalomyelitis
(D) myasthenia gravis
(E) multiple sclerosis

5. Which of the following areas is most likely to be affected by the chronic inflammation that is characteristic of Sjögren's syndrome?

(A) Thyroid glands
(B) Isles of Langerhans
(C) Prostate gland
(D) Nasal passages
(E) Skin

6. A 49-year-old man has been placed on methyldopa for a recently diagnosed hypertension. He returns to his primary care physician complaining of a low-grade fever and fatigue. He is jaundiced and has splenomegaly. Laboratory results include marked hemoglobinuria. He is diagnosed with autoimmune hemolytic anemia. Which of the following statements describes the antibodies etiologically associated with this disease?

(A) Cause agglutination at 4°C but not at 37°C
(B) Primarily consist of IgM
(C) Avidly fix complement
(D) Demonstrate specificity for red blood cell antigen I
(E) Can be detected by antiglobulin (Coombs') test

7. Which of the following statements is true about autoimmuĺne diseases in general?

(A) They have a tendency to occur more frequently in men
(B) Hypogammaglobulinemia is common
(C) No hereditary pattern has been noted
(D) Autoantibodies are usually found in the serum
(E) Elevated serum complement levels are common

8. Renal failure is a common cause of death in patients with

(A) Sjögren's syndrome
(B) Rheumatoid arthritis
(C) Rheumatic fever
(D) Pemphigus vulgaris
(E) Systemic lupus erythematosus (SLE)

9. Rheumatoid factor is an antibody directed against determinants on the immunoglobulin molecule's

(A) γ chain
(B) μ chain
(C) J (joining) chain
(D) λ chain
(E) κ chain

ANSWERS AND EXPLANATIONS

1. The answer is D [II A 2]. This patient has ankylosing spondylitis, a form of rheumatoid arthritis that causes spinal deformity, primarily in older men. Rheumatoid arthritis is an autoantibody disease. There is no evidence that T-cell immunity is involved; hence, the T cells would not go into mitosis on contact with autoantigens. Elevated serum gamma globulin levels are one of the general signs of autoimmune disease that may be of diagnostic importance. Other signs include depressed levels of serum complement, lesions detected on biopsy, and the presence of immune complexes in the serum.

2. The answer is C [II M 2 c]. Paroxysmal cold hemoglobinuria is a rare type of autoimmune hemolytic disease that is associated with the Donath-Landsteiner antibody, a cold antibody of the IgG class directed against red blood cell antigen P. Cold-antibody hemolytic anemia involves antibodies of the IgM class that are optimally reactive in the cold. Warm-antibody hemolytic anemia involves primarily IgG antibodies that are optimally reactive at 37°C. Idiopathic thrombocytopenic purpura (ITP) results from antibody-mediated platelet destruction. Pernicious anemia results from defective red blood cell maturation due to immunologically mediated faulty absorption of vitamin B_{12}.

3. The answer is B [Table 10–3]. Systemic lupus erythematosus (SLE) is a systemic autoimmune disease. Some autoimmune diseases are organ-specific: The immune response is directed against just one organ or tissue type, as in Hashimoto's thyroiditis (target = thyroid); pernicious anemia (target = gastric tissue); multiple sclerosis (target = myelin basic protein); and myasthenia gravis (target = acetylcholine receptor). Other autoimmune diseases are systemic. The target antigens are widespread throughout the body, as in SLE (target = cell nuclear material) and rheumatoid arthritis (target = IgG). In the case of organ-specific disease, the lesions generally are restricted because the antigen in that organ is the target of the immunologic attack. In systemic autoimmune diseases, lesions affect more tissues because antigen–antibody complex deposition is more disseminated.

4. The answer is C [II D 1]. In acute disseminated encephalomyelitis, both in humans and in the animal models, there is perivascular accumulation of lymphocytes and other cells throughout nervous tissue, along with variable demyelination. The latter appears to be triggered via a T-cell-mediated response to myelin basic protein.

5. The answer is D [II C 1 b]. The prostate gland is not affected by Sjögren's syndrome, which is characterized by dry eyes (keratoconjunctivitis sicca) and dry mouth (xerostomia). Secretions that lubricate the nasal passages and the vagina are decreased as well. Salivary and lacrimal glands are infiltrated with plasma cells, B cells, and T cells, suggesting an immunologic etiology. Patients also demonstrate hypergammaglobulinemia and several types of autoantibodies such as rheumatoid factor, antinuclear antibodies, and antibodies to salivary duct epithelium.

6. The answer is E [II M 2 a]. The "warm" antibodies of autoimmune hemolytic disease react with red blood cells at 4°C or at 37°C, although they show optimal reactivity at 37°C. In contrast, "cold" isoagglutinins react optimally at 4°C. The most common type of autoimmune hemolytic disease involves warm antibodies, which are primarily IgG, are poor at complement fixation, and can be detected by the antiglobulin (Coombs') test. Warm antibodies are directed primarily against Rh antigens on the red blood cells.

7. The answer is D [I B 2, C 4 a, E 1]. Complement levels usually are depressed in autoimmunity, not elevated, because of the presence of immune complexes in the serum. Most autoimmune diseases are more common in women; for example, approximately 85% of patients with systemic lupus erythematosus (SLE) are women. This implies that sex hormones may play a precipitating (estrogens) or controlling (androgens) role. Certain autoimmune diseases have an increased incidence in association with particular human leukocyte antigens (HLAs), especially antigens coded for in the HLA-DR locus. Most diagnostic tests rely on examination of serum for decreased complement levels and for increases in immune complexes and gamma globulin.

8. The answer is E [II B]. Systemic lupus erythematosus (SLE) is a chronic inflammatory systemic (multiorgan) disease triggered by the deposition of immune complexes on the basement membrane of blood vessels. Renal failure is a common cause of death because immune complex deposition occurs in blood vessels of the renal glomeruli, leading to glomerulonephritis.

9. The answer is A [II A 2 a (2)]. Rheumatoid factor is an antibody that has specificity for the γ heavy chain. Rheumatoid factor usually is of the IgM class; however, rheumatoid factors that are IgG or IgA have been described. These molecules occur in a high percentage (70%–90%) of patients with rheumatoid arthritis. Other autoimmune diseases [e.g., systemic lupus erythematosus (SLE), Sjögren's syndrome] also can induce rheumatoid factor in the patient's serum. Rheumatoid factor also is found in patients with leprosy, tuberculosis, and other nonautoimmune diseases.

Chapter 9

Immunodeficiency Disorders

Vignette

An 18-month-old white female is brought to the pediatrician's office for evaluation of a recurrent fever, runny nose, and cough. According to the mother, the child has been "sickly," frequently contracting colds and illnesses from other children. The child suffers from diarrhea several times each month, but the mother has attributed this to new or different foods that the child eats. The illnesses first started when the child was 7 months of age, when the family moved from California to Texas.

Gestation and birth were both without complications. From the mother's description, the child is reaching the developmental milestones appropriately. The child has had no previous surgeries or hospitalizations. There are no known food or drug allergies, and she is not taking any medications. The mother states that the child is eating solid foods three times a day and taking mid-morning and afternoon snacks.

During the physical examination, the patient is alert and playful. Her blood pressure is 94/68 mm Hg, her pulse is 90 beats/min, her respirations are 24 breaths/min, and her temperature is 101.2°F. The child's weight is 9 kg, her length is 82 cm, and her head circumference is 48 cm. The child has a clear nasal discharge, her posterior pharynx is moderately erythematous, and her tympanic membranes are clear. Her cardiac, pulmonary, and abdominal examination results are benign. The pediatrician suspects that there may be an immunodeficiency causing the child's symptoms, and he orders blood tests.

1. What is the significance of the onset of symptoms at 7 months of age?
2. The predominance of upper respiratory and gastrointestinal complaints suggests what sort of immunodeficiency?
3. What is the most remarkable finding from the physical examination, and how is it explained?

A complete blood count (CBC) with differential and an immunologic profile with quantitative serum IgG, IgA, and IgM are performed. Suspecting that the child has a viral upper respiratory illness, the pediatrician prescribes medications for symptomatic relief and instructs the mother to return in 1 week to discuss the laboratory results.

The CBC and immunoglobulin profile reveal the following:

WBCs = 14,000/mm^3 (normal is 6,000–17,000/mm^3)
Neutrophils = 32% (normal is 40%–60%)
Eosinophils = 2% (normal is 1%–3%)
Basophils = 1% (normal is 0%–1%)
Monocytes = 5% (normal is 4%–8%)
Lymphocytes = 60% (normal is 20%–40%)
Hemoglobin = 12.2 g/dl (normal is 10.5–13.5 g/dl)
Hematocrit = 36% (normal is 33%–39%)
Platelets = 225,000/mm^3 (normal is 150,000–300,000/mm^3)
IgG = 750 mg/dl (normal is 550–950 mg/dl)
IgM = 50 mg/dl (normal is 30–80 mg/dl)
IgA = 5 mg/dl (normal is 30–70 mg/dl)

4. What is the final diagnosis?
5. What is the child's prognosis?

I. **GENERAL CONSIDERATIONS.** In view of the complex nature of the immune response, it is not surprising that a wide array of immunodeficiencies exists. An estimated 1 in every 500 people in the United States is born with an immune system defect. Many more acquire transient or permanent immunologic impairments later in life that may have serious consequences.

A. **Clinical evaluation**

1. **Signs** of immunodeficiency disorders primarily include recurrent infections, chronic infections, unusual (opportunistic) infecting agents, and poor response to antimicrobial treatment. Other manifestations such as hepatosplenomegaly or diarrhea occasionally occur (Table 9-1).

2. When an immunodeficiency syndrome is suspected on the basis of persistent and recurrent infections, the work-up should include an evaluation of the patient's native and acquired immune capabilities (Table 9-2).

B. **Management of the immunodeficient patient**

1. **Treatment** of immunodeficiency disease has **two goals.**
   a. **Minimize the occurrence and impact of infections** by:
      (1) **Avoidance** of people with contagious diseases
      (2) Close **monitoring** of patients for infections
      (3) Prompt and vigorous use of **antibiotics** when appropriate
      (4) Active (or passive) **immunization** if possible
   b. **Replace the defective component** of the immune system by passive transfer or transplantation. Specific measures include:
      (1) Administration of pooled **gamma-globulin** to patients with certain immunoglobulin deficiencies
      (2) Infusions of **cytokines** such as interleukin-2 (IL-2), granulocyte–monocyte colony-stimulating factor (GM-CSF), and gamma interferon (IFN-γ) in people with particular diseases
      (3) **Transfusions**
         (a) Neutrophils in the treatment of phagocytic defects
         (b) Autologous lymphocytes that have been transfected with the adenosine deaminase (ADA) gene for treatment of one form of severe combined immunodeficiency
      (4) **Transplantation** of fetal thymus tissue or of bone marrow stem cells in attempts to restore immune competence

2. Other aspects of management are mentioned later under specific disorders.

TABLE 9-1. Clinical Features Associated with Impaired Immune Function

Highly suggestive features
Infections, recurrent or chronic, characterized by:
Unusual etiologies (opportunists)
Normal flora
Common environmental organisms
Slow recovery or poor response to treatment
Features frequently seen
Failure to thrive
Chronic diarrhea
Hepatosplenomegaly
Autoantibodies or autoimmune disease

TABLE 9-2. Tests Used in the Initial Evaluation of a Patient with Suspected Immunodeficiency Disease

Area of Immune Competence Evaluated	Test	Function of Test
Complement	Radial immunodiffusion	Quantitates complement proteins
	Hemolytic assay	Assesses functional activity
Phagocytic functions	Differential with complete cell count	Quantitates cells
	Chemotaxis	Determines cell mobility
	Nitroblue tetrazolium reduction	Measures PMN production of toxic oxygen metabolites
	Microbicidal activity	Determines cells' ability to kill
Lymphocytic functions	Flow cytometry	Quantitates cells using monoclonal antibodies to specific CD antigens (e.g., CD19 or CD20 for B cells; CD2, CD3, or CD5 for T cells) (CD4 and CD8 can be used for T-cell subsets)
	Differential with complete blood count	Measures total lymphocytes
	Mitogen assays	Determines fuctional status of B and T cells
	Skin tests	Measures functional status of T cells
	Radial immunodiffusion	Measures immunoglobulin levels that reflect B-cell function

PMN = polymorphonuclear neutrophils; *CD* = cluster of differentiation.

II. PHAGOCYTIC CELL DEFECTS. Although defects can occur in most phagocytic cells, polymorphonuclear leukocytes are emphasized here.

A. Quantitative defects

1. In **neutropenia** or **granulocytopenia,** the total number of normal circulating cells is suppressed as a result of decreased production or increased destruction.
   a. **Causes of decreased neutrophil production**
      (1) Administration of bone marrow depressant drugs (e.g., cancer chemotherapeutic drugs)
      (2) Leukemia
      (3) Inherited conditions in which development of all bone marrow stem cells, including myeloid precursors (e.g., reticular dysgenesis), appears to be defective
      (4) Spontaneously arising autoantibody that inhibits granulopoiesis
   b. **Causes of increased neutrophil destruction**
      (1) Autoimmune phenomena following the administration of certain drugs (e.g., quinidine, oxacillin) that may induce antibodies capable of opsonizing normal neutrophils
      (2) Hypersplenism characterized by exaggeration of the destructive functions of the spleen with resultant deficiency of peripheral blood elements

2. **Asplenia,** whether congenital, surgical, or due to organ destruction by malignancy or

sickle cell disease, can result in an increased incidence of infections, particularly septicemia caused by *Streptococcus pneumoniae* and enterobacteria.

B. **Qualitative defects.** In qualitative disorders, the phagocytic cells fail to engulf and kill microorganisms. The defect may involve any of the phagocytic activities: chemotaxis, ingestion, or intracellular killing.

1. **Chronic granulomatous disease (CGD)** is characterized by recurrent infections with various microorganisms, both gram negative (e.g., *Escherichia, Serratia, Klebsiella*) and gram positive (e.g., *Staphylococcus*). CGD is primarily an X-linked recessive disorder that appears in the first 2 years of life. Only 200–250 cases have ever been reported in the United States.
   a. **Clinical and immunologic features**
      (1) Granuloma formation occurs in many organs, and it appears to reflect the body's attempt to mount a T-cell response to compensate for the inability of the neutrophils to kill the organism.
      (2) An enzymatic inability to generate toxic oxygen metabolites such as hydrogen peroxide during the oxygen consumption activity of the hexose monophosphate (HMP) shunt is evident.
         (a) This is a result of a defect in neutrophilic **cytochrome b,** which is part of an heterodimeric complex containing nicotinamide adenine dinucleotide phosphate **(NADPH) oxidase** that catalyzes the one-electron reduction of oxygen to superoxide. This defect leads to suppression of intracellular killing of ingested microorganisms.
         (b) There are several genetic forms of CGD, X-linked as well as autosomal.
      (3) The neutrophils of patients with CGD are unable to kill bacteria such as *Staphylococcus aureus* and *Pseudomonas aeruginosa* that produce the enzyme catalase.
         (a) The catalase breaks down the small amount of hydrogen peroxide produced in the cells and protects the microbe.
         (b) Catalase-negative bacteria are less of a problem as they do not metabolize hydrogen peroxide themselves.
      (4) B- and T-cell function and complement levels usually are normal.
   b. **Diagnosis** depends on the in vitro demonstration of defective killing by neutrophils, or the inability to form hydrogen peroxide and other toxic oxygen metabolites.
   c. **Treatment**
      (1) The use of antibiotics appropriate for the infectious agent is essential.
      (2) Temporary maintenance with neutrophil infusions from a family member may be of value.
      (3) IFN-γ may activate the cells and enhance their killing ability via oxygen-independent mechanisms (e.g., lysosomal enzymes).

2. **Glucose-6-phosphate dehydrogenase (G6PD) deficiency** is an X-linked immunodeficiency disease with a clinical picture similar to that of CGD. In G6PD deficiency, however, hemolytic anemia also is present. The disorder is believed to result from the deficient generation of NADPH, which is a necessary reducing equivalent for the oxidase.

3. **Myeloperoxidase deficiency** is found in some patients with recurrent microbial infections. This enzyme is an important microbicidal agent in normal neutrophils. A susceptibility to *Candida albicans* and *S. aureus* infections is the chief problem in affected people.
   a. Superoxide and hydrogen peroxide are formed in normal amounts, but because the myeloperoxidase enzyme is lacking, neutrophil killing is impaired.
   b. Treatment involves the use of appropriate antimicrobial agents.

4. **Chédiak-Higashi syndrome** is a relatively rare disease of humans.
   a. **Clinical and immunologic features**
      (1) This syndrome is characterized by recurrent, severe, pyogenic infections, which are primarily streptococcal and staphylococcal in etiology. Prognosis is poor, and most patients die in childhood.

(2) The patient's neutrophils contain abnormal giant lysosomes, which can apparently fuse with the phagosome but are impaired in their ability to release their contents, thus resulting in a delayed killing of ingested microorganisms.

b. Diagnosis. Neutrophil chemotaxis and killing are abnormal, natural killer (NK) cell activity is decreased, and lysosomal enzyme levels are depressed. Oxygen consumption, hydrogen peroxide formation, and HMP activity are normal.

c. Treatment involves the use of antibiotics appropriate for the type of infection.

5. Job's syndrome

a. Clinical features. This syndrome is characterized by recurrent "colds" (i.e., lacking the normal inflammatory response) staphylococcal abscesses, chronic eczema, and otitis media.

b. Immunologic features and **diagnosis**

(1) Neutrophils demonstrate normal ingestion and killing activity but defective chemotaxis.

(2) Serum levels of immunoglobulin E (IgE) are extremely high.

(3) Eosinophilia may be present.

c. Treatment consists of the administration of antibiotics appropriate for the infectious agent.

6. "Lazy leukocyte" syndrome

a. Clinical and immunologic features. This condition is characterized by susceptibility to severe microbial infections. Patients exhibit neutropenia, a defective chemotactic response by neutrophils (hence the name of the disorder), and an abnormal inflammatory response.

b. Treatment involves the use of suitable antimicrobial drugs.

7. Leukocyte adhesion deficiency is another rare immunodeficiency disorder, characterized by recurrent bacterial and mycotic infections and impaired wound healing.

a. Immunologic features

(1) The leukocytes of patients with this disorder have defects of adhesion to endothelial surfaces and to each other (aggregation), as well as poor chemotactic and phagocytic activities.

(2) Cytotoxicity mediated by neutrophils, NK cells, and T lymphocytes also is depressed.

b. Treatment involves the administration of antimicrobial drugs to combat the infectious agent.

III. B-CELL DEFICIENCY DISORDERS (Table 9-3)

A. **Bruton's X-linked hypogammaglobulinemia** manifests as recurrent bacterial infections in patients that are extremely compromised in their ability to synthesize immunoglobulins. Cellular immunity is normal. It is estimated that this disease occurs in 1 in 100,000 people.

1. Clinical features. Infections (e.g., sinusitis, pneumonia, meningitis) caused by organisms such as *Streptococcus, Haemophilus, Staphylococcus,* and *Pseudomonas* begin when infants are 5–9 months of age.

2. Immunologic findings

a. Low serum levels of all classes of immunoglobulins

b. Lack of circulating B cells with surface immunoglobulins (sIg), although pre-B cells containing cytoplasmic mu (μ) chain are found in the bone marrow and in lymphoid tissues

c. Absence of germinal centers and plasma cells in lymph nodes

d. Hypoplastic tonsils and Peyer's patches

e. Intact T-cell functions

3. Immunogenetic features. Gene mapping indicates that the genetic defect is on the long

TABLE 9-3. Key Features of Selected B-Cell and T-Cell Immunodeficiency Diseases

Disease	Cellular Defect	Functions Affected
B-cell disorders		
X-linked agammaglobulinemia	Pre-B-cell maturation	All antibodies
Common variable hypogammaglobulinemia	B-cell maturation	Various antibodies
Transient hypogammaglobulinemia of infancy	Unknown; Th-cell maturation in some patients	IgG, IgA
Selective IgA deficiency	IgA B-cell maturation	IgA
Secretory component deficiency	Mucosal epithelial cell	sIgA
T-cell disorders		
DiGeorge syndrome	Dysmorphogenesis of third and fourth pharyngeal pouches	T cells
Chronic mucocutaneous candidiasis	No T-cell receptor for *Candida* antigens	T cells
Combined B- and T-cell disorders		
SCID		
X-linked form	T-cell maturation	T cells and antibody
Autosomal recessive form	T- and B-cell maturation	T cells and antibody
ADA deficiency	Toxic metabolite accumulation	T cells and antibody
PNP deficiency	Toxic metabolite accumulation	T cells and antibody
Nezelof's syndrome	Unknown	T cells and antibody
Immunodeficiency associated with other defects		
Ataxia-telangiectasia	B and T cells; suspected defect in DNA repair	T cells and antibody [with abnormal gait (ataxia), vascular malformations (telangiectasia)]
Wiskott-Aldrich syndrome	Glycosylation of membrane proteins	T cells and antibody (with thrombocytopenia and eczema)

ADA = adenosine deaminase; MHC = major histocompatibility complex; PNP = purine nucleotide phosphorylase; SCID = severe combined immunodeficiency disease; sIgA = secretory IgA; Th = helper T cell.

arm of the X chromosome. The disease is presumably a result of a block in the maturation of pre-B cells into lymphocytes with surface IgM.
  a. The protein tyrosine kinase is defective or absent in B cells.
  b. Pre-B cell V/D/J rearrangement and μ chain production are normal.
  4. Treatment consists of intramuscular or intravenous injections of pooled human gammaglobulin, which usually are administered monthly. Intravenous immunoglobulins (IVIG) are preferred as they deliver a higher level of antibodies to the patient. Avoidance of infection and administration of appropriate antibiotics are essential.

B. Other hypogammaglobulinemias

  1. Transient hypogammaglobulinemia of infancy results when the onset of immunoglobulin synthesis, particularly IgG synthesis, is delayed. The cause is unknown but may be associated with a temporary deficiency of helper T (Th) cells.

    a. Clinical and immunologic features

        (1) Most infants go through a period of hypogammaglobulinemia between the fifth and seventh months of life. Many children suffer from recurrent respiratory infections during this time period.

        (2) A few infants experience a developmental delay in the ability to synthesize IgG.

            (a) Infants have recurrent pyogenic gram-positive infections (e.g., in the skin, meninges, or respiratory tract).

            (b) The situation resolves on its own, usually by 16–30 months of age.

    b. Treatment involves the administration of antibiotics, gamma-globulin, or both.

2. Common variable hypogammaglobulinemia (acquired hypogammaglobulinemia) resembles Bruton's hypogammaglobulinemia except that symptoms (e.g., repeated pyogenic infections) first appear when the patient is 15–25 years of age.

    a. Immunologic findings. The disorder is associated with a high incidence of autoimmune diseases.

        (1) Although the number of sIg-positive circulating B cells is normal, the ability to synthesize and/or secrete immunoglobulin is defective. Serum levels of immunoglobulins decrease as the disease progresses.

        (2) Cell-mediated immune functions, which usually are intact, are sometimes defective.

    b. Treatment is the same as that for Bruton's hypogammaglobulinemia.

C. **Selective immunoglobulin deficiency (dysgammaglobulinemia)** is a decrease in the serum level of one or more immunoglobulins but with normal or increased levels of others. **Selective IgA deficiency,** which affects about 1 in 700 people, is the most common form of any immune deficiency disorder.

1. Clinical features

    a. Clinical findings include recurrent **sinopulmonary and gastrointestinal infections.** This reflects the absence of sIgA protecting these mucous membrane surfaces. Patients also have an increased incidence of autoimmune diseases, malignancy, and allergy.

    b. Many people may be asymptomatic, however. Those with associated IgA–IgG2 deficiencies are more likely to be symptomatic.

2. Immunologic findings

    a. Serum levels of IgA are low, but levels of IgG and IgM are normal or increased.

    b. IgA-bearing B cells are present, but they are defective in their ability to secrete this immunoglobulin.

3. Treatment. These patients should not be treated with pooled human gamma-globulin preparations because an anaphylactic sensitivity may be induced in the recipient by infusion of the missing immunoglobulin. Aggressive antibiotic therapy to control the infectious agent must be used.

IV. **T-CELL DEFICIENCY DISORDERS** (see Table 9-3)

A. **DiGeorge syndrome** is the eponymic name for congenital thymic hypoplasia.

1. Etiology

    a. DiGeorge syndrome is caused by **faulty development of the third and fourth pharyngeal pouches during embryogenesis.** Absence or hypoplasia of both the thymus and parathyroid glands results.

    b. The basis for the developmental abnormality is not known.

2. Clinical features

    a. Thymus aplasia (or hypoplasia) results in cellular immunodeficiency with profoundly impaired T-cell function, which is manifested by recurrent infection with viral, fungal, protozoan, and mycobacterial agents.

    b. Hypoparathyroidism leads to hypocalcemic tetany.

    c. The facial appearance is abnormal, with a fish-shaped mouth and low-set ears.

    d. Cardiac anomalies usually are present as well.

  3. Immunologic findings

    a. Lymphocytopenia usually is found. T cells are reduced in number. The lymphopenia usually is detected by flow cytometry techniques (see Chapter 6 IV C 1 b).

    b. Delayed hypersensitivity reactions and the ability to reject allografts are impaired.

    c. Most patients have normal immunoglobulin levels. In some patients, however, the levels of circulating antibody are low, at least to certain antigens, because of the reduced numbers of Th cells.

  4. Treatment

    a. Transplantation of a thymus can result in permanent reversal of the syndrome, with the production of functioning T cells.

    b. Hypocalcemia can be controlled by administration of calcium and vitamin D.

    c. In most patients, the condition improves with age, even without thymus transplants. Patients are relatively normal by the age of 5 or 6 years. Extrathymic sites probably serve as areas for T-cell maturation, or typical thymic and parathyroid tissues develop ectopically.

B. **Chronic mucocutaneous candidiasis** is a syndrome of skin and mucous membrane infection with *C. albicans*. It is associated with a unique defect in T-cell immunity.

  1. Immunologic findings

    a. The total lymphocyte count appears to be normal. The presence of T cells is confirmed through enumeration of CD3+ cells.

    b. However, the T cells show an impaired ability to produce macrophage migration-inhibiting factor (MIF) in response to *Candida* antigen, although their response to other antigens may be normal. The delayed hypersensitivity skin reaction to *Candida* antigen also is negative.

    c. The antibody response to *Candida* antigen is normal.

  2. Treatment. Attempts at therapy with various antifungal agents and with thymus transplantation have met with varying degrees of success. Patients must be observed carefully for the onset of endocrine dysfunction, particularly Addison's disease, which is the major cause of death.

V. **COMBINED B-CELL AND T-CELL DEFICIENCY DISORDERS** (see Table 9-3)

A. **Severe combined immunodeficiency disease (SCID)** is an X-linked recessive or autosomal recessive disease that involves a combined defect in both humoral and cell-mediated immunity. Patients usually die within the first or second year of life from overwhelming microbial infection.

  1. Immunologic findings

    a. Classically, SCID is associated with lymphopenia and hypoplasia of the thymus gland. Affected people have no T cells and are unable to mount a humoral immune response.

    b. The autosomal recessive form of SCID often involves an enzyme deficit.

      (1) Approximately **50%** of patients with the autosomal recessive form of the disease (about 20% of the total) have an **ADA deficiency.**

        (a) This deficiency leads to the accumulation of metabolites that are toxic to lymphocytes because they block DNA synthesis.

        (b) DNA synthesis is impaired by an intracellular accumulation of deoxyadenosine triphosphate that inhibits ribonucleotide reductase. Depletion of deoxyribonucleoside triphosphates results.

(2) Another form of SCID is caused by a **deficiency of purine nucleotide phosphory-lase (PNP),** an enzyme involved in purine catabolism. This defect also leads to the accumulation of metabolites toxic to DNA synthesis.

    c. The X-linked form of the disease is due to a stem cell defect.

2. Treatment

    a. Specific antibiotics and gamma-globulin are helpful, but successful immunologic reconstitution requires transplantation of histocompatible bone marrow for the X-linked disease.

    b. ADA deficiency was the first human disease to be successfully treated using gene therapy.

        1. The patient's peripheral blood T lymphocytes are transfected with a retroviral vector containing the ADA gene. After the T-cell population is expanded by in vitro culture, the cells are infused into the original donor.

        2. The resultant clinical improvement is transient because of the limited half-life of the transfused cells. Thus, the procedure needs to be repeated periodically or autologous bone marrow stem cells can be used.

B. **Nezelof's syndrome** is a group of disorders that have similar immunologic features. All patients with this syndrome are susceptible to recurrent microbial infections of diverse etiology.

1. Immunologic findings

    a. **T-cell immunity is markedly reduced.**

    b. **B-cell deficiency varies.** Levels of specific immunoglobulin classes may be low, normal, or elevated **(dysgammaglobulinemia).** The antibody response to specific antigens usually is low or absent.

2. Treatment. Thymus transplantation or thymic hormone administration has been somewhat successful. Aggressive treatment of infections with specific antibiotics and gamma-globulin is useful.

C. **Wiskott-Aldrich syndrome** has three features: thrombocytopenia, eczema, and recurrent infections caused by encapsulated microbes.

1. Immunologic findings

    a. Serum IgM levels are low, with normal levels of IgG and elevated levels of IgA and IgE. Isohemagglutinins are present in small amounts or absent.

    b. The number of B cells is normal. Any apparent B-cell deficit seems to be associated with a failure to make antibodies in response to polysaccharide antigens.

    c. T-cell immunity usually is intact in the early phases of the disease but wanes as the disease progresses.

2. Treatment involves vigorous use of antibiotics and bone marrow transplantation.

D. **Ataxia–telangiectasia** is an autosomal recessive disease that involves the nervous, endocrine, and vascular systems.

1. Clinical features

    a. Ataxia–telangiectasia is characterized by uncoordinated muscle movements (ataxia) and by dilation of small blood vessels (telangiectasis) that is readily observed in the sclera of the eye.

    b. This disease first appears in children younger than 2 years of age and is associated with repeated sinopulmonary infections. Older patients develop carcinomas.

2. Immunologic findings

    a. **Selective IgA deficiency is apparent,** with variable abnormalities affecting other immunoglobulins.

    b. T-cell deficiency is variable.

3. Treatment of sinopulmonary infection with antibiotics is essential. Intravenous immunoglobulin (IGIV) may decrease the number of infections.

VI. **SECONDARY IMMUNODEFICIENCY CONDITIONS.** Several disorders are associated with secondary immunodeficiency, which can lead to an increased susceptibility to opportunistic infections.

A. **Measles and other viral infections** can affect the body's defenses in several ways.

1. These conditions can induce a transient suppression of delayed hypersensitivity. The number of circulating T cells is decreased, and lymphocytic response to antigens and mitogens is reduced. Similar effects may be seen after measles immunization.

2. Viral infections also can adversely affect macrophages.

B. **Acquired immune deficiency syndrome (AIDS)** is caused by a retrovirus called **human immunodeficiency virus (HIV).** Viral transmission occurs through sexual intercourse and contact with blood. AIDS is contracted primarily, but not exclusively, by male homosexuals, intravenous drug abusers, people who receive transfusions, and infants born of infected mothers.

1. **Clinical features**
   a. The **initial infection** may be accompanied by a mild mononucleosis-like illness with fever and malaise.
   b. After an **incubation period** of months to years, the infected person may show weight loss, fever, lymphadenopathy, oral candidiasis, and diarrhea.
   c. **Full-blown AIDS** develops years after the initial infection with HIV.
      (1) Patients demonstrate pronounced suppression of the immune system and contract severe, life-threatening opportunistic infections by such microbes as *Pneumocystis, Mycobacterium, Toxoplasma,* and *Candida.*
      (2) They also experience recrudescence of diseases caused by several herpes viruses, including herpes simplex, Epstein-Barr, varicella, and cytomegalovirus.

2. **Immunologic findings**
   a. HIV has a tropism for cells bearing the CD4 surface marker. A surface glycoprotein, **gp120,** attaches the virus to this specific T-cell marker.
      (1) This causes a reduction in the level of Th and Tdth cells.
      (2) The result is a marked lymphopenia.
   b. T lymphocytes cannot produce the normal amount of IL-2, delayed hypersensitivity is diminished, and the activity of NK cells is reduced.
   c. Specific antibody production may also be disrupted.

3. **Treatment**
   a. **Zidovudine [azidothymidine (AZT)] is a potent reverse transcriptase inhibitor**.
      (1) AZT **interferes with DNA synthesis and blocks viral replication.** However, more drug-resistant strains of increasing virulence are being observed.
      (2) **Dideoxyinosine (DDI), dideoxycytosine (DDC) and 3-thiacytosine (3-TC)** are nucleoside analogues that also block reverse transcriptase with resultant inhibition of DNA synthesis, are used in combination with AZT or in patients who are unable to tolerate AZT.
   b. **Protease inhibitors such as ritonavir, saquinavir, and indinavir** are also used in treatment of HIV infection. These agents block the viral protease enzyme that is needed to cleave viral polyproteins into functional units (e.g., reverse transcriptase).
   c. **Combined drug therapy** with AZT, 3-TC, and a protease inhibitor is used in treatment of **pregnant mothers** and has been shown to protect the infant from acquiring HIV transplacentally or during the birth process.
      (1) Treatment begins in the second trimester and continues daily throughout the pregnancy and then the infant is similarly treated for 6 weeks postpartum.
      (2) Similar three-drug therapy is used to treat individuals who have been accidentally exposed to the virus. In this case, the therapy lasts for about 2 months.
   d. Drugs that **mimic the CD4 target** are promising, and **recombinant CD4** has been shown to inhibit HIV replication in vitro.

e. **Antimicrobial agents** are of value in the management of opportunistic infections and may significantly prolong the life of patients with AIDS.

VII. COMPLEMENT DEFICIENCIES. Deficiencies of complement components or functions have been associated with increased incidence of infections and autoimmune diseases [e.g., systemic lupus erythematosus (SLE)].

A. **C1 esterase inhibitor (C1 INH) deficiency** is associated with **hereditary angioedema,** a disorder that is characterized by transient but recurrent localized edema.

1. The defect leads to uncontrolled C1s activity and resultant production of a kinin that increases capillary permeability. C2a and C4a are also generated in these patients and can contribute to the local edema by causing histamine release from mast cells in the vicinity of the local trauma.

2. The skin, gastrointestinal tract, and respiratory tract may be affected. Laryngeal edema may be fatal.

B. **C2 and C4 deficiencies** can cause a disorder similar to SLE, possibly as a result of a failure of complement-dependent mechanisms to eliminate immune complexes.

C. **C3 deficiency** can result in severe, life-threatening infections, particularly with pyogenic organisms such as streptococci and staphylococci. Absence of the C3 component means that the chemotactic fragment C5a is not generated. C3b is not deposited on membranes, and impaired opsonization results.

D. **C5 deficiency** leads to increased susceptibility to bacterial infection associated with impaired chemotaxis.

E. **C6, C7, and C8 deficiencies** can result in increased susceptibility to meningococcal and gonococcal septicemias because complement-mediated lysis is a major control mechanism in immunity to *Neisseria.* In patients with these protein deficiencies, the severity of the neisserial infection is greater, and the incidence of sepsis, arthritis, and disseminated intravascular coagulopathy is increased.

Vignette Revisited

1. At approximately 6 months of age, maternal IgG that crossed the placenta during gestation diminishes to the point that it no longer offers protection to the child. For this reason, many immunodeficiencies go unrecognized during the first year of life.
2. The frequency of upper respiratory and gastrointestinal complaints suggests a deficiency in the protection of mucus membranes, which is provided by secretory IgA.
3. The child's vital signs are within normal range, and her height and head circumference are in the 50th percentile. Her weight, however, is in the 5th percentile, despite her mother describing adequate caloric intake. Given the history of repeated infections, the most likely scenario is one in which the child is directing all available calories to fighting off the invading pathogens. Other causes, such as malabsorption, inadequate caloric intake, and failure to thrive, also should be considered.
4. The hemoglobin, hematocrit, and platelets are all within normal range, decreasing the likelihood of a catastrophic bone marrow disorder. Her elevated white blood cell count with lymphocytosis supports the diagnosis of an acute viral infection. The discovery of a severely diminished serum IgA level with normal circulating amounts of IgG and IgM supports the diagnosis of selective IgA deficiency.
   Selective IgA deficiency is the most frequently recognized selective hypogammaglobulinemia, with an estimated 1 in 700 white persons affected. Both serum and se-

cretory IgA are decreased or absent. The inheritance pattern is variable; some patterns are autosomal dominant, and others are autosomal recessive. Patients commonly have an associated autoimmune disease.

5. The clinical appearance of IgA deficiency varies. Some patients have no symptoms, some have occasional respiratory infections and diarrhea, and rarely, patients have severe, recurrent infections leading to permanent intestinal and airway damage. Treatment with commercial immune globulin is ineffective because IgA is not present in the preparation. Infusions of plasma containing IgA are dangerous because anti-IgA antibodies may develop, leading to systemic anaphylaxis or serum sickness. Some cases of IgA deficiency may spontaneously remit. The mainstay of treatment is avoidance of sick contacts and treating infections aggressively.

1. Bruton's hypogammaglobulinemia is indicative of a deficiency of what cell type?

(A) B cell
(B) Macrophage
(C) T cell
(D) Monocyte
(E) Neutrophil

2. Job's syndrome is thought to result from

(A) a B-cell deficit
(B) suppressed IgE production
(C) a defect in macrophage killing
(D) a defect in neutrophil chemotaxis
(E) suppressed IgA production

3. Chronic granulomatous disease (CGD) is a result of which one of the following immunodeficiency conditions?

(A) Hypocomplementemia
(B) A defect in T-cell number
(C) A defect in T-cell function
(D) A defect in B-cell function
(E) A defect in neutrophil function

4. Which one of the following is a complement defect that could result in immunodeficiency with increased incidence of opportunistic infections?

(A) Impaired chemotaxis
(B) Insufficient hexose monophosphate (HMP) shunt (glucose) metabolism
(C) Depressed C3aR levels
(D) Defective opsonization
(E) Defective C1 esterase inhibitor

5. Chronic granulomatous disease (CGD) is characterized by which of the following conditions?

(A) Delayed chemotactic response
(B) Recurrent fungal and viral infections
(C) Eczema and thrombocytopenia
(D) Defective oxidative burst by neutrophils
(E) Inability to respond to *Candida albicans* antigens

6. A 3-year-old boy has a history of repeated sinopulmonary infections. He has also had several episodes of diarrheal disease. Phagocytic functions and T-cell numbers are reported as normal. Complement levels are normal, as are IgG and IgM levels. There is a selective IgA deficiency and some T-cell functional deficits detected by laboratory analysis. Which is the most likely diagnosis?

(A) Acquired immune deficiency syndrome (AIDS)
(B) Common variable hypogammaglobulinemia
(C) C3 deficiency
(D) Ataxia–telangiectasia
(E) Bruton's hypogammaglobulinemia

7. A 46-year-old male drug abuser has had recurrent pulmonary infections and a chronic case of oral candidiasis. Diarrheal disease has also been a problem. Laboratory evaluation reveals marked lymphopenia associated with reversal of CD4:CD8 T-cell ratio. Which one of the following diagnoses is most likely correct?

(A) Acquired immune deficiency syndrome (AIDS)
(B) Ataxia-telangiectasia
(C) Chronic mucocutaneous candidiasis
(D) DiGeorge syndrome
(E) Nezelof's syndrome

8. A 16-year-old boy presents to his physician with a history suggestive of systemic lupus erythematosus (SLE). The patient has a rash, arthralgia, and mild proteinuria. Serologic evaluation detects no antibodies of diagnostic value. Which one of the following diseases is most likely to be diagnosed in this patient?

(A) Rheumatoid arthritis
(B) Common variable hypogammaglobulinemia
(C) C2 deficiency
(D) Sjögren's syndrome
(E) Wegener's granulomatosis

9. An 18-month-old boy has been troubled with repeated pulmonary infections. He has also had boils three different times. Complement and phagoctyic functions are reported as normal. The child contracted chickenpox at 9 months of age and had a normal recovery from that viral infection. Which one of the following diseases is the most likely diagnosis?

(A) Acquired immune deficiency syndrome
(B) Bruton's hypogammaglobulinemia
(C) Common variable hypogammaglobuline- mia
(D) DiGeorge syndrome
(E) Chronic granulomatous disease

10. A 19-year-old previously healthy female patient presents with the complaint of repeated, chronic pulmonary infections. Laboratory evaluation reveals normal numbers of circulating B cells but defective synthesis and/or secretion of immunoglobulins. What is the most likely diagnosis?

(A) Thymic and parathyroid dysgenesis
(B) Common variable hypogammaglobuline- mia
(C) A complement protein deficiency
(D) Bruton's hypogammaglobulinemia
(E) Wiskott-Aldrich syndrome

1. The answer is A [III A]. Patients with Bruton's hypogammaglobulinemia are deficient in B cells and plasma cells, and therefore have low serum levels of all classes of immunoglobulins. T cells and phagocytes are normal in number and function.

2. The answer is D [II B 5]. Job's syndrome (hyper-IgE syndrome) is characterized by "cold" staphylococcal abscesses, chronic eczema, and extremely high serum levels of IgE. It is related to defective neutrophil chemotaxis. The ingestion and killing of microorganisms by neutrophils appear to be normal.

3. The answer is E [II B 1]. Chronic granulomatous disease (CGD) reflects an inability of neutrophils to respond to phagocytosis with the normal oxidative burst; apparently it is caused by a defect in nicotinamide adenine dinucleotide phosphate (NADPH) oxidase. The most common form of the disease is X-linked (63% of cases) and is due to a defect in cytochrome b component of the enzyme. The result is suppression of intracellular killing of ingested microorganisms. B-cell, T-cell, and natural killer (NK) cell functions, as well as complement levels, usually are normal. The mortality rate can be reduced considerably by early diagnosis and aggressive therapy.

4. The answer is D [VII C]. Opsonization could be compromised if there were a deficit in the third component of the complement cascade. This could result in lower amounts of C3b being produced during the response to an infecting agent. This potent opsonin can be generated without the participation of antibodies via the alternative pathway of complement activation. A defect in chemotaxis could cause immune deficiency by blocking the ability of phagocytes to migrate to the site of inflammation. However, this would be a problem with the phagocytic system not a complement deficiency, although it is true that C5a is a potent chemotaxin. If hexose monophosphate (HMP) shunt activity is insufficient, the phagocytic cell would not have the energy required for chemotaxis or for new membrane synthesis, which is an essential part of phagocytosis. Depressed levels of C3a receptors in basophil

and mast cell membranes would interfere with histamine release from these cells but would not likely contribute to increased incidence of infections. Deficits in the C1 esterase inhibitor result in hereditary angioneurotic edema.

5. The answer is D [II B 1]. In patients with chronic granulomatous disease (CGD), chemotactic responses are normal. CGD is an immunodeficiency syndrome with onset in the first 2 years of life; it is inherited primarily as an X-linked trait. Characteristics include recurrent bacterial infections, hepatosplenomegaly, lymphadenopathy, and granuloma formation, which appears to reflect faulty phagocytosis. Neutrophils fail to respond to phagocytosis with the normal oxidative burst, apparently due to defects in nicotinamide adenine dinucleotide phosphate (NADPH) oxidase. Chemotactic responses are normal, as is the patient's ability to respond to candidal antigens. Eczema and thrombocytopenia are part of the clinical presentation of patients with Wiskott-Aldrich syndrome; these individuals have trouble with encapsulated bacterial pathogens.

6. The answer is D [V D]. Immune deficits in ataxia–telangiectasia include variable T-cell deficiency, selective IgA deficiency with variable abnormalities in other immunoglobulins, and an occasional inhibited antibody response to certain antigens. Ataxia–telangiectasia is an inherited immune deficiency characterized by uncoordinated muscle movements (ataxia) and dilated small blood vessels in the sclera of the eye (telangiectasia). Acquired immune deficiency syndrome (AIDS) is caused by a retrovirus—human immunodeficiency virus (HIV)—which causes a marked reduction in CD4+ cells and a marked reversal of the CD4:CD8 T-cell ratio to less than 0.5 (the normal ratio is at least 1.5). This leads to pronounced suppression of the immune system, with resultant susceptibility to opportunistic infections. A deficiency in complement component C3 may manifest itself as a disorder similar to Bruton's disease with an increase in bacterial infections (e.g., boils, pneumonia, and diarrhea). The patients with a C3 deficit have particular difficulty with pyogenic organisms such as staphylococci and streptococci.

In common variable hypogammaglobuline-mia, levels of circulating B cells are normal, but the ability to synthesize or to secrete immunoglobulin is defective. The defect may be caused by a population of suppressor T (Ts) cells that inhibit B-cell maturation.

7. The answer is A [VI B]. Acquired immune deficiency syndrome (AIDS) is caused by a retrovirus—human immunodeficiency virus (HIV)—which causes a marked reduction in CD 4+ cells and a marked reversal of the CD4:CD8 T-cell ratio to less than 0.5 (the normal ratio is at least 1.5). This leads to pronounced suppression of the immune system, with resultant susceptibility to opportunistic infections. Immune deficits in ataxia–telangiectasia include variable T-cell deficiency, selective IgA deficiency with variable abnormalities in other immunoglobulins, and an occasional inhibited antibody response to certain antigens. Ataxia–telangiectasia is an inherited immune deficiency characterized by uncoordinated muscle movements (ataxia) and dilated small blood vessels in the sclera of the eye (telangiectasia). Chronic mucocutaneous candidiasis is a peculiar immunologic deficit wherein the patient has a single impairment: they cannot respond to antigens of *Candida albicans* and thus have chronic, unremitting infections caused by this agent. Fortunately they are usually cutaneous and do not become systemic. The patients usually respond to antifungal therapy with drugs like nystatin, flucytosine, or fluconazole. DiGeorge syndrome is a T-cell deficiency caused by hypoplasia of the thymus gland due to faulty embryogenesis. The parathyroid is also hypoplastic. The affected individuals have recurrent viral, fungal, and mycobacterial infections. The parathyroid deficit is evidenced by hypocalcemic tetany. Nezelof's syndrome also is evidenced by T-cell deficit. Gamma globulin levels are variable.

8. The answer is C [VII B]. A deficiency in complement component C2 may manifest itself as a disorder similar to systemic lupus erythematosus (SLE), possibly because of a failure of complement-dependent mechanisms to eliminate immune complexes. Most patients with rheumatoid arthritis have several antibodies (most notably the anti-IgG antibody known as rheumatoid factor). Similarly, Sjögren's patients are diagnosed by detection of antibodies to exocrine gland duct epithelium. Patients

with Wegener's granulomatosis have antineutrophil cytoplasmic autoantibodies. Common variable hypogammaglobulinemia will evidence itself by the occurrence of repeated bacterial infections.

9. The answer is B [III A]. Patients with Bruton's disease have an increase in bacterial infections (e.g., boils, pneumonia, and diarrhea). Their primary deficit is in a tyrosine kinase enzyme; the result of this deficiency is an inability to form immunoglobulin molecules in the endoplasmic reticulum. The patients can synthesize mu heavy chains but cannot complete the steps needed to make intact IgM antibody molecules and to display them in the cell membrane. They have pre-B cells in the bone marrow but lack mature B cells with surface immunoglobulins in peripheral lymphoid tissues. Acquired immune deficiency syndrome (AIDS) is caused by a retrovirus—human immunodeficiency virus (HIV)—which causes a marked reduction in CD4+ cells and a marked reversal of the CD4:CD8 T-cell ratio to less than 0.5 (the normal ratio is at least 1.5). This leads to pronounced suppression of the immune system, with resultant susceptibility to opportunistic infections. In common variable hypogammaglobulinemia, levels of circulating B cells are normal, but the ability to synthesize or to secrete immunoglobulin is defective. The defect may be caused by a population of suppressor T (Ts) cells that inhibit B-cell maturation. DiGeorge syndrome is a T-cell deficiency caused by hypoplasia of the thymus gland due to faulty embryogenesis. The parathyroid gland also is hypoplastic. The affected individuals have recurrent viral, fungal, and mycobacterial infections. The parathyroid deficit is evidenced by hypocalcemic tetany. Nezelof's syndrome also is evidenced by T-cell deficit; gamma globulin levels are variable. In patients with chronic granulomatous disease (CGD), chemotactic responses are normal. CGD is an immunodeficiency syndrome with onset in the first 2 years of life. It is inherited primarily as an X-linked trait. Characteristics include recurrent bacterial infections, hepatosplenomegaly, lymphadenopathy, and granuloma formation, which appears to reflect faulty phagocytosis. Neutrophils fail to respond to phagocytosis with the normal oxidative burst, apparently because of a defect in nicotinamide adenine dinucleotide phosphate (NADPH) oxidase.

10. The answer is B [III B 2]. In common variable hypogammaglobulinemia, levels of circulating B cells are normal, but the ability to synthesize or to secrete immunoglobulin is defective. The patients gradually lose the ability to respond to antigens and become susceptible to bacterial opportunistic agents. Thymus and parathyroid dysgenesis (DiGeorge syndrome) is a T-cell deficiency caused by hypoplasia of the thymus gland due to faulty embryogenesis. The parathyroid also is hypoplastic. The affected individuals have recurrent viral, fungal, and mycobacterial infections. The parathyroid deficit is evidenced by hypocalcemic tetany. Complement deficiencies are evidenced by either an increase in pyogenic infections (C3 deficit), neisserial sepsis (C5–C8), or autoimmune phenomena (C1, 2, 4). Patients with Bruton's disease have an increase in bacterial infections (e.g., boils, pneumonia, diarrhea). Their primary deficit is in a tyrosine kinase enzyme; the result of this deficiency is an inability to form immunoglobulin molecules in the endoplasmic reticulum. The patients can synthesize mu heavy chains but cannot complete the steps needed to make intact IgM antibody molecules and to display them in the cell membrane. They have pre-B cells in the bone marrow but lack mature B cells with surface immunoglobulins in peripheral lymphoid tissues. Eczema and thrombocytopenia are part of the clinical presentation of patients with Wiskott-Aldrich syndrome. These individuals have trouble with encapsulated bacterial pathogens. They can synthesize most antibodies but characteristically have a low level of IgM.

Chapter 10

Transplantation and Tumor Immunology

Vignette

A 38-year-old man with a 20-year history of insulin-dependent diabetes mellitus presents for a routine examination by his physician. Despite tight insulin control of his blood glucose, the man's renal function has diminished from diabetic nephropathy, and his blood urea nitrogen and creatinine levels have gradually risen over the last few years. His physician believes it is time to initiate the transplantation process and begin the search for a suitable donor.

1. What is the difference in graft survival rates between living related donor grafts versus cadaveric donor grafts?

The patient's sister has volunteered to donate one of her kidneys for transplantation. Blood samples from the brother and sister are found to match at human leukocyte antigen (HLA)-A, HLA-B, and HLA-D loci, and they both have blood type O. The patient is started on cyclosporine and given multiple blood transfusions before the operation.

2. What are the mechanism of action and potential side effects of cyclosporine?
3. What is the purpose of multiple blood transfusions just before grafting?

Both the harvest operation and the transplant procedure are completed without complications for both the patient and his sister. The sister will be discharged from the hospital in less than 1 week. The patient will need to remain in the hospital for several weeks to monitor the function of his new kidney and to ensure that the graft is not rejected by his immune system.

4. What are some of the short- and long-term complications of organ transplantation?

I. TRANSPLANTATION

A. Introduction

1. **Types of grafts**
   a. **Syngrafts,** or **isografts,** involve the transfer of normal tissue between **genetically identical (syngeneic)** individuals (i.e., identical twins or animals of the same inbred line).
   b. **Autografts** are grafts removed from and placed in the same individual (e.g., skin graft from a person's leg to his face).
   c. **Allografts,** or **homografts,** involve the transfer of normal tissue between **allogeneic** individuals (i.e., genetically different individuals of the same species).
   d. **Heterografts,** or **xenografts** (also called **xenogeneic** grafts), are tissues transferred between animals of two different species (e.g., baboon liver transplanted into a human).

2. **Prognosis**
   a. Generally, isografts and autografts survive for an indefinite period of time.
   b. Allogeneic and xenogeneic grafts result in some degree of immune rejection, which may be prevented or aborted by the use of immunosuppressive agents.

3. **Organ transplantation in humans.** The National Institutes of Health reports that the demand for transplants far exceeds the number of organs available for transplantation. In April 2000, almost 80,000 patients were awaiting transplant organs (Table 10-1).
   a. **Kidneys** are the most frequently transplanted organs (see Table 10-1). In 1987, nearly 158,000 Medicare patients had end-stage renal disease; the only available treatment for this condition is maintenance dialysis or a kidney transplant.

TABLE 10-1. Incidence of Selected Organ Transplants, United States, 1998

Organ	Number of Transplants	Number of People Awaiting Transplants
Kidney	12,166	44,974
Heart	2,345	4,143
Lung	862	3,588
Heart/lung	47	208
Liver	4,487	15,164
Pancreas	248	896

Source = http://www.unos.org/frame_default.asp? Category = news data. Data as of April 2000.

TABLE 10-2. Diseases Treatable by Bone Marrow Transplantation*

Genetic Diseases	Malignancies
Sickle cell anemia	Acute lymphoblastic leukemia
Thalassemia major	Acute myelogenous leukemia
Wiskott-Aldrich syndrome	Chronic myelogenous leukemia
Chédiak-Higashi syndrome	Lymphoma
Ataxia–telangiectasia	Myeloma
Severe combined immunodeficiency	Solid tumors:
Chronic granulomatous disease	Breast
Mucocutaneous candidiasis	Lung
Fanconi's disease	Ovary
Aplastic Anemia	Testicle

*Both allogeneic and autologous bone marrows can be used.

    b. Bone marrow transplantation is used in the treatment of several diseases (Table 10-2).

B. **Histocompatibility gene complex**

  1. Characteristics of histocompatibility antigens

    a. Histocompatibility antigens, or **transplantation antigens,** are antigens expressed on cell surfaces that determine the compatibility or incompatibility of transplanted tissue.

    b. These antigens induce the immune response in the host that may cause rejection of transplanted tissue.

    c. The most important histocompatibility antigens are products of genes of the **major histocompatibility complex (MHC).** These antigens are termed **human leukocyte antigens (HLAs)** because they are found in high concentrations on lymphocytes and other white blood cells. HLAs also occur on other nucleated cells in the body (e.g., macrophages and hepatocytes).

    d. The **ABO antigens** of the red blood cell system also act as strong transplantation antigens. ABO compatibility between donor and recipient must exist or graft survival is compromised.

    e. Minor histocompatibility antigens, such as those coded for on the Y chromosome, can also contribute to graft rejection.

2. MHC and histocompatibility genes
   a. Description. The MHC is a closely linked complex of genes that governs the production of the major histocompatibility antigens.
      (1) In **mice,** this complex (designated H-2) is found on chromosome 17.
      (2) In **humans,** the MHC is located on the short arm of chromosome 6. A portion of the MHC codes for the HLA histocompatibility antigens (Figure 10-1).
   b. Composition. A population varies considerably in its histocompatibility makeup because of the multiplicity of HLA molecules.
      (1) There are **six major groups of classical HLAs.**
         (a) HLA-A, HLA-B, and **HLA-C** are encoded by the HLA-A, B, and C loci of the MHC complex (see Figure 10-1).
         (b) HLA-DR, HLA-DQ, and **HLA-DP** are encoded by gene loci in three subregions (DR, DQ, and DP) of the HLA-D region of the MHC complex (see Figure 10-1). In addition, some HLA-D antigens are not the product of specific gene clusters; instead, they are the result of gene mixing between antigens encoded by the three major D subregion loci.
      (2) Most of the HLA genes are **highly polymorphic** (i.e., multiple alleles occurring at a single HLA locus).
         (a) According to the HLA Informatics Group of The Anthony Nolan Bone Marrow Trust, currently locus HLA-A has 124 recognized alleles; loci DR, C, DQ, and DP have 265, 74, 58, and 99, respectively; and locus B has 258. Thus, the number of potential antigen combinations in the population is astronomical (at least $124 \times 265 \times 74 \times 58 \times 99 \times 258$).
         (b) In the HLA-D subregions, especially HLA-DR, many of the HLA molecules have two or three functional β-chain genes (but only one α chain).
            (i) This allows a single cell to express more than two allelic forms of each DR molecule.
            (ii) Additional variants are hybrids of the α chain of one allele and the β chain of the other allele within an HLA-DR locus. Such hybridization leads to the formation of the HLA-D molecules.
      (3) The HLA genes are **codominant** in expression.
         (a) When an individual is heterozygous for a particular HLA locus (as in Figure 10-2; case B, locus B), both alleles at that locus are expressed. Therefore, in the heterozygote, both antigens encoded by these alleles are present on the tissue cells.
         (b) In contrast, in a homozygous individual, the alleles of the locus on both chromosomes are identical (as in Figure 10-2; case B, locus A), and only one HLA is specified.
         (c) Usually, one individual expresses a dozen or more different DR, DQ, and DP gene products per cell. This greatly expands the population of molecules that can act as epitope presenters in the process of MHC restriction.

3. Class I and class II MHC antigens
   a. Classification. The classical HLA molecules encoded by genes of the MHC fall into two categories.
      (1) HLA-A, HLA-B, and **HLA-C** are class I antigens.
      (2) HLA-DP, HLA-DQ, and **HLA-DR** are class II antigens.
   b. Location. Both class I and class II antigens are surface-expressed components of the cell, though secreted forms of class I molecules are also found in the circulation. The expression of class II molecules on the cell surface is one of the most widely used markers of T-cell activation (Figure 10-3).
      (1) Class I antigens occur on all nucleated human cells (except sperm) and on platelets. (In the mouse, however, the corresponding H-2 MHC antigens also are present on erythrocytes).
      (2) Class II antigens are found chiefly on the surfaces of immunocompetent cells, including dendritic cells, macrophages, monocytes, resting T cells (in low amounts), activated T cells, and B cells.

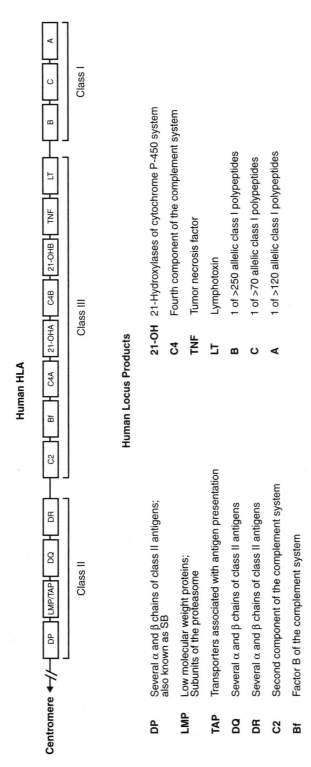

Figure 10-1. Schematic map of the major histocompatibility gene complex (MHC) in humans and the gene products associated with each locus. The immune response (Ir)-associated genes are located in the human leukocyte antigen (HLA)-D region, which contains the DP, DQ, and DR loci. There is not a single locus for each component but rather clusters of several loci encoding the α and β chains of each of the class II antigens (see Figure 10-4). Genes for tumor necrosis factor (TNF) are between the class III and class I genes.

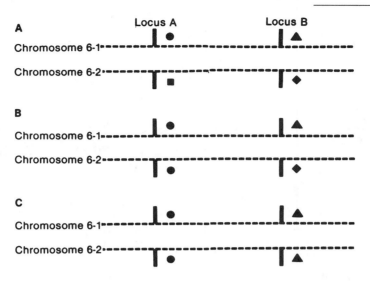

Figure 10-2. Schematic representation of codominant alleles. In the human leukocyte antigen (HLA) complex on chromosome 6, each gene is codominant in expression; that is, in an individual having different alleles at corresponding loci of the two chromosomes, both alleles are expressed. ●, ■, ▲, ◆, represent HLA antigens expressed by each locus on both chromosomes. In case (*A*), four different antigens are expressed (● ■ ▲ ◆); in case (*B*), three antigens are expressed (● ▲ ◆); and in case (*C*), two antigens are expressed (● ▲). The haplotype is the set of alleles present on a single chromosome; thus, in case (*A*) the haplotype of chromosome 6–1 is ● ▲ and the haplotype of chromosome 6–2 is ■ ◆. The ● ▲ haplotype is also found in chromosome 6–1 in case (*B*) and in both chromosomes in case (*C*).

    c. Structure. Class I and class II antigens are each molecules composed of two polypeptide chains, α and β, which are held together by noncovalent bonds (Figure 10-4). The chains are 90% protein and 10% carbohydrate.

       (1) Class I antigens

          (a) The α chain (44 kDa) has three domains, carries the antigenic specificity, and is anchored in the cell membrane. The α_1 and α_2 domains form a basket-like structure, or groove, distal to the cell membrane that holds a peptide epitope 8 to 10 amino acids long.

          (b) The β chain (12 kDa) is a β_2-microglobulin (i.e., it is a small protein that migrates with the beta-globulins in serum electrophoresis). It is not encoded by the MHC, is not polymorphic, and does not have a transmembrane region.

       (2) Class II antigens

          (a) The α chain (34 kDa) and the β chain (29 kDa) each consist of two extracellular domains (α_1, α_2, and β_1, β_2, respectively), a transmembrane region, and a cytoplasmic tail. The α_1 and β_1 domains form a membrane-distal groove that holds a peptide epitope 15 to 23 amino acids long.

          (b) Both chains are encoded in closely linked HLA-D region gene clusters.

          (c) Most of the HLA antigen-specific epitopes (i.e., the antigenic determinant regions) are found in the β chain.

    d. Functions

       (1) Both class I and class II MHC molecules are important in **controlling immunologic responses** by a process known as **MHC restriction.**

          (a) The class II antigens play a role in **antigen presentation** by professional antigen presenting cells (APC), including macrophages, dendritic cells, and B cells, to T cells. The epitope of the antigen is presented to its homologous receptor on the T cell, thus triggering activation of the latter cell (See Chapter 5, II B 1 and C 1, 2).

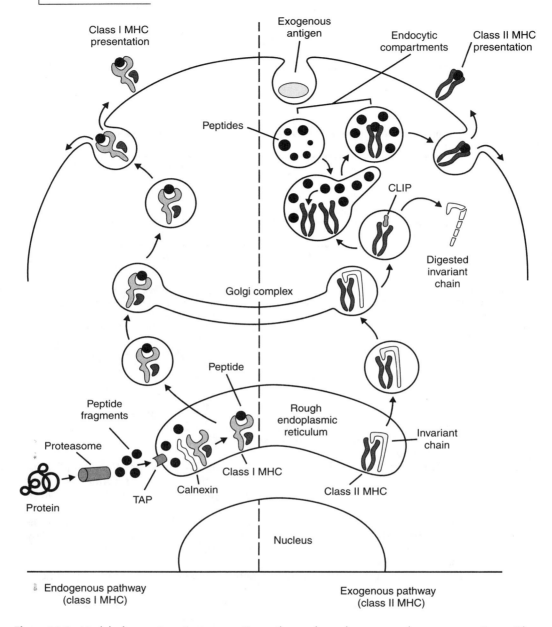

Class I MHC
presentation

Exogenous
antigen

Endocytic
compartments

Class II MHC
presentation

Peptides

CLIP

Digested
invariant
chain

Golgi complex

Peptide

Peptide
fragments

Rough
endoplasmic
reticulum

Invariant
chain

Proteasome

Class I MHC

Class II MHC

Protein

TAP

Calnexin

Nucleus

Endogenous pathway
(class I MHC)

Exogenous pathway
(class II MHC)

Figure 10-3. Model of separate antigen-presenting pathways for endogenous and exogenous antigens. The mode of antigen entry into cells and the site of antigen processing appear to determine whether antigenic peptides associate with class I MHC molecules in the rough endoplasmic reticulum or with class II molecules in endocytic compartments. Some elements of this model have not been experimentally demonstrated. *CLIP* = Class II-associated Invariant Chain Peptide; *MHC* = major histocompatibility complex; *TAP* = transporter associated with antigen presentation (Redrawn from Kuby J: *Immunology,* 3rd edition. New York, W.H. Freeman and Co., 1994, p. 257)

(b) Both class I and class II MHC antigens are involved in the **sensitization phase** of **cell-mediated cytotoxicity** [also called **cell-mediated cytolysis (CMC)**], which is mediated by cytotoxic T (Tc) lymphocytes.

   (i) Class I and class II antigens both occur on the APC. Class I antigens react with the CD8 molecule on the Tc-cell precursor. Class II antigens react

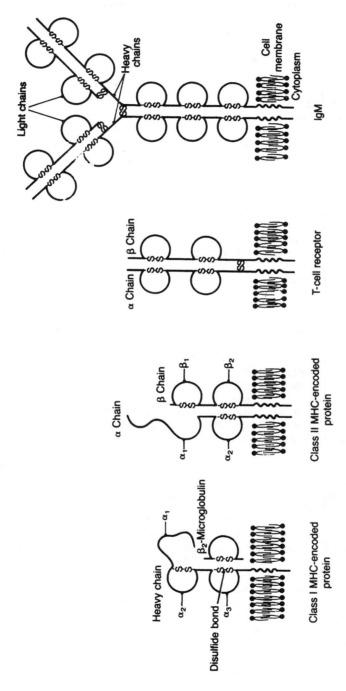

Figure 10-4. Molecular structures of the class I and class II proteins encoded by the major histocompatibility complex (MHC), the T-cell receptor, and the monomeric immunoglobulin molecule. Note the structural similarity; the molecules also share similar sequences of amino acids. The molecules are characterized by loops (domains) made up of about 70 amino acids within each chain. (Adapted with permission from Marrack P, Kapler J: The T cell and its receptor. *Sci Am* 254:36B45, 1986.)

with the CD4 molecule on the helper T (Th) cell, thus ensuring the presence of lymphokines that enhance the proliferation and maturation of the Tc-cell precursor.

(ii) Class I antigens are involved in MHC restriction of CMC, primarily in virus-infected or malignant cells.

(c) MHC restriction is not found in hyperacute graft rejection nor in some antitumor processes, both of which are mediated by antibodies. It also is absent from the effector phase of acute and chronic graft rejection.

(2) Class I and class II MHC antigens also can serve as targets of the immune response.

(a) In **CMC,** HLA alloantigens are recognized by Tc cells. Therefore, they serve as important target antigens in graft rejection.

(i) Class I HLA-A and HLA-B antigens and class II HLA-DR antigens are termed major transplantation antigens because they are among the principal antigens recognized by the host during the process of graft rejection.

(ii) The CMC assay is an *in vitro* correlate of graft rejection.

(b) Class II antigens are believed to be the antigens principally responsible for the **graft-versus-host (GVH) reaction.**

e. **Identification**

(1) The **mixed lymphocyte reaction** is often used to identify and define **class II antigens.** This lymphocyte reaction is an *in vitro* correlate of the GVH response.

(2) The **lymphocytotoxicity test** can identify both **class I and class II antigens.**

(3) **Serologic assays** can be used to find DR-encoded class II antigens.

(4) **DNA typing** also can be performed to molecularly define both **class I and class II antigens.**

4. **Other types of MHC molecules**

a. **Intracellular antigen-processing proteins** are less polymorphic than the classic molecules.

(1) **Low-molecular-weight proteins (LMPs)** incorporate into the proteasome, which degrades intracellular proteins for binding in the class I groove. Two LMPs, **LMP2 and LMP7,** are encoded within the HLA-D region centromeric to HLA-DQ. LMP2 and LMP7 expression is induced by γ-interferon (IFN-γ).

(2) **Transporters associated with antigen processing (TAPs)** convey peptides produced by the proteasome into the endoplasmic reticulum (ER). They are dimers of two products, **TAP1 and TAP2,** that are encoded within the same region of HLA-D as LMP2 and LMP7.

(3) **Tapasin** is a chaperone protein for loading peptides into class I molecules in the ER. It is encoded centromeric to HLA-DP.

b. **Nonclassic class I and class II antigens** are less polymorphic than the classic molecules. They sometimes exhibit more limited tissue distribution as well.

(1) Class I variants include **HLA-X, HLA-E, and HLA-J** (located between the HLA-C and HLA-A loci); and **HLA-H, HLA-G, and HLA-F** (located telomeric to HLA-A).

(a) **HLA-E** is expressed on most tissues and appears to be a ligand of certain natural killer (NK) cell inhibitory and stimulatory receptors.

(b) **HLA-G** is expressed on trophoblast cells of the placenta (as well as in some malignant cells) and also exhibits NK cell inhibitory properties.

(c) The other variants are considered **pseudogenes** because the functions of their gene products are currently unknown.

(2) Class II variants include **HLA-DMα and HLA-DMβ**; and **HLA-DNα and HLA-DOβ. HLA-DMα and HLA-DMβ** form dimeric molecules, as do **HLA-DOβ and HLA-DNα.** These antigens play specialized roles in class II peptide loading.

(a) The **HLA-DMα/HLA-DMβ** molecule catalyzes peptide loading in the class II groove.

(b) The **HLA-DNα/HLA-DOβ** molecule inhibits the action of the **HLA-DMα/HLA-DMβ** molecule.

       (c) The **HLA-DNα/HLA-DOβ** molecule is expressed in the thymus and on B cells. Numerous pseudogenes are also present in the HLA-D region.

  c. Class III antigens

    (1) Some loci on chromosome 6 are associated with certain complement components (C2, C4, and factor B of the alternative pathway), with tumor necrosis factors α and β (TNF-α and TNF-β), and with two hydroxylase enzymes (see Figure 10-1). These molecules are known as class III MHC antigens, although they are not involved in histocompatibility.

    (2) Class III antigens do not participate in MHC restriction or graft rejection.

  d. Immune response (Ir) genes

    (1) Specific Ir genes are found in the MHC of inbred lines of animals, indicating that the response to particular antigens is genetically controlled. Thus, strain 2 guinea pigs and the F-1 hybrid respond to phenylated poly-L-lysine (DNP-PLL), whereas strain 13 does not.

    (2) These genes occur in the HLA-D region in humans and encode the DR, DP, and DQ antigens (class II antigens).

5. Diseases associated with MHC alleles

  a. Many diseases have a statistical association with molecules of the MHC. For example, several autoimmune diseases, such as systemic lupus erythematosus, occur more frequently in individuals with the HLA-DR3 antigen (see Table 8-2).

  b. Most HLA-associated diseases are connected to haplotypes of HLA-B and HLA-D subregions (particularly DR and DQ).

C. **Clinical transplantation immunology**

1. Overview of the donor–recipient work-up. The compatibility of donor and recipient must be determined before transplantation to optimize graft survival and minimize the likelihood of a rejection reaction.

  a. ABO blood group compatibility is first established.

  b. Tissue typing to identify **HLAs** is then performed.

  c. Cross-matching is used to test the recipient's serum for **preformed antibodies** against the donor's HLAs.

  d. When the recipient's serum does not kill donor lymphocytes (as when the donor–recipient pair are HLA-identical siblings), the mixed lymphocyte reaction may be used to determine if the donor cells stimulate blastogenesis in the recipient's lymphocytes.

2. Blood group antigens

  a. General considerations

    (1) These very strong cell-surface antigens are found on many other tissues of the body as well as on the surface of red blood cells. They represent very potent transplantation antigens because antibodies against the blood group antigens (**isohemagglutinins**) occur naturally in humans (Table 10-3).

    (2) Therefore, both the donor's and the recipient's blood groups must be established before a transplantation procedure or a transfusion.

TABLE 10-3. ABO Blood Group Genetics and Occurrence

Phenotype	Genotype	Isohemagglutinin Present	Occurrence of Phenotype (%)*
A	AA or AO	Anti-B	40
B	BB or BO	Anti-A	10
O	OO	Both	45
AB	AB	Neither	5

*Figures represent percentage of United States population.

    b. The **four blood groups**
       (1) The four antigenic phenotypes (blood groups) of the ABO system are A, B, AB, and O (see Table 10-3).
       (2) The various phenotypes are determined by different **allelic combinations.** The ABO gene has three alleles: A, B, and O. The A and B alleles are dominant over O. The latter carbohydrate is, in fact, usually not immunogenic.
          (a) People in blood groups A or B can be either homozygous (AA, BB) or heterozygous (AO, BO).
          (b) Those in blood group O are homozygous (OO).
          (c) Those in blood group AB are heterozygous (AB).
    c. **Tests for ABO blood group compatibility.** Both recipient's and donor's blood types are established by agglutination tests.
       (1) Red blood cells are tested with standard anti-A and anti-B antisera.
       (2) The presence of preformed antibodies (anti-A or anti-B isohemagglutinins) is determined by assays using known blood group A and B cells.

3. Histocompatibility testing
    a. **Sources of cells and typing sera**
       (1) **Cells.** The best cells for detecting HLAs are lymphocytes obtained from the peripheral blood and from lymph nodes, the spleen, or the thymus. These cells are used for two reasons: because of their availability, and because they have the highest concentration of HLAs on the cell surface.
       (2) **Sera.** The typing sera used in the lymphocytotoxicity assay come from several sources.
          (a) **Multiparous women**
             (i) During pregnancy, fetal lymphoid cells can cross the placenta into the mother's circulation.
             (ii) The fetal antigens derived from the father's genetic contribution are foreign to the mother and sensitize her, much as they do in Rh sensitization (see Chapter 7). No fetal disease has been associated with HLA sensitization.
          (b) **Patients who have received multiple transfusions.** The white blood cells and platelets in the transfused blood provide the sensitizing antigens.
          (c) **Volunteers who have been sensitized** by blood transfusions, white blood cell inoculations, or tissue grafts
          (d) **Patients who have rejected a transplanted organ**
    b. **Lymphocytotoxicity test.** This test can identify both class I and class II antigens.
       (1) Purified lymphocytes to be tested are incubated with a battery of antisera of known HLA specificity. If a test antiserum contains an antibody to one of the HLAs on the cell, the antibody binds to the cell membrane.
       (2) Complement is then added, and incubation is continued. If the cell has antibody bound to its membrane, it is killed by complement activation.
       (3) Trypan blue or eosin, which is specifically absorbed by damaged or dying cells, is then added.
       (4) Dead cells are stained, whereas live cells do not take up the dye, thus indicating whether a particular serum–complement combination is cytotoxic for the lymphocytes. The HLAs on a cell can be determined by noting which antiserum caused cell lysis.
    c. **Mixed lymphocyte reaction (blastogenesis assay).** This test uses DNA synthesis to detect the incompatibility of class II antigens i.e., those coded by HLA-D region genes. Over 420 antigens are encoded by this region, and all can be detected by mixed lymphocyte reactions.
       (1) This assay is a mitotic response of T cells to HLAs.
          (a) When antigens such as HLA molecules on the membranes of other cells interact with lymphocytes, they stimulate lymphocyte mitosis. Small lymphocytes are transformed into blast cells in response to foreign HLAs.
          (b) To identify any HLA-D antigen, it is necessary to use lymphocytes that are sensitized to the antigen in question.

(2) Procedure
  (a) If the lymphocytes from a donor and a recipient are mixed in tissue culture, both sets of lymphocytes undergo blastogenesis and proliferate if they are histoincompatible (**two-way test**).
  (b) The mixed lymphocyte reaction usually is performed as a **one-way procedure** (i.e., only one of the cell populations in the mixture can respond).
    (i) Donor lymphocyte division is prevented by irradiating the cells or treating them with mitomycin C, which cross-links DNA. Thus, the donor cells cannot undergo blast transformation but can still act as stimulating cells.
    (ii) The recipient's cells still undergo blastogenesis if there is HLA-D region incompatibility. Histocompatibility varies inversely with the number of blast cells produced.
  (3) If there are several potential donor-recipient pairs or donors, the donor selected should have **lymphocytes that stimulate the recipient the least.**
d. DNA typing. Histocompatibility tests can be done in numerous ways. Two example approaches use specific polymerase chain reaction (PCR) primers and then either oligonucleotide probes or sequencing to identify class I and class II antigens.
  (1) DNA is prepared from peripheral blood leukocytes of donor and/or recipient origin. It is then amplified by PCR using gene-specific primers.
  (2) If **single-stranded oligonucleotide (SSO) probe hybridization** is used, then a series of oligonucleotides that bind to certain known HLA allele sequences are hybridized with the PCR product to obtain the HLA type of an individual.
  (3) In the case of **direct DNA sequencing,** the PCR product is used as a template in sequencing reactions with locus-specific primers. The sequences obtained for the loci of donor and recipient can then be compared.
  (4) Direct DNA sequencing is advantageous over SSO analysis because it is not dependent on prior knowledge of specific allelic polymorphisms (which is required to make the SSO probes). Therefore, new alleles are often identified by direct DNA sequencing.

4. Cross-matching
  a. The recipient's serum may have **preformed antibodies** against the donor's HLAs as a result of multiple blood transfusions, an earlier transplantation, or multiple pregnancies.
  b. Cross-matching may be performed by complement-dependent lymphocytotoxicity using the donor's lymphocytes as targets for the recipient's preformed antibodies.
    (1) Samples of the patient's serum are collected over a period of time. All of the serum samples must be cross-matched against the donor's lymphocytes because the antibody titer may change over time and thus may be detectable in only one serum sample.
    (2) If even one cross-matching test kills the donor's lymphocytes, transplantation is not performed.

5. Host response to transplantation
  a. Graft survival rates
    (1) When kidney transplants come from HLA-identical siblings, transplant recipients have a 5-year survival rate of more than 80%.
    (2) When two HLAs match, the graft survival rate is 70%.
    (3) When more than two HLAs are mismatched, the chances for graft survival are considerably lower.
    (4) When kidney transplants come from cadavers, regardless of matching, the 5-year survival rate is 33% to 50%. These figures are improving, however, as a result of better management practices and the use of new immunosuppressive drugs.
  b. Rejection reactions
    (1) Types of reactions. At least three types of rejection reactions can take place after transplantation.
      (a) Hyperacute rejection. This rejection pattern may occur when the donor and

recipient have not been matched for ABO blood group antigens or when the recipient has preformed antibodies to other donor antigens.

- **(i)** As soon as the vascular supplies between the recipient and the donor organ are linked, the antibodies start attacking the organ; they may sensitize donor cells to complement-mediated lysis or to destruction by NK or phagocytic cells.
- **(ii)** In certain cases, the organ fails to show any blood flow. Vascular occlusion occurs after a rapid vascular spasm, and the organ is never perfused by the recipient's blood.

- **(b) Acute or accelerated rejection.** Acute rejection is believed to be caused by sensitized T lymphocytes. This type of reaction occurs 10 to 30 days after transplantation. Because the recipient has not been previously sensitized, it takes time to develop sensitized lymphocytes, which then increase in number and attack the graft. This is the typical picture of a cell-mediated immune response.
  - **(i)** The graft (especially around small blood vessels) is infiltrated with small lymphocytes and mononuclear cells, along with some granulocytes, causing destruction of the transplanted tissue.
  - **(ii)** If an antigenically identical graft is made in this sensitized recipient, very rapid rejection occurs. This event, which is referred to as the **second-set phenomenon,** actually is an example of the anamnestic response.

- **(c) Chronic rejection.** This may be a cellular immune response, an antibody response, or a combination of the two.
  - **(i)** In chronic rejection, a slow loss of tissue function occurs over a period of months or years.
  - **(ii)** The antigens that evoke chronic rejection may be weak antigens of the HLA system or antigens in minor histocompatibility loci such as those on the Y chromosome.

- **(2) Non-MHC restriction.** The initial recognition of allogeneic (nonself) cells-that is, the recipient's immunologic recognition of the donor's cells-is not MHC restricted.
  - **(a)** T lymphocytes can react with foreign HLAs without the necessity for antigen presentation in association with self class I MHC molecules.
  - **(b)** This phenomenon, termed **alloreactivity,** is a reflection of the T lymphocytes' innate ability to recognize foreign MHC molecules. These T cells are those stimulated in the mixed lymphocyte reaction.
    - **(i)** Alloreactive $CD8^+$ Tc cells are stimulated by target cells that bear class I MHC molecules.
    - **(ii)** Alloreactive $CD4^+$ Th cells are stimulated by target cells that carry class II MHC molecules.
  - **(c)** If this alloreactivity did not exist, and rejection were MHC restricted, the mixed lymphocyte reaction would not take place. It has been estimated that as many as 10% of circulating T lymphocytes can react with any given allograft antigen.

- **(3) MHC restriction.** Because MHC restriction plays a role in the **induction of antigraft antibodies** and **Tc cells,** it contributes to graft rejection. However, the expression (or attack) phase of Tc activity must occur in the absence of self MHC molecules on the target cell. In fact, if the target cell is self, there is no reaction against it.

6. Postoperative immunosuppressive therapy
  a. General principles
  - **(1)** Immunosuppressive therapy, which is required by **all transplant recipients,** is directed primarily at blocking the induction or expression of cell-mediated immunity.
  - **(2)** The only **exception** to the need for immunosuppressive therapy is the case in which the donor and recipient are **identical twins** (i.e., are autotolerant).

  b. Immunosuppressive drugs. These agents and their mechanisms of action are discussed more fully in Chapter 5.

    (1) Corticosteroids are used for maintenance therapy or are given in a bolus at the time of a rejection crisis.

        (a) These anti-inflammatory agents reduce the number of circulating lymphocytes.

        (b) In addition, corticosteroids interfere with the production of lymphokines, thus blocking the expansion of the immune response to the graft.

    (2) Antimetabolites and **alkylating agents** exert their immunosuppressive effects by interfering with DNA and RNA function. This in turn causes death of rapidly dividing cells such as lymphocytes, particularly those undergoing immunologic induction.

        (a) Azathioprine is a commonly used antimetabolite. The body converts this drug to the purine analogue mercaptopurine.

        (b) Cyclophosphamide, a cyclic nitrogen mustard, is a popular alkylating agent.

    (3) Cyclosporine (cyclosporin A), a cyclic peptide antibiotic produced by various fungi, is very effective in inhibiting the T-cell component of the rejection process.

        (a) This drug binds to the active site of **cyclophilin,** a cellular enzyme that catalyzes the correct folding of proteins and inhibits the transcription of the interleukin-2 (IL-2) gene.

        (b) In addition, cyclosporine blocks the secretion of the lymphokine **IFN-γ.** This effect is important to graft survival because IFN-γ has several **antigraft** properties, including:

          (i) Increased expression of MHC (target) antigens on graft tissues

          (ii) Activation of macrophages that participate in the rejection process

        (c) Studies have shown that two new **macrolide antibiotics** are potent immunosuppressants that act synergistically with cyclosporine to block T-cell responses.

          (i) FK-506 disrupts transcription of genes for IL-2, IL-3, and IL-4; IFN-γ; and TNF.

          (ii) Rapamycin, another fungal metabolite, also blocks interleukin signal transduction in lymphocytes.

        (d) Cyclosporine and other antibiotics are not toxic to white blood cell precursors and thus do not cause leukopenia.

    (4) Antibody preparations. Antilymphocyte globulin and **antithymocyte globulin** are capable of destroying human T cells by sensitizing them to phagocytosis or complement-mediated lysis. Most of these preparations are monoclonal products.

        (a) These antisera, which are used most frequently as prophylactics, are administered postoperatively for about 2 weeks to block the induction of graft sensitization.

        (b) They also are used in the management of acute rejection episodes.

  c. Problems in postoperative management

    (1) Infection often occurs with the use of high doses of immunosuppressive drugs. About 25% of the deaths that occur after kidney transplantations are the result of sepsis.

    (2) Malignancy develops in about 6% of all transplant patients.

        (a) Some are common malignancies, such as carcinoma of the skin; however, about half are lymphomas or reticuloendothelial cell sarcomas.

        (b) This excessive susceptibility to malignancy may be explained by a drug-induced impairment in immunosurveillance. Ordinarily, the immune system checks out the body for mutated cancerous cells. When the immune system is suppressed, however, such cells are allowed to escape and proliferate.

7. Special graft situations

  a. Privileged tissues. Immunologically privileged tissues are tissues from different anatomic locations that are not rejected no matter where they are transplanted.

    (1) Bone, cartilage, tendon, and **sections of major blood vessels** are privileged, probably because of their low content of HLAs.

    (2) The **fetus** also can be considered privileged tissue, although the mechanisms for its survival are complex and poorly defined. The womb also may represent a privileged site.

(3) **Nonvascularized tissue** also may serve as privileged tissue. The use of this tissue as a graft ordinarily eliminates immune rejection.

(a) For example, the **cornea** can restore vision when transplanted under acceptable surgical conditions and when the vascular bed is not damaged.

(b) However, if the cornea is placed in vascularized tissue or if trauma at the transplant site causes inflammation and vascularization, the graft is rejected.

b. **Privileged sites**

(1) Certain areas, such as the **brain** and the **anterior chamber of the eye,** are privileged sites. These sites tolerate grafting without sensitization of the recipient.

(2) This is most likely the result of little or no lymphatic drainage in these tissues.

c. **GVH disease**

(1) **Etiology and pathogenesis**

(a) GVH reactions are an expression of T-cell function. When an **immunologically competent graft** is transplanted into an **immunologically compromised host,** the graft tissue can mount an immunologic attack on the recipient. This is termed **graft rejection of the host.**

(b) This condition occurs when the donor and the immunologically compromised recipient are antigenically different.

(2) **Affected tissues**

(a) GVH disease is a major limiting factor in allogeneic **bone marrow transplantation.** It also can involve grafts of the **skin, alimentary tract,** and **liver** if the engrafted tissue contains immunocompetent T cells.

(b) GVH reactions do not affect heart or kidney transplantations because these organs usually are flushed to remove donor T cells.

(3) **Clinical expression.** GVH disease is characterized by liver abnormalities, a measles-like skin rash, diarrhea, wasting, and death.

(4) **GVH disease in bone marrow transplantation**

(a) GVH disease follows a bone marrow transplant when the recipient possesses specific histocompatibility antigens that are not present in the immunocompetent donor. In this case, the transplanted bone marrow contains immunocompetent lymphocytes that become sensitized to the recipient's antigens and mount an immunologic attack.

(b) Therefore, bone marrow transplantation should be performed only between histocompatible individuals—preferably between histoidentical siblings, if possible.

(c) In addition, if the T cells are removed from the bone marrow before bone marrow engraftment (e.g., by use of antithymocyte serum plus complement), the incidence and severity of GVH disease can be markedly reduced.

(d) Vigorous immunosuppression is used in bone marrow recipients at the first sign of GVH disease. However, this treatment often leads to serious, life-threatening infections. Approximately 20% of bone marrow recipients die of recrudescence of prior cytomegaloviral infections.

II. TUMOR IMMUNOLOGY

A. **Introduction.** There is considerable clinical evidence suggesting that **tumors are immunogenic** and that the **human body responds immunologically to tumors in a manner similar to the response to transplanted foreign tissues.**

1. The presence of a **mononuclear cell infiltrate** *in situ* in inflammatory carcinomas correlates with improved survival rates. For example, a person with a breast carcinoma accompanied by an inflammatory response seems to do better than someone whose carcinoma is not associated with an inflammatory process.

2. **Metastatic cells** commonly are present in patients with cancer, but the frequency of their implantation and growth is low, which is demonstrated by several findings.
   a. After cancer surgery, it is common to detect malignant cells in the blood; however, metastatic implantation is much more rare.
   b. Cancer patients readily demonstrate **immediate and delayed hypersensitivity** to autologous tumor-cell extracts in skin reaction tests.
   c. The **incidence of malignancy** is highest in the neonatal period and in old age, when the immune system functions less effectively. In addition, patients with depressed cell-mediated immunity have an increased incidence of certain malignancies.
   d. The patient with AIDS is particularly likely to have Kaposi's sarcoma (a rare tumor in people with an intact cell-mediated immunity) and other malignancies.
   e. Children with certain congenital immunodeficiencies are at increased risk for cancer. For example, lymphomas and acute myelogenous leukemia occur in 10% to 30% of children with Wiskott-Aldrich syndrome.
   f. In general, there is a three-fold increase in the incidence of cancer in allograft recipients when compared to age-matched controls. This is due to the use of immunosuppressive drugs in these patients to prevent graft rejection.

B. | **Tumor-associated antigens (TAAs)**

1. **A distinct feature of tumor immunology is that the tumor-bearing host is interacting with a source of antigen that is constantly changing.**
   a. The antigenic profile of the cells is altered such that normally occurring antigens may be lost, whereas new epitopes (**neoantigens**) emerge. Some human malignancies secrete large amounts of hormones. For example, certain forms of testicular cancer produce large amounts of human chorionic gonadotropin (hCG).
   b. A list of antigens associated with human malignancies is presented in Table 10-4.

2. **TAAs may be completely unique to a particular tumor in a specific person.** The emergence of these completely unique TAAs often accompanies **carcinogen-induced cancers.**
   a. **The carcinogen acts as a mutagen.** The tumors induced in different people by a single carcinogen do not have similar antigens, as do malignancies of viral etiology, because of the random occurrence of the mutation.
   b. More commonly, **TAAs are similar in all people carrying a particular tumor;** such antigens are commonly termed **tumor-specific antigens (TSAs),** although in fact they may be found in more than one type of tumor or even in nonmalignant diseases. For example, prostate-specific antigen is found in elevated amounts in the blood of individuals with prostate cancer and in patients with prostatitis.
   c. **Some tumors express normal antigens in excessive amounts.**
      (1) Thus, **myeloma proteins** are the immunoglobulin product of the particular B cell that went "out of control" and became malignant. Patients with this disease (myeloma) also excrete light-chain dimers known as Bence Jones proteins in their urine.
      (2) Similarly, the **common acute lymphoblastic leukemia antigen (CALLA)** is abundant in the blood of patients with this most common form of childhood leukemia. Normally, CALLA is expressed only on B-cell progenitors, which comprise less than 1% of normal bone marrow cells.

3. **Oncofetal antigens** are present during normal fetal development but are lost during differentiation of fetal tissue, and they apparently are not synthesized by adults. Oncofetal antigens, however, may reappear during regeneration of the appropriate tissue (e.g., liver) or they may appear as TAAs with the development of malignancy. Two of the most widely studied oncofetal antigens are the **α-fetoprotein (AFP)** and **carcinoembryonic antigen (CEA).**
   a. **AFP** is an alpha globulin that is synthesized and secreted by fetal liver cells. It has 40% homology with serum albumin (i.e., 40% of its amino acid sequence matches that of albumin). It reaches fetal concentrations of 3 mg/ml and can be detected in umbilical cord blood and occasionally in the mother's serum.

TABLE 10-4. Antigens Associated with Human Malignancy*

Antigen	Tumor
Viral	
Hepatitis B	Primary liver cancer
Human papilloma viruses 16 and 18	Cervical carcinoma
Epstein-Barr	Burkitt's lymphoma Nasopharyngeal cancer
Human T-cell leukemia virus I (HTLV–1)	Adult T-cell leukemia
Oncofetal	
Carcinoembryonic	Colorectal carcinoma Pancreatic carcinoma
α-Fetoprotein	Primary liver cancer Testicular and ovarian cancer Gastric and pancreatic cancer
Other	
Myeloma proteins	Multiple myeloma
Prostate-specific antigen	Prostatic cancer
Prostatic acid phosphatase	Prostatic cancer
S–100 calcium-binding protein	Melanoma[†]
CA–125 glycoprotein	Ovarian cancer
CA19–9 glycoprotein	Pancreatic cancer
15–3 Glycoprotein	Breast and lung cancer

*These antigens are found in a high incidence in patients with the tumors listed but are found in other conditions as well, therefore, they are not tumor specific. They are used for diagnostic or prognostic purposes.

†There have been over 40 different melanoma–membrane-associated antigens defined with the use of monoclonal antibodies.

(1) **AFP has been reported to be immunosuppressive,** which may be important in the induction of neonatal tolerance to autoantigens. In cell culture, AFP has several effects on T cells: it decreases Th-cell activity and enhances Ts-cell activity.

(2) **Most but not all hepatomas secrete large amounts of AFP.** However, its presence is not diagnostic of hepatoma but is merely suggestive, because AFP also has been detected in the serum of patients with prostatic and gastric carcinomas, teratomas, and embryonal carcinoma of the testes. AFP also may be found in certain nonmalignant conditions, such as cirrhosis of the liver and hepatitis.

(3) Monitoring the changes in the AFP content of a cancer patient's serum provides a **prognostic index** (or marker) after surgery or chemotherapy. For example, a dramatic increase in the serum concentration of AFP after surgery or chemotherapy signals recurrence of the malignancy.

b. **CEA** is detected in the gut, liver, and pancreas of the fetus during the second trimester of pregnancy. It is also found in low levels in the serum of healthy adults.

(1) **CEA is associated with several types of cancer.** About 70% of patients with **carcinoma of the colon** have high serum levels of CEA. An even higher association (90%) occurs in patients with **pancreatic carcinoma.** CEA has also been detected in significant quantities in cancers of the lung, breast, and prostate gland.

(2) **CEA also occurs in several nonmalignant states.** Approximately 15% of heavy smokers have elevated serum CEA levels. Serum CEA levels also may be elevated in patients with **cirrhosis of the liver** or **chronic lung disease.** As in the case of AFP, the utility of CEA lies in its prognostic potential.

4. **Virus-induced TAAs** are either component proteins or new enzymes that are induced in the cell to aid in the replication of the virus.
   a. **Epstein-Barr virus (EBV) antigens** have been found in the cells of patients with Burkitt's lymphoma and nasopharyngeal carcinoma. These patients have high levels of specific antibodies to EBV antigens, which further indicates that Burkitt's lymphoma and nasopharyngeal carcinoma are induced by this viral agent.
   b. **Other RNA and DNA viruses** (e.g., adenoviruses, papovaviruses, herpesviruses, retroviruses) also may induce TAAs.

5. **Tumor-specific transplantation antigens (TSTAs)** are a subpopulation of TAAs that can induce a **protective immune response** in the host if they occur in the membrane of the malignant cell.
   a. **An appropriate immune response against these immunogens favors the control of a malignancy and elimination of the cancer cells from the body.** As a general rule, the cell-mediated immune response is the most efficient tumoricidal mechanism. Occasionally, cytocidal antibodies also are demonstrable in the host.
   b. **Most human tumors of a given histologic type have at least one TSTA in common.** Thus, the lymphocytes and antibodies from neuroblastoma patient A will react with and try to destroy tumor cells from neuroblastoma patient B, but not with other cells from patient B. The cells from patient A also will not react with tumor cells from patients suffering from other types of malignancies; that is, they have **immunologic specificity.**

C. **Immune response to tumor antigens.** Because the tumor cells have acquired new antigens, they are recognized by the host as foreign. The immune response attempts to rid the body of the tumor cells. However, the tumor produces soluble antigens, which tend to neutralize these protective responses. In addition, some antibodies may actually enhance tumor growth (Figure 10-5).

1. **Immune surveillance.** By this mechanism, the body is continuously purging itself of potentially cancerous cells, which are thought to arise frequently during a person's life span.

2. **Mechanisms of tumor rejection.** Both specific and nonspecific immune responses—humoral and cell-mediated—are believed to be involved in the rejection of a tumor (Table 10-5).
   a. **TSTA-specific sensitized T cells** constitute the major immunologic barrier against cancer.
      (1) **Tc cells** appear in response to antigens such as TSAs or viral antigens. Tc cells can kill tumor cells by direct contact through the actions of several cytotoxic products (see Table 1-9, Chapter 1).
      (2) **The cells of delayed-type hypersensitivity** are also important in antitumor immunity. These cells release lymphokines following contact with tumor antigens. The lymphokines attract macrophages and activate these cells to enhance their tumoricidal activity.
   b. **Specific antibodies** may rid the body of tumor cells.
      (1) **Complement-dependent cytotoxicity** can be mediated by antibodies, particularly IgM. When antibody binds to the surface of a tumor cell, the classic complement pathway is triggered, which leads to the eventual destruction of the tumor cell via lysis, opsonization and intracellular destruction, or release of toxic metabolites and lysosomal contents with resultant tumor cell destruction.
      (2) The antibodies also may function by **"arming" macrophages and neutrophils** so that these cells can then react with and destroy the tumor cells. This is exemplified in **antibody-dependent cellular cytotoxicity (ADCC),** in which the effector **NK cells** have enhanced affinity for the tumor "target" due to the adhesive action of the antibody molecule.
         (a) NK cells have an Fc receptor on the cell surface (FcγRIII, or CD16); the antibody involved is IgG1 or IgG3.
         (b) When NK cells encounter a tumor cell that has IgG molecules on its surface, the NK cells interact with the "sensitized" tumor cell and destroy it through release of cytotoxic molecules (see Table 1-9).

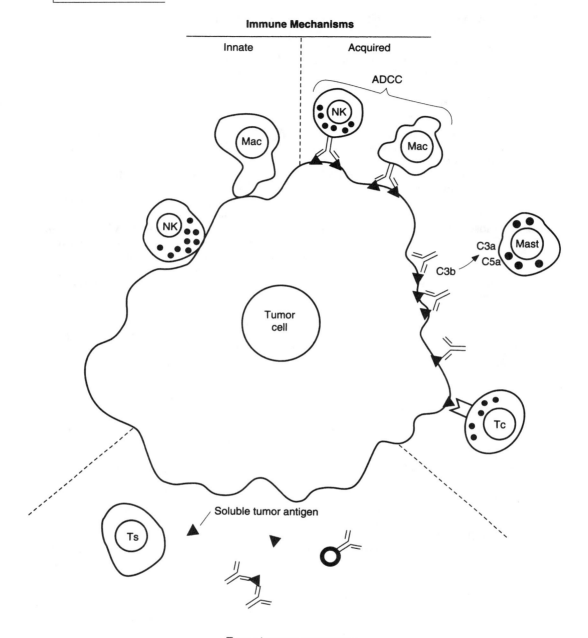

Figure 10-5. Potential immune responses to tumors. At the *top* of the figure are responses that are protective. The *innate* resistance to malignancy is exemplified by the natural killer (*NK*) and macrophage (*Mac*) cells. The *acquired* immune responses are demonstrated by cytotoxic T (*Tc*) cells, antibody-dependent cellular cytotoxic (*ADCC*) cells, complement-activating antibodies, the opsonic (*C3b*) and chemotactic (*C3a, C5a*) split products of complement activation that enhance inflammation via release of histamine from mast cells, and the radionuclide-labeled antitumor antibodies that can deliver ionizing radiation directly to the tumor. Tumor escape mechanisms are depicted in the *bottom* portion of the figure. Soluble tumor antigen and tumor antigen–antibody complexes can neutralize effective immune mechanisms before they reach the tumor target; that is, tumor-specific suppressor (*Ts*) cells and suppressive substances (e.g., prostaglandins) and antibodies cannot activate complement and cannot sensitize ADCC cells for tumor target killing (e.g., enhancing antibodies).

TABLE 10-5. Host Antitumor Factors that Are Operative in Immune Surveillance, Interfere with the Development of Malignancy, and Aid in Recovery from Cancer

Innate Immune Processes
  Macrophages
  Natural killer cells

Acquired Immunities
  Humoral
    Opsonic antibodies
    Complement-activating antibodies
    Antibody-dependent cellular cytotoxicity
  Cell mediated
    Cytotoxic T cells
    dth T cells
  Soluble mediators
    Interferon-γ
    Tumor necrosis factors α and β

c. In addition to their role in ADCC, **NK cells** can also kill tumors by direct contact. This activity is non-MHC restricted, and the cells require neither prior experience with the tumor nor antigen presentation by accessory cells.
   (1) Once target cell contact has been made, the NK cell releases soluble cytotoxic factors such as perforin, proteases, nucleases, and TNF-α by a process very much like that of the Tc cell.
   (2) NK cells can be activated by IFN-γ.
d. In their normal state, **macrophages** are not very cytotoxic. However, they can kill tumor cells when activated.
   (1) Antibodies to TSAs may bind simultaneously to tumor cells and macrophages through the antigen-binding site on the former and the FcγRI and FcγRII receptors on the latter. This forms a bridge that activates macrophage-mediated cytotoxicity, which leads to death of the tumor cell.
   (2) *In vivo,* sensitized T cells are triggered to release **macrophage-activating factors,** which interact with macrophages, changing their metabolism and making them potent killers of tumor cells. The two major activators are IFN-γ and TNF-α.
   (3) Activated macrophages do not rely on interacting with any specific tumor antigen; however, like NK cells, they do seem to distinguish malignant from normal cells.
   (4) Macrophages produce many **antitumor products,** including:
      (a) Hydrolytic enzymes that degrade connective tissue and activate several complement components and coagulation factors
      (b) IFN-α, which acts indirectly by activating NK cells
      (c) TNF-α (also called cachectin), which is a protein that induces other cells to release IL-1, IL-6, IL-8, and IFN.
         (i) Locally, TNF-α increases T-cell adhesion to the vascular endothelium and activates these cells to heightened cytotoxicity.
         (ii) Systemically, TNF-α causes fever and synthesis of acute-phase proteins (see Table 5-3, footnote).
      (d) Hydrogen peroxide, and other oxidative products of the glycolysis that accompanies phagocytosis, can be directly toxic to tumor cells by disturbing the cell membrane.
      (e) Nitric oxide (NO) has been shown to be toxic to tumor cells and bacteria and may be of major importance in controlling parasitic infections, such as toxoplasmosis. For optimal expression of this pathway, macrophages need to be stimulated by both IFN-γ and TNF. Oxygen is combined with the guanidino nitrogen of L-arginine to produce NO by the enzyme **nitric oxide synthetase.**

D. **Immunologic factors favoring tumor growth**

1. **Tumor cell attributes often allow a tumor to escape immune destruction** (Table 10-6).
   a. **Tumor antigenic heterogeneity** facilitates tumor survival.
   b. Modulation of tumor antigenicity (**antigenic modulation**) occurs when antibody to the tumor cell reacts with the appropriate antigens on the tumor cell surface. If the antibody is cytotoxic, tumor cells expressing the homologous antigen are destroyed. This favors the emergence of tumor cells whose membranes have a different antigenic mosaic.
   c. Tumors release **immunosuppressive factors** such as AFP and prostaglandin E_2.

2. **Blocking factors** also may enhance tumor growth. The serum of cancer patients often contains soluble TSTA or TSTA-antibody complexes, which react with (i.e., "block") the tumor-specific receptors on sensitized T cells, thereby preventing their cytotoxic interaction with tumor cells.
   a. Ordinarily, TSTA in the groove of a class I MHC molecule interacts with the tumor antigen recognition site on the T-cell surface. This triggers the cytotoxic activity of the T cell.
      (1) Free tumor antigen could interact with the T-cell receptor and actually not trigger the T cell but prevent it from recognizing and attacking the tumor cell.
      (2) Soluble TSTA also can react with cytotoxic antibody before the cytotoxic antibody can attach to the tumor cell and sensitize it to ADCC killing.
   b. The most potent blocking factors in serum are the **tumor-specific immune complexes.** These antigen-antibody complexes act like free tumor antigen, masking the tumor recognition sites of T cells, which prevents the T cells from recognizing and attacking the tumor cells. These complexes paralyze the T cells in a state of nonreactivity.

3. **Immune enhancement** is a form of blocking in which specific antibodies in the serum may protect tumor cells from cell-mediated destruction. The effector antibodies, known as **enhancing antibodies,** usually are noncomplement-fixing antibodies that react with TSTAs in the cell membrane and protect them from a cytotoxic interaction with complement-fixing antibodies, ADCC cells, or Tc cells.

4. **Other factors favoring tumor growth**
   a. **Ontogenic status.** The immune response is poorly developed or very weak in people

TABLE 10-6. Mechanisms by which Tumors Escape the Immune Response of the Host

Mechanism	Effect
Tumor is nonimmunogenic	No immune response occurs
Tumor modulates its surface antigens	Tumor changes antigens to avoid immune destruction
Loss of class I MHC molecules	Tumor cannot be destroyed by MHC-restricted cytotoxic T cells
Loss of adhesion molecules	Cytotoxic T cells cannot attach effectively to tumor cell membrane
Tumor secretes immunosuppressive molecules	Immune response is down-regulated
Tumor induces an immune response that protects the tumor cell from destruction	Tumor–growth-enhancing antibodies react with tumor TSTAs and prevent the interaction of these TSTAs with protective immune factors; suppressor cells interfere with the induction of a protective immune response

MHC = major histocompatibility complex; *TSTA* = tumor-specific transplantation antigens.

at certain times of life. Neonates and the elderly have the highest incidence of malignancy.

  b. **Immunologic deficiency** may be hereditary or may be induced by such means as irradiation, infection (e.g., with HIV), or immunosuppressive drugs. The incidence of malignancy is greatly increased in immunodeficient people.

E. Immunotherapy

1. **Principles of treating humans with tumors** include:
   a. Reduction of the tumor "load" by surgery, chemotherapy, or both
   b. Modification of tumor cells to enhance their antigenicity and eliminate their viability
   c. Activation of the immune response through the use of adjuvants

2. **Immunotherapeutic modalities** being tried for the treatment of humans with tumors include the following.
   a. **Immunotoxins.** Tumor-specific monoclonal antibodies conjugated to tumoricidal substances, such as radionuclides or toxins (e.g., diphtheria toxin, ricin), are administered by injection. The monoclonal antibodies carry the therapeutic agent directly to the tumor, which lowers toxicity to normal tissues.
   b. **Macrophage-activating compounds.** Administering macrophage-activating compounds has been explored extensively as a mode of cancer immunotherapy (Table 10-7). Because activated macrophages are such potent killers, there is much interest in treating tumor patients with compounds that are known to activate macrophages. These include:
      (1) **Bacille Calmette-Guérin (BCG),** the mycobacterial vaccine used to immunize people against tuberculosis
      (2) **IFN-γ**, which activates most cells of the immune system and increases the expression of class I MHC molecules on tumor cells, thus rendering them more susceptible to destruction by Tc lymphocytes
      (3) **Muramyl dipeptide,** a synthetic peptide that mimics the action of mycobacteria
      (4) **Cytokine genes,** which have been shown to increase the immunogenicity of cancer cell vaccines in experimental animals
         (a) The gene encoding granulocyte-macrophage colony stimulating factor promotes the development of dendritic cells at the site of vaccine deposition. The dendritic cells initiate the most potent T-cell response. The genes cause production of large amounts of the protein locally.
         (b) Introduction of the **IL-12 gene** into cancer cell vaccines also enhances the de-

TABLE 10-7. Cytokine Therapy for Tumors*

Cytokine	Tumor Type	Results	Comments
Interferon α and β	Hairy cell leukemia	Prolonged remission	Cytostatic; Increased MHC class I expression
Interferon-γ	Ovarian carcinoma	Remission	Cytostatic; T-cell activation; Increased MHC classes I and II expression
Tumor necrosis factor-α (TNF-α)	Varied	Reduction in tumor mass	Cytostatic; Lymphocyte activation
Interleukin-2 (IL-2)	Melanoma	Remission	T- and natural killer (NK) cell activation
IL-2 and interferon-γ	Renal carcinoma	Remission	T-cell and NK-cell activation

*These cytokines all activate macrophages to high tumoricidal activity. The usual regimen calls for systemic administration in high dosage.

MHC = major histocompatibility complex

velopment of cell-mediated immune responses. The genes cause production of large amounts of the protein locally.

   c. **Heat shock proteins** purified from bacterial cells have been shown to be excellent adjuvants when mixed with TSTAs.

Vignette Revisited

1. Before the discovery of cyclosporine (cyclosporin A), patients took a combination of corticosteroids and azathioprine. With this therapy, the survival rate of unrelated donor grafts was 50% to 60% at 1 year. The introduction of cyclosporine has increased survival of unrelated donor grafts to approximately 80%. Survival of living related donor grafts before and after the use of cyclosporine remains at approximately 90%.

2. Cyclosporine is a cyclic polypeptide derived from a fungus. It interferes with the secretion of interleukin-2 by T lymphocytes, which results in a potent blockade of T-cell proliferation and thereby inhibits T-cell–mediated immune responses.

   The major side effects of cyclosporine are renal and, to a lesser degree, hepatic toxicity. This results in the need to carefully balance the dose of drug to maximize the level of immunosuppression while minimizing the toxic effects. Distinguishing declining renal function caused by rejection from decreased renal function caused by cyclosporine toxicity may be difficult. Clarification is usually accomplished by histopathologic examination of biopsy specimens of the transplanted organ.

3. The administration of multiple blood transfusions before grafting has been shown to significantly prolong graft survival. The prolonged graft survival is presumed to be due to tolerance induction of some kind, but the exact mechanism is unclear. In addition, patients are immunosuppressed at the time of surgery secondary to uremia from their kidney failure, which causes a degree of immunologic anergy.

4. Transplant recipients receiving immunosuppressive therapy are particularly susceptible to infection, especially those of viral origin. Cytomegalovirus is common and may be fatal in immunosuppressed patients. Cytomegalovirus, Epstein-Barr virus, hepatitis B virus, and HIV may all be transmitted from donor to recipient. Prevention requires extensive pretransplant serologic testing.

   Transplant patients also have a propensity to develop certain tumors. B-cell lymphomas from Epstein-Barr virus infection, squamous cell carcinoma of the skin secondary to human papillomavirus, and Kaposi's sarcoma, which is also virally mediated, are all commonly seen in this patient population.

1. Several types of immunologic rejection reactions can occur after organ transplantation. The rejection reaction that is caused by the presence of preformed antibodies in the recipient is referred to as

(A) acute
(B) hyperacute
(C) chronic
(D) immediate
(E) accelerated

2. Class I human leukocyte antigens (HLAs) can be best described as

(A) cell-surface proteins that contain HLA-A, HLA-B, and HLA-C determinants
(B) substances involved in macrophage interactions with B cells
(C) complement components
(D) antigens involved in the inductive (sensitization) phase of cell-mediated cytolysis (CMC)
(E) antigens principally responsible for the graft-versus-host (GVH) reaction

3. As compared to T cells, B-cell membranes are rich in which of the following antigens?

(A) Class I human leukocyte antigens (HLAs)
(B) Class II HLAs
(C) Class III HLAs
(D) HLA-B antigens
(E) Complement-activating antigens

4. Antilymphocyte globulin and antithymocyte globulin are effective in suppressing allograft rejection because of their ability to

(A) suppress cell-mediated immunity
(B) suppress humoral immunity
(C) block lymphocyte transformation
(D) react with antigens in the graft
(E) mimic anti-idiotype antibodies induced during graft rejection

5. Efficient T-cell–mediated killing of virus-infected cells requires that the T cells and the target cells be identical with respect to which of the following?

(A) ABO blood group antigens
(B) Rh blood group antigens
(C) Class I human leukocyte antigens (HLAs)
(D) Class II HLAs
(E) Class III HLAs

6. An immune response to foreign tissue is suppressed in which of the following phenomena?

(A) Immune tolerance
(B) Immune enhancement
(C) Immune surveillance
(D) Immune deviation
(E) Immune complex reactions

7. Which of the following tests can be used for typing of class I histocompatibility antigens?

(A) Cell-mediated lympholysis
(B) Donor-recipient mixed lymphocyte response
(C) Primed lymphocyte typing
(D) Mixed lymphocyte response with homozygous typing cells
(E) Antibody- and complement-mediated cytotoxicity

8. Chronic graft rejection may be caused by

(A) T cells
(B) antibodies
(C) T cells and antibodies
(D) T cells and macrophages
(E) Natural killer cells

9. Graft-versus-host (GVH) disease would occur from a poorly matched bone marrow transplant rather than from a similarly matched kidney transplant because the kidney

(A) expresses few donor class I human leukocyte antigens (HLAs)
(B) expresses few donor class II HLAs
(C) contains few donor erythrocytes
(D) contains few donor B cells
(E) contains few donor T cells

10. Donor-recipient graft compatibility is determined through evaluation of which of the following?

(A) Class I human leukocyte antigens (HLAs), ABO blood group, and antibodies to donor lymphocytes
(B) Class II HLAs, ABO blood group, and antibodies to donor lymphocytes
(C) Both class I and class II HLAs, ABO blood group, and antibodies to donor lymphocytes
(D) Class III HLAs, ABO blood group, and antibodies to donor lymphocytes
(E) ABO blood group and antibodies to donor lymphocytes

11. The cornea is considered to be privileged tissue because

(A) it contains few human leukocyte antigens (HLAs)
(B) it contains abundant HLAs
(C) it is nonvascularized tissue
(D) it is vascularized tissue
(E) it is coated with enhancing antibodies

12. Which of the following transplants involves a transfer of skin from the thigh to the face?

(A) Allogeneic
(B) Autologous
(C) Heterogenic
(D) Idiotypic
(E) Syngeneic

13. A cadaver kidney transplant can be characterized as which of the following types of transplants?

(A) Allogeneic
(B) Autologous
(C) Heterogenic
(D) Idiotypic
(E) Syngeneic

14. Which of the following human viruses is associated with cervical cancer?

(A) Human immunodeficiency virus (HIV)
(B) Cytomegalovirus (CMV)
(C) Human papilloma viruses (HPV)
(D) Human T-cell leukemia virus I (HTLV I)
(E) Epstein-Barr virus

15. Which of the following anti-tumor compounds is produced primarily by macrophages?

(A) Interferon-γ
(B) Perforin
(C) Nucleases
(D) Nitric oxide
(E) Proteases

16. When cytotoxic materials, such as radioactive nuclides, are conjugated to tumor specific monoclonal antibodies, what are the immunotherapeutic reagents called?

(A) Adjuvants
(B) Immunotoxins
(C) Cytokines
(D) Defensins
(E) Enhancing factors

17. Which of the following interleukin genes has been incorporated into cancer cell vaccines to enhance the production of a protective immune response?

(A) Interleukin 1 (IL-1)
(B) IL-2
(C) IL-4
(D) IL-8
(E) IL-12

18. Which of the following is the monoclonal protein seen in the plasma of patients with multiple myeloma?

(A) Surface antigen of the hepatitis B virus
(B) Surface antigen of the B cell infected with Epstein-Barr virus
(C) Surface antigen of the T cell infected with human immunodeficiency virus
(D) Immunoglobulin produced by a malignant B cell
(E) Immunoglobulin light chain dimer which is secreted throught the kidney.

ANSWERS AND EXPLANATIONS

1. The answer is B [I C 5 b (1) (a)]. Hyperacute rejection of a transplanted organ occurs when the recipient's preformed antibodies attack the donor organ, causing a rapid vascular spasm, vascular occlusion, and lack of organ perfusion by the recipient's blood. This could occur in the case of an ABO blood group mismatch, in which a donor organ containing blood group A or group B antigens is transplanted into a patient who has preformed anti-A or anti-B antibodies. This is avoided by blood group matching before transplantation. A similar hyperacute rejection reaction can result with human leukocyte antigen (HLA) mismatch, in which the recipient has preformed antibodies to a HLA in the donor organ.

2. The answer is A [I B 3 a, b]. Class I histocompatibility antigens are cell surface membrane proteins that contain human leukocyte antigen (HLA)-A, HLA-B, or HLA-C determinants. These antigens are involved in the effector phase of cell-mediated cytolysis (CMC) and in graft rejection. In both these processes, class I antigens are the major antigens by which the effector cells, cytotoxic T (Tc) cells, recognize target tissues. Class II antigens are the histocompatibility antigens involved in the presentation of antigen to T cells and B cells by macrophages. By a principle referred to as major histocompatibility complex (MHC) restriction, the macrophage must bear a class II antigen identical to that expressed on the B-cell membrane. Class III antigens include, among other substances, complement components C2, C4, and factor B; class III antigens are not involved in histocompatibility.

3. The answer is B [I B 3 b]. B-cell membranes are rich in class II human leukocyte antigens (HLAs), which also are found in macrophage membranes and in the membranes of activated peripheral blood T cells. Class I HLAs, including HLA-B antigens, are found on all lymphocytes and macrophagesCin fact, class I HLAs are found on all nucleated cells except sperm and trophoblasts. Class III HLAs are not involved in histocompatibility but are complement components, specifically C2, C4, and factor B; class III genes also code for tumor necrosis factors α and β (TNF-α and TNF-β) and for cytochrome hydroxylases.

4. The answer is A [I C 6 b (4)]. Antilymphocyte and antithymocyte globulins destroy T cells, thereby suppressing cell-mediated immunity and promoting graft survival. Antilymphocyte serum also might suppress antibody formation. Lymphocyte transformation could actually be triggered by antilymphocyte serum (in the absence of complement) if the serum was directed to the proper membrane component (e.g., to the phytohemagglutinin or lipopolysaccharide receptors). Non--complement-fixing antibodies could react with transplantation antigens and block cytotoxic T (Tc)-cell interaction with the grafted tissue.

5. The answer is C [I B 3 d (1); Chapter 5 IV C 1 b]. Class I histocompatibility antigens [i.e., human leukocyte antigens (HLA)-A, -B, and -C] are involved in cell-mediated immune functions. In cell-mediated cytotoxicity, the target cell and the cytotoxic T (Tc) cell must be identical with regard to the HLAs coded at the A, B, and C loci. The HLA in the membrane of the virally infected target cell is recognized as "self" by the CD8 molecule in the membrane of the Tc cell, thus allowing destruction of the altered host cell bearing class I molecules with viral protein-derived peptides bound in their grooves. This requirement for cellular recognition is known as major histocompatibility complex (MHC) restriction; it is important because it ensures that Tc cells will attack infected cells rather than attacking free virus particles that may be at a site distant from the source of the virus (or its antigens). Class II identity is a similar prerequisite for the cellular interactions that occur during the inductive (sensitization) phase of an immune response.

6. The answer is A [I C 6; Ch 5 X A 2]. In immune tolerance, an immunologically competent host does not react to specific antigen produced by the graft. In such situations, the graft can survive almost indefinitely. In contrast to immune tolerance, immune enhancement involves antibodies on cells in the graft that block efficient antigen presentation by the graft.

7. The answer is E [I C 3 b]. Class I antigens are also called serologically defined antigens because they can be identified by serologic tests. Class I antigens are detected by incubating lymphocytes with antisera specific to human leukocyte antigens (HLA)-A, -B, or -C. In the presence of complement, the antibody-sensitized cells are killed and the resultant membrane changes can be detected by the uptake of eosin or trypan blue, both of which are excluded from live cells.

8. The answer is C [I C 5 b (1) (c)]. Chronic graft rejection may be caused by specific antibody, sensitized cytotoxic T (Tc) cells, or both. Rejection of the graft may be total or partial, with recovery of graft function. The antigens involved in chronic graft rejection usually are antigens in minor histocompatibility loci [i.e., weak antigens not coded for by the human leukocyte antigen (HLA) complex].

9. The answer is E [I C 8 c (2) (b)]. The kidney contains practically no T lymphocytes and, therefore, it is not likely to induce graft-versus-host (GVH) disease. After the organ is removed from the donor, it is perfused to remove all donor blood in its vasculature before its implantation. The bone marrow cannot be similarly purged of donor blood and must instead be treated with antithymocyte serum to remove the immunologically reactive cells.

10. The answer is C [I B 4 a; I C 1, 2, 3]. Class III human leukocyte antigens (HLAs) code for nonhistocompatibility antigens such as C2 and C4 of the complement system and are not involved in the graft rejection. The ABO blood group antigens are significant in the determination of histocompatibility. ABO blood group compatibility must exist between donor and recipient; crossing the blood group barrier compromises graft survival and may lead to hyperacute rejection. Typing of class I and class II HLAs also must be performed in the evaluation of donor-recipient compatibility. This is done through cytotoxicity assays, including the lymphocytotoxicity test. In this test, cytotoxic antibodies in serum from a sensitized recipient react with cell-surface antigens on donor lymphocytes, so that the lymphocyte cell membrane disintegrates and the cell dies. The reaction is detectable because dye is specifically absorbed by damaged and dying cells. Such a reaction would negate the use of that particular donor. In the blastogenesis assay, which is based on the mixed lymphocyte reaction, lymphocytes from both the prospective donor and the recipient are cultured and observed for reactions. Histocom-

patibility is assumed to exist if blastogenesis does not occur.

11. The answer is C [I C 7 a (3) (a)]. The cornea is "privileged" tissue only when the transplant procedure is conducted in a manner such that its nonvascularized status is not breached. The eye chamber is considered overall to be a privileged site in that all of its contents remain sequestered from T lymphocytes circulating in the vasculature. Even in the absence of corneal transplantation, an autoimmune attack (i.e., sympathetic ophthalmia) can result if the eye is traumatized and the T cells of an individual are allowed to enter the chamber.

12. The answer is B [Chapter 2 II B; Chapter 10 I A 1]. The transfer of skin from the thigh to the face in the same person is an autograft, which involves the transfer of autologous tissue. Autografts are done in plastic surgery to repair burn wounds, for example. Bone is commonly used in autograft procedures to promote healing of nonunited fractures, to restore structural integrity to the skeleton, and to facilitate cosmetic repair, as in facial reconstruction, where pieces of bone from the hip are used to rebuild portions of the face damaged by accident or malignancy. Allogeneic bone grafts also are performed; these involve the transfer of bone between genetically dissimilar members of the same species. For this purpose, the bone is aseptically removed, sterilized by ethylene oxide or gamma irradiation, and frozen. Freezing is used for all bone tissue transplants except fresh autografts because it reduces immunogenicity.

13. The answer is A [Chapter 2 II B; Chapter 10 I A 1]. Transplanting a cadaver kidney is a relatively standard procedure that uses allogeneic tissue to replace a patient's diseased organ. People awaiting a cadaver kidney transplant often receive blood transfusions to treat anemia and to increase graft survival. Untransfused patients have approximately 40% to 50% graft function after 2 years, whereas patients who have received transfusions have a 60% to 80% chance of long-term graft function. Mechanisms of this transfusion effect include the elimination of immunologic responders who demonstrate donor-specific cytotoxic antibodies in the pregraft screening, the development of suppressor T (Ts) cells, and the generation of blocking or anti-idiotypic antibodies.

14. The answer is C [Table 10-4]. Human papilloma viruses (HPVs) of serotypes 16 and 18 are etiologically associated with cervical carcinoma, penile, and laryngeal cancer in humans. Human immunodeficiency virus (HIV) is not an oncogenic virus, nor is cytomegalovirus (CMV). Human T-cell leukemia virus I (HTLV I) is a retrovirus that causes T cell leukemia in adults. Epstein-Barr virus causes infectious mononucleosis in the United States but is associated with Burkitt's lymphoma seen primarily in adolescent males in central Africa.

15. The answer is D [II C 2 d (4) (e)]. Macrophages are a rich source of nitric oxide, which is a potent antitumor agent that also has antimicrobic activities. Production is stimulated by gamma interferon and tumor necrosis factor. An enzyme is activated, nitric oxide synthetase, that adds oxygen to the guanidino nitrogen of L-arginine to produce nitric oxide. Macrophages produce interferon-α, not interferon-γ. Natural killer cells and cytotoxic T cells are the major sources of perforin and the granzymes (proteases and nucleases).

16. The answer is B [II E 2 a]. Immunotoxins are produced in the laboratory by coupling cytotoxic molecules such as toxins (e.g., diphtheria toxin or ricin, both of which are potent inhibitors of protein synthesis) or radioactive isotopes to antibodies specific for the tumor cell. The antibodies are monoclonal (i.e., of a single specificity) to assure that the lethal "hit" will kill only the cancer cells. Adjuvants are immunostimulants that enhance the immune response in a nonspecific manner. Cytokines are proteins made by cells that affect the behavior of other cells. Two have found some success in the treatment of human malignancies, interferon-γ and interleukin 2. Defensins are antimicrobial products of phagocytic cells. Enhancing factors such as soluble tumor specific transplantation antigens and non-complement activating antibodies will help tumor cells avoid the immune response.

17. The answer is E [II E 2 b (4) (b)]. Introduction of the interleukin 12 (IL-12) gene into cancer cell vaccines enhances the development of cell-mediated immune responses (i.e., cytotoxic and delayed hypersensitivity T cells). The genes are taken up and expressed by cells in the vicinity of the injection. The cytokine they release (IL-12) acts in synergy with interleukin 2 from the T helper 1 cell to channel the immune response toward cellular elements rather than antibodies.

18. The answer is D [II B 2 c (1)]. The myeloma protein which is detected in the plasma of patients with multiple myeloma is an immunoglobulin molecule produced by that particular malignant B cell. It is called monoclonal because only that clone (i.e., the progeny of that single mutated cancer cell) secretes that particular protein. Bence Jones protein is a light chain dimer from the same cell and it is secreted through the kidneys and will be found in high concentrations in the urine. It is a pyroglobulin and will be irreversibly precipitated when the temperature is elevated to 56 degrees Celsius. There is no known virus associated with multiple myeloma.

CASE STUDIES IN CLINICAL DECISION-MAKING

Case 1

Mrs. Watson brings her 2-year-old son Tommie to the family medicine clinic for a checkup following a recent bout of pneumonia. Although Tommie is subjectively better, with his pulmonary infection responding well to oral penicillin therapy and his lung fields clearing on chest radiograph, three days after treatment he developed dermatitis involving his trunk and extremities.

QUESTIONS

1. *What organisms are most likely to cause pneumonia in otherwise healthy children?*
2. *What is the possible significance of the timing of the appearance of Tommie's rash and the initiation of penicillin therapy?*

DISCUSSION

Common organisms causing pneumonia in otherwise healthy individuals include pneumococcus, streptococcus, staphylococcus, haemophilus, and *Mycoplasma pneumoniae*. All but *M. pneumoniae* and penicillinase- producing haemophilus and staphylococcus species are readily treated with penicillin G. The pneumococcus is beginning to show some resistance to penicillin G; in these cases, vancomycin, erythromycin, or chloramphenicol have been used with success. Uncommon organisms that may present as pneumonia in immunocompromised individuals include parasites (*Pneumocystis carinii*), fungi (Aspergillus and Candida species), viruses (cytomegalovirus, herpes simplex), gram-negative enteric bacteria, anaerobic bacteria, and bacteria considered to be nonpathogenic in healthy individuals. The appearance of the rash several days after the start of penicillin therapy is highly suggestive of penicillin allergy. However, patients with Epstein-Barr virus (EBV) infections almost universally develop a rash if given ampicillin or penicillin.

Results of laboratory studies drawn on Tommie's initial visit 3 days ago are now available and reveal a mildly elevated white blood cell count and a differential cell count with an increase in the polymorphonucleocytes and several "bands" also present. The induced sputum Gram stain contained many white blood cells and few squamous epithelial cells, indicating a good sample was obtained. The sputum culture has grown out *Staphylococcus epidermidis*, an organism considered nonpathogenic in healthy children.

QUESTIONS

3. *What is the significance of the increase in polymorphonuclear leukocytes?*
4. *How do the culture results alter further management and therapy?*
5. *What questions does Mrs. Watson need to address?*

DISCUSSION

An increase in polymorphonuclear leukocytes on peripheral blood smear along with an increase in the total white blood cell count is suggestive of bacterial infection. The presence

195

of band forms indicates an acute process. An increase in lymphocytes would suggest a viral infection.

A positive culture from an adequate sample that grows an otherwise nonpathogenic organism in healthy individuals should alert the investigator to the possibility of an immunodeficiency problem. Antibiotic therapy should cover a broad spectrum of organisms, and further tests should focus on ruling out various immunologic dysfunctions.

Mrs. Watson should be asked to provide an extensive, detailed previous medical history for Tommie. A history of family allergies would be useful as well as the general health history of other family members.

Upon further questioning, Mrs. Watson reports that there is a family history of allergies. Tommie has three older sisters who are healthy. His only brother died of bacterial pneumonia at 4 years of age. Tommie had been a colicky baby and had repeated episodes of diarrhea. He contracted German measles from his sister at the age of 14 months, which resolved without complications. Suspecting a possible immunodeficiency disorder based on the history provided and the culture results, the physician draws another blood sample and orders the following tests: immunoglobulin profile, nitroblue tetrazolium reduction assay, phagocytic index, and intraphagocytic killing curve.

The antibiotics are changed to a third-generation cephalosporin, and, as a precautionary measure, a swab of fluid exuding from a skin lesion is sent to the microbiology lab.

QUESTIONS

6. *What does the history of healthy daughters and sickly sons imply?*
7. *What is gained by switching from penicillin to a third-generation cephalosporin?*

DISCUSSION

An inheritance pattern affecting all males and sparing most females is characteristic of an X-linked recessive genetic disorder. Females are usually carriers unless they are homozygous for the allele and would therefore express the trait.

A third-generation cephalosporin adds coverage against penicillinase-producing strains of staphylococcus and streptococcus species as well as broad gram-negative coverage.

One week later, when the laboratory results return, the physician notes that *Serratia marcescens,* an opportunistic pathogen, was isolated from the skin lesions. Tommie is slightly hypergammaglobulinemic, but there is no elevation of immunoglobulin E (IgE). The nitroblue tetrazolium reduction assay was negative (i.e., there was no reduction of the dye), the phagocytic index was within normal limits, and the intraphagocytic killing curve was depressed.

Mrs. Watson was asked to return to discuss the test results and for further genetic counseling.

QUESTIONS

8. *Based on the test results, what is the most likely cause for Tommie's frequent infections?*
9. *How should therapy be directed in the future?*
10. *What are the implications of these findings for Tommie's sisters?*

DISCUSSION

The results of the phagocytic studies indicate that Tommie most likely has chronic granulomatous disease (CGD). His cells were unable to reduce the nitroblue tetrazolium dye during phagocytosis. The phagocytic index was normal but the intraphagocytic killing curve was depressed, indicating that the neutrophils were able to engulf the test organism but were unable to kill the ingested microbes. Mrs. Watson was asked to return for appropriate counseling as to the genetic implications of the disease, its management, potential complications, and prognosis. The physician also stressed the need for early diagnosis and aggressive therapy in future infections.

A hallmark of diseases of impaired immunity, such as CGD, is recurrent infection by agents normally considered to be nonpathogenic. The physician was suspicious of a phagocytic defect because Tommie had normal levels of antibodies and intact cell-mediated immunity (i.e., his gamma globulin level was normal and he had no trouble with German measles). His white blood cells were morphologically normal, thus the defect had to reside in the biochemical events that occur during phagocytosis.

CGD is an inherited, most commonly X-linked disease of male children and infants, characterized by recurrent infections and death at an early age. Tommie's mother was a carrier, and half of her daughters may also be carriers. Fortunately, the carrier state can be detected by the same test used to diagnose the disease. Carriers have lowered nitroblue tetrazolium dye reduction and intraphagocytic killing abilities.

Case 2

A 25-year-old white man presents to the clinic complaining of fatigue and a sore throat of 2 weeks' duration. The patient denies having nausea, vomiting, diarrhea, cough, chest pain, and weight loss, but believes he has had a fever. His medical history is unremarkable, and he knows of no contact with a sick person. Of note on physical examination are an oral temperature of 101°F, marked bilteral, tender, mobile, anterior and posterior cervical adenopathy, a gray–white exudative tonsillitis, and a palpable spleen. A complete blood count with differential is ordered and reveals a white blood cell count of 14,000 with 63% atypical lymphocytes.

QUESTIONS

1. *Formulate a differential diagnosis at this point.*
2. *What is the significance of atypical lymphocytes (also known as Downey cells), given the patient's signs and symptoms?*

DISCUSSION

The differential diagnosis based on the patient's signs and symptoms includes Epstein-Barr virus (EBV), cytomegalovirus (CMV), secondary syphilis, HIV infection, lymphoma, and Hodgkin's disease. A high percentage of patients with infectious mononucleosis who are given ampicillin or amoxicillin will develop an extensive morbilliform rash. If this occurs and EBV infection has not been suspected, and therefore not tested for, the incorrect conclusion may be drawn that the patient is allergic to penicillin.

Downey cells are abnormal lymphocytes that have a foamy cytoplasm. They are characteristic of infectious mononucleosis and are T lymphocytes responding to the EBV-infected B cells. EBV is one cause of infectious mononucleosis. In response to the virus, the patient produces several different antibodies, some of which will neutralize the virus and hasten recovery. One of the antibodies produced during the infection agglutinates sheep erythrocytes because of the presence of a shared (heterophil) epitope between the red blood cell and the virus. A related virus, CMV, causes a similar disease but does not induce the production of these same antibodies.

A monospot test is requested, and the results are positive. A diagnosis of infectious mononucleosis is made. The patient is sent home for bed rest and is counseled to eat properly and to not exert himself.

QUESTIONS

3. The diagnosis relies on a serologic procedure called the heterophile test. What does this mean?

4. Are there other infectious diseases in which similar antigenic relationships are involved in serologic diagnosis?

DISCUSSION

Heterophilic antibodies are those that are induced by one immunogenic stimulus and react with the inducing agent as well as with unrelated antigens because of the presence of common (shared) epitopes. Heterophilic relationships are useful in the serologic diagnosis of various infectious diseases and represent a more convenient and usually less expensive test than would be possible using the infectious agent itself. Two commonly used antigens are cardiolipin, used in the diagnosis of syphilis (which is caused by the spirochete *Treponema pallidum,* which cannot be cultivated in a laboratory) and the *Proteus vulgaris* antigens that react with antibodies in rickettsial disease, such as Rocky Mountain spotted fever. Rickettsial pathogens also are difficult to grow.

Another heterophil antigen is thought to be involved in the production of blood group A isoagglutinins.

QUESTION

5. What is this antigen, and how might it induce the production of these antibodies in individuals with blood groups O and B?

DISCUSSION

The Forssman antigen could be responsible for the production of anti-A isoagglutinins in individuals with blood groups O and B. For example, this heterophil antigen is present in corn and could be immunogenic once absorbed from the intestinal tract. Another possible stimulus could come from bacteria that have the Forssman antigen in their cell walls. If these microbes colonize the mucous membranes of the body, they could induce an anti-A response. The A antigen is not found in people with blood group O or B; therefore, these individuals would respond to the antigen by producing homologous isoagglutinin.

Case 3

A middle-aged man who works for an American oil company on an offshore drilling rig located in the Gulf of Mexico has been flown by helicopter to the emergency department after slipping from a ladder and injuring his femur. On examination, there is obvious swelling and deformity to the right femur, but pedal pulses are intact. After determination that there are no other injuries, radiographs of the right femur and hip are ordered and blood is drawn in preparation for an operation to set his obviously fractured femur.

QUESTIONS

1. As an emergency physician, what would be the primary concern about the patient's fracture?

2. What preoperative laboratory studies would be appropriate to order?

DISCUSSION

Femur fractures are easily diagnosed. Due to the proximity of major neurovascular structures, their integrity must be ascertained. Because a closed femoral fracture can hide a loss of 4–6 units of blood into the thigh, blood should be replaced as needed. Surgical fixation is the definitive treatment for these fractures.

Appropriate preoperative laboratory studies include complete blood count (CBC) with platelets, blood type and crossmatch, serum electrolytes with blood urea nitrogen (BUN) and creatinine, and coagulation studies.

While awaiting the results of the ordered studies, a more detailed history is obtained from the patient. He explains that his health has been slipping for almost 2 years. He has become weaker and tires more easily but attributes these signs, and his low back pain, to advancing age. Constipation has become a problem recently, and his gums bleed when he brushes his teeth. Twice in the past year he has been hospitalized with pneumonia.

The laboratory results come in and reveal the following values: White blood cell count (WBC) = 3500/mm^3, hemoglobin = 9.5 g/dl, hematocrit = 28%, platelets = 9000/mm^3, BUN = 60 mg/dl, creatinine = 4 mg/dl, and bleeding time is 7 minutes. The prothrombin time (PT) and partial thromboplastin time (PTT) are within normal limits. The radiographs show a fracture of the femoral neck, bordered both proximally and distally by an osteolytic lesion. A second osteolytic lesion is identified in the fifth lumbar vertebra.

QUESTIONS

3. *What is the significance of the patient's history coupled with the laboratory findings?*
4. *Formulate a differential diagnosis based on the given information.*

DISCUSSION

A 2-year history of progressive weakness and fatigue with a moderately low hematocrit should direct the clinician to consider the many causes of chronic anemia. The additional findings of low white blood cell (WBC) and platelet counts indicate a pancytopenia and a probable ongoing process in the bone marrow. The patient's bleeding gums and recent infections can be attributed to his thrombocytopenia and neutropenia, respectively. Elevated BUN and creatinine values reveal his renal insufficiency and need further investigation. The presence of osteolytic lesions is perhaps the most significant clue to the diagnosis at this point. The lesions also may cause hypercalcemia, leading to constipation and contributing to the patient's weakness.

A bone malignancy, specifically myeloma, is suspected, and other disease processes must be ruled out because the treatment and prognosis may be vastly different. Myeloma must be distinguished from benign monoclonal gammopathy, polyclonal hypergammaglobulinemia, and other malignant lymphoproliferative diseases such as Waldenström's macroglobulinemia, lymphomas, and primary amyloidosis.

Traction is applied to the patient's fracture, and he is admitted to the hospital for an extensive work-up. Over the next several days, the results of the additional ordered studies become available. The patient's calcium is elevated at 12.1 mg/dl and is being managed with aggressive fluid therapy. The erythrocyte sedimentation rate (ESR) is elevated, and the reticulocyte count is depressed. The bone series reveals three more punched-out osteolytic lesions in his skull. The bone marrow aspirate shows increased numbers of plasma cells and large multinucleated cells. The serum protein electrophoresis (SPEP) demonstrates a large spike in the gamma region, and the urine protein electrophoresis (UPEP) shows kappa light

chains, or Bence-Jones proteins, in the urine. His creatinine clearance is decreased to 30 ml/min. Renal biopsy reveals interstitial infiltrates of abnormal plasma cells and protein casts in the distal convoluted and collecting tubules. A diagnosis of IgG myeloma is made, and appropriate therapy is started.

QUESTIONS

6. *Explain the recent laboratory findings.*
7. *How should future therapy be directed?*
8. *What is the patient's prognosis?*

DISCUSSION

Multiple myeloma is a type of cancer that arises from a malignant mutation of a single plasma cell. This cell rapidly multiplies in the body and metastasizes to the bone marrow. The cancerous cells overproduce the immunoglobulin of the class they were destined to produce (IgG in this case) and, in addition, produce excess light chains. The light chain dimers (Bence Jones proteins) are usually detected in the urine because kidney lesions are a common part of the disease picture. The pancytopenia and depressed reticulocyte count are a result of the plasma cell proliferation in the bone marrow, which interferes with erythropoiesis. The elevated sedimentation rate reflects the increase in protein content in the blood, which makes it hyperviscous.

The optimal chemotherapy regimen for myeloma has not been determined. Most recently, combination chemotherapy with alkylating agents has been used. Bone marrow transplantation has been attempted in young patients with promising results but is still considered experimental treatment. The current goal of treatment of symptomatic myeloma is palliation. Localized radiotherapy may be useful for relief of bone pain or for eradicating the tumor at the site of pathologic fracture.

The median survival of patients with myelomas is 3 years. Life expectancy is markedly shortened in those patients with high paraprotein spikes, renal failure, hypercalcemia, or extensive bone disease. Recurrent infection with encapsulated bacteria, especially *Streptococcus pneumoniae* and *Haemophilus influenzae,* is the primary cause of death in these patients.

Case 4

The patient is a 14-year-old female prostitute who, 4 days ago, experienced an episode of shaking chills followed by perspiration and fever. These symptoms abated later that day but have recurred daily since. She has recently developed tenderness in her right wrist and a small sore on her right index finger. The patient says she has not experienced vaginal discharge, diarrhea, dysuria, swollen joints, sore throat, jaundice, or abdominal pain.

Physical examination reveals a well-developed young woman with fever (her temperature is 40.3°C), a shaking chill, and regular respiration of 20. Her blood pressure is 110/70, and her heart rate is 135. The lesion on the index finger is brown at the center, is slightly raised, and is surrounded with a small erythematous ring. Extension of the thumb causes pain and palpable crepitus. Thickening and redness are noted around the wrist. The remainder of the physical examination is unremarkable.

Laboratory data reveal the following values: normal urinalysis; complete blood count (CBC) with Hct 35%, Hgb 11.4 g/dl, and white blood cells (WBCs) 19,500/mm^3 with polymorphonuclear leukocytes (PMNs) 90%, bands 5%, lymphocytes 4%, and monocytes 1%; normal radiologic and chemical studies.

QUESTIONS

1. *Which of the above data are helpful?*
2. *How is the data helpful?*

DISCUSSION

At this point, the diagnosis is unclear. The most important finding is the elevated white cell count, with 90% PMNs and 5% bands, which suggests an acute infection.

The patient is placed on antibiotics and is admitted to the hospital. Specimens are sent to the laboratory for culture and sensitivity assays. *Neisseria gonorrhoeae* is isolated from the cervix and the blood.

QUESTIONS

3. *What treatment is recommended?*
4. *Is there any underlying problem that contributed to the severity of this infection?*

DISCUSSION

The patient has gonorrhea, and because she is high risk, she may well have more than one infection. Her infection is caused by a penicillinase-producing *N. gonorrhoeae* (PPNG). The organism is susceptible to ceftriaxone, and this is the drug of choice. Tetracycline or doxycycline may be added to the treatment to combat *Chlamydia trachomatis,* an organism that commonly coinfects with gonococcus.

Gonococcal infections are usually asymptomatic in women and are restricted to urethritis or cervicitis in the few women who are symptomatic. The patient in question has an underlying complement deficiency, which has compromised her ability to deal with this infectious agent. Complement deficiencies are associated with a breakdown in host resistance to microorganisms. Complement (C) is involved in host defense mechanisms as an opsonin (C3b), a chemotaxin (C5a), a lytic system (C5–C9), and in altering vascular permeability (C3a, C4a, C5a).

Deficiencies in the C proteins of the membrane attack complex are associated with increased frequency and severity of infections by encapsulated bacteria, particularly members of the genus *Neisseria* (i.e., the gonococcus and meningococcus species). It is of interest that deficiencies of C5 through C8 are involved in this association; C9 deficiency does not seem to predispose to neisserial disease.

Deficiencies in other C proteins are associated with recurrent pyogenic infections (particularly C3) and autoimmune (immune complex) diseases. A deficiency in the C1 esterase inhibitor regulatory protein is the most common C protein deficiency known and is associated with hereditary angioneurotic edema.

Case 5

A boy scout troop has recently returned from the national jamboree in a national park in Tennessee. Shortly after their return, one of the scouts began to feel ill. He initially complained only of a decreased appetite and easy fatigability. Two days later, he developed a severe headache, muscle and joint pain, and intermittent chills and fever. The appearance of a diffuse maculopapular rash prompted his mother to bring him to the physician's office.

QUESTIONS

1. What is the relevance of the recent trip and the onset of the scout's illness?
2. Are there any characteristics of the rash that should prompt the physician to seek more information?

DISCUSSION

The patient's recent camping trip and the onset of his symptoms are likely more than coincidence. Additional questioning should focus on camp conditions, illness in any of the other campers, drinking water sources, and the occurrence of any animal or insect bites. Many infectious rashes evolve through various stages. Knowing the time of onset along with the initial location and appearance can provide important diagnostic clues.

According to the patient's mother, none of the other children from the trip have become ill. The patient tells you that the campers drank either bottled or chlorinated water, none from wells or streams. Everyone slept in tents and went on daily hikes in the woods. One scout was scratched by a raccoon and another sprayed by a skunk. Many of the hikers came back from the woods with ticks, but "the scout masters pulled them all off."

On physical examination, the patient looks acutely ill. His temperature is 103.4°F, pulse 120 beats per minute and regular, respiratory rate is 24 breaths per minute, and blood pressure is 106/60 mm Hg. Cardiac, pulmonary, and abdominal examination results are all benign. He has a diffuse maculopapular rash covering his trunk and proximal extremities. Distally, there is a gradual transition to a petechial rash. The patient explains that his rash first appeared around his wrists and ankles then spread up his arms and legs to the rest of his body. Neurologically, he appears slightly lethargic, but there are no meningeal signs.

Based on the history and the physical examination alone, the physician feels fairly certain about a diagnosis. However, because of his high fever and change in mental status, the physician decides to admit the patient to the hospital for a few days of intravenous antibiotics and a thorough diagnostic work-up.

QUESTIONS

3. What is the differential diagnosis at this point?
4. What type of antibiotic should the patient be given initially?
5. What laboratory tests should be ordered on the patient's admission to the hospital?

DISCUSSION

A differential diagnosis based solely on the rash limits the etiology to only a handful of possible agents. Measles, typhoid, certain rickettsial species, and meningococcemia may all produce rashes that may be confused with the presentation seen in the patient. A suspicion of the latter requires blood cultures and cerebrospinal fluid (CSF) analysis.

Because a specific agent has not yet been identified, giving the patient a broad-spectrum antibiotic at this point would be prudent. A third-generation cephalosporin, such as ceftriaxone or cefotaxime, would be appropriate and should be started as soon as possible, preferably after samples needed for cultures have been drawn.

Laboratory tests performed on admission should include a complete blood cell count (CBC) with differential and platelets; urinalysis; blood, throat, and urine cultures; serum chemistries; certain specific febrile agglutinins; coagulation studies; and CSF analysis and culture.

Once in the hospital, the patient does well. Over the next few days his fever resolves, the rash has progressed to a petechial phase and now involves his palms as well, and his arthralgias and myalgias no longer bother him. The initial studies that the physician ordered revealed the following:

white blood cells (WBCs) = 18,000/mm³ with 65% lymphocytes, 30% neutrophils, and 5% monocytes; platelets = 110,000/mm³; prothrombin time (PT) = 9 sec, partial thromboplastin time (PTT) = 20 sec; urine with 2+ protein and moderate red blood cells (RBCs); all cultures negative to date; serum and CSF chemistries within normal limits; febrile agglutinins to *Proteus* OX2 and *Proteus* OX19 at 1:10 and 1:20, respectively.

The patient is switched to an oral antibiotic and discharged. At his 1-week follow-up visit, a convalescent serum sample is drawn, and febrile agglutinins to *Proteus* OX2 and *Proteus* OX19 are both 1:320.

QUESTIONS

6. *What is the final diagnosis?*
7. *What is the first-line antibiotic of choice?*
8. *Explain the low platelet count and the shortened PT/PTT.*

DISCUSSION

The patient had Rocky Mountain spotted fever. The causative agent, *Rickettsia rickettsii,* is transmitted by the bite of ticks. In the United States, most cases occur in the eastern third of the country during the late spring and summer months. The mortality rate of Rocky Mountain spotted fever varies with age. In the untreated elderly, it may be as high as 70%; in children, less than 20%. The usual cause of death is pneumonitis and respiratory or cardiac failure.

The rickettsial organisms penetrate deeply into the blood vessel walls. This endothelial damage results in loss of the integrity of the lumen wall, thereby causing passing platelets to adhere (which lowers the platelet count) and activate the coagulation pathways. The PT is a measure of the extrinsic coagulation pathway and measures factors X, VII, V, II, and I. The PTT measures the intrinsic pathway and factors XII, XI, IX, VIII, X, VI, II, and I. Because these pathways are activated throughout the body by the infection secondary to the endothelial damage, the tendency to form microscopic clots is increased (thus, the platelet count is decreased), and the PT and PTT times are shortened. Leukocytosis, proteinuria, and hematuria are also common. In some patients, there is splenomegaly, hepatomegaly, jaundice, gangrene, myocarditis, or uremia.

The antibiotics of choice for this condition are chloramphenicol (oral or intravenous) or oral tetracycline, both of which are more specific to rickettsial organisms. Tetracyclines inhibit protein synthesis by binding to the 30S subunit of the bacterial ribosome and prevent binding of aminoacyl–transfer RNA. Chloramphenicol inhibits bacterial protein synthesis by binding to the 50S ribosomal subunit and prevents peptide bond formation. Rickettsial organisms have yet to show resistance to either one.

R. rickettsii shares an antigen with the bacterium *Proteus vulgaris,* allowing useful serological diagnosis by checking the febrile agglutinins to *Proteus* OX19 and OX2. When the titer is low (e.g., 1:10, 1:20), there is not much antibody made against the Proteus organism. The ratio signifies the highest dilution of the patient's serum in which antibody could be detected. After the patient had been infected by the rickettsial organism for a period of time, he should have formed antibodies if his immune system was working properly. At his 1-week follow-up visit, his serum could be diluted as far as 1:320 and still agglutinate the bacteria, which indicated that his immune system was fighting the infection well.

Case 6

A 57-year-old homeless man presents to the emergency department complaining of shortness of breath. He says he has been feeling poorly for several months and went to the public health clinic several weeks ago, where he received an injection that did nothing to relieve his symptoms. His breathing became labored over the weekend, and now he is having trouble walking more than a few yards before having to stop to catch his breath. He denies having chest pain, dizziness, peripheral edema, orthopnea, or hemoptysis. He states that he has been sweating profusely, especially at night, and thinks he has had a fever. His clothing seems to fit more loosely, and his "smoker's cough" has progressively worsened.

His previous medical history is negative for cardiac events, and he has no cardiac risk factors other than smoking a pack of cigarettes every 2 days. He was hospitalized several years ago for 3 days after being struck by a car but denies having any sequelae or operations. He takes no prescribed medications and has no known drug allergies.

The patient usually sleeps in the city parks at night but occasionally stays at one of the local shelters when the weather is bad. He admits to drinking a pint of bourbon and 2 or 3 quarts of beer daily. He denies recent intravenous drug abuse and claims to have abstained from any drug abuse for 2 years.

QUESTIONS

1. *What is the differential diagnosis at this point?*
2. *Aside from the patient's dyspnea, what other health care issues need to be addressed when this patient is admitted?*

DISCUSSION

Despite this patient's lack of chest pain and significant cardiac risk factors, an acute myocardial infarction must be ruled out. A 12- or 15-lead electrocardiogram (ECG) and serial creatine kinase isoenzyme studies are appropriate at this point. A significant pneumonia or bacterial endocarditis could also explain the patient's current symptoms. Pneumothorax should also be suspected if there is history of recent trauma or if the patient has advanced chronic obstructive pulmonary disease (COPD), in which case an emphysematous pulmonary bulla may have spontaneously ruptured. Lung cancer also should be considered and ruled out, if possible. A chest radiograph would rule out pneumothorax, help identify and localize any masses or pneumonias, and confirm any suspicion of cardiomegaly found on physical examination.

Once the cause of the patient's dyspnea is found and treatment is started, several other issues must be managed. A recent history of illicit drug use places him at high risk for human immunodeficiency virus (HIV) infection. His daily alcohol intake not only places him at risk for acute withdrawal on admission to the hospital, it almost guarantees that the patient will be malnourished and have multiple electrolyte abnormalities. Being homeless increases his exposure to certain pathogens and makes follow-up care difficult.

During the physical examination, the patient appears older than his stated age. He is thin-limbed with a protuberant abdomen and is slightly tachypneic while reclining on the stretcher. His vital signs are blood pressure = 115/68 mm Hg; pulse = 84 beats/min; and respirations = 30 breaths/min. He has good dentition, no obvious lymphadenopathy, and a normal cardiac examination. Auscultation of his lung fields reveals diffusely scattered rales, which do not clear after he coughs. The result of abdominal examination is benign. Neurologic examination is nonfocal, and the patient is alert and oriented to person, place, and time.

A pulse oximeter was placed and showed an oxygen saturation of 85% on room air. Arterial blood gases were measured, and the patient was placed on supplemental oxygen at 4 L/min, which improved his saturation to 92%. His respirations slowed to 16/min, and he appeared to be more comfortable. His ECG was normal with no signs of ischemia. An intravenous line was started, and blood was drawn for a complete blood count, electrolyte evaluation, liver function tests, and coagulation studies. Consent was obtained for an HIV test. A chest radiograph revealed diffuse pulmonary infiltrates in both lungs. The patient was able to produce a purulent sputum sample, which was sent to the laboratory for Gram and acid-fast staining, as well as routine and mycobacterial cultures.

The attending physician decided to start the patient on empiric broad-spectrum antibiotics until an organism is identified via culture. He also placed the patient on a benzodiazepine taper to prevent delirium tremens. As the patient was being wheeled upstairs to his room, a medical student asked the attending physician if it would be beneficial to perform a Mantoux test with purified protein derivative (PPD) and control antigens to rule out tuberculosis. The physician agrees and instructs the student to do it himself and report the results in 3 days.

QUESTIONS

3. *Is an oxygen saturation of 92% acceptable in this patient?*
4. *Why is it necessary to place control antigens with the PPD?*
5. *Why is the student instructed to report the results after 3 days?*

DISCUSSION

The preferred oxygen saturation in a healthy individual is 98% to 100%. In patients with compromised pulmonary function, the percentage is naturally lower. Those with a saturation of 90% have a Po_2 of only 60 mm Hg and require immediate care. Patients with an extensive smoking history may have COPD manifestations and rely on an oxygen respiratory drive as opposed to the normal CO_2 drive. Administering too much supplemental oxygen to these patients suppresses their respiratory drive and causes them to become more hypoxic. Considering that this patient has an active pulmonary process as well as a smoking history to inhibit his oxygen saturation, placing him on low amounts of supplemental oxygen will decrease his respiratory rate while increasing his saturation and making him more comfortable. He should be closely monitored over the next several hours to ensure that his respiratory drive does not become inhibited.

Placing control antigens, such as *Candida* or *Trichophyton,* with the PPD helps to differentiate between a negative PPD result and an anergic response. Patients who are immunocompromised, malnourished, or who have an overwhelming infection may not be able to mount an adequate immunologic response to an antigen challenge. If the PPD and controls fail to react after 72 hours, a chest radiograph should be ordered to check for various radiographic manifestations of tuberculosis. A Ghon complex, a calcified granuloma typically seen in the upper pulmonary lobes, may be seen as residual evidence of a healed primary tuberculosis infection.

The PPD skin test is an example of a type IV (delayed) hypersensitivity reaction. These reactions peak 24–48 hours after exposure to antigen. Measuring the width of induration at 48–72 hours after antigen exposure ensures that the reaction has peaked. Typically, reactions larger than 10 mm in healthy patients are considered to be positive for mycobacterial exposure. Immunosuppressed patients with induration greater than 5 mm and people in close contact with tuberculosis patients should be started on drug therapy.

During the night, the patient's laboratory tests are reported to be within normal limits except for an elevated white blood cell count secondary to his infection and a low albumin level, which confirms his poor nutritional status. His arterial blood gas showed a metabolic acidosis with respiratory compensation caused by his infection and resulting tachypnea. The sputum Gram stain contained many white blood cells and few squamous epithelial cells. The acid-fast stain revealed many organisms. Because of the combination of a positive acid-fast stain; history of weight loss, fatigue, and night sweats; and his homelessness putting him at increased risk for tuberculosis, the patient is immediately placed in respiratory isolation and started on multidrug therapy for tuberculosis. A dietary consultation was requested to manage his poor nutritional status, and social services was contacted to help arrange long-term care and follow-up. Neither the PPD nor the controls ever showed any reaction, which was likely to be secondary to his malnourished state. His HIV test eventually returned negative.

QUESTIONS

6. *Does an acid-fast stain confirm the diagnosis of tuberculosis?*
7. *How long does it take to receive final results for acid-fast cultures?*

8. *What drugs are currently used to treat tuberculosis?*
9. *Are there any specific side effects to any of the medications that will be used to treat this patient?*

DISCUSSION

Acid-fast bacilli on sputum stain do not confirm the diagnosis of tuberculosis. The specimen may become contaminated with saprophytic nontuberculous mycobacteria that colonize the oropharynx. Typically, multiple sputum specimens are needed to identify acid-fast bacilli.

Mycobacterial cultures are notoriously slow growing and may require 6–8 weeks for final interpretation. For this reason, patients are started on chemotherapy based on the history, physical examination, and radiographic findings, and acid-fast stains. With the emergence of drug-resistant strains of *Mycobacterium tuberculosis,* sensitivity studies are frequently performed on the positive cultures.

First-line antituberculosis drugs include isoniazid, rifampin, pyrazinamide, ethambutol, and streptomycin. Standard therapy currently consists of isoniazid, rifampin, and pyrazinamide daily for 2 months followed by isoniazid and rifampin twice weekly for 4 additional months. If resistance to isoniazid is suspected, ethambutol may be substituted until sensitivity studies are reported.

All of the first-line drugs have side effects that must be monitored. Isoniazid, rifampin, and pyrazinamide are all hepatotoxic. Isoniazid may cause a peripheral neuritis, which can be prevented with oral pyridoxine. Rifampin causes urine and body secretions to turn orange. Pyrazinamide can cause hyperuricemia. Ethambutol causes an optic neuritis, so that red–green color discrimination and visual acuity must be tested before starting therapy. Streptomycin is ototoxic and nephrotoxic, so that hearing and renal function must be monitored.

Case 7

Pauline (age 4) and her family were driving to Yellowstone National Park and stopped at a motel in Sheridan, Wyoming. The entire family went swimming, had dinner, and returned to their room to watch television. During the evening, Pauline developed a cough and began wheezing. She became progressively worse throughout the night despite the antihistamines and cough syrup her mother gave her. Early the next morning, her parents took her to the emergency department of the local hospital because her breathing had become labored.

Physical examination on admission revealed an anxious and tired 4-year-old in acute respiratory distress. Her nostrils were flared, her trachea shifted up and down with each breath, and she was actively using her accessory muscles of respiration. Her pulse was 120 beats per minute, and her respirations were 42 per minute. On auscultation, she had diminished breath sounds throughout her lung fields, and only minimal wheezes could be heard apically. The remainder of the physical examination was within normal limits.

Fearing severe respiratory compromise, arterial blood was drawn and sent to the laboratory for analysis, and β-agonist nebulized treatments and supplemental oxygen were initiated. The blood gas results returned showing a PaO_2 of 63 (normal is 80 to 100 mm Hg), a $PaCO_2$ of 55 (normal is 35 to 45 mm Hg), and a pH of 7.35 (normal is 7.35 to 7.45).

QUESTIONS

1. *Based on the physical findings alone, how serious is Pauline's condition?*
2. *Should the arterial blood gas values cause concern?*

DISCUSSION

Based on the initial physical examination, Pauline is critically ill. The recruitment of accessory muscles (intercostal and scalene) to breathe and her tachypnea are ominous signs. The observation that she appears tired indicates that she has been struggling for many hours and may soon slip into pulmonary arrest. Decreased breath sounds in virtually all lung fields should inform the clinician that a significant degree of bronchoconstriction is present, resulting in poor oxygen exchange in the alveoli.

In a normally hyperventilating patient, a high-normal PaO_2, a low $PaCO_2$, and relative alkalosis secondary to the "blowing off" of CO_2 would be expected. In Pauline's case, she has grown weary to the point that she is moving very little volume through her lungs. This leads to CO_2 retention and the lowered pH. If definitive care is not begun immediately and her blood gases do not improve quickly, she will need to be intubated to manage her airway.

Pauline's father reports that her respiratory problems first appeared when she was 9 months of age, and they were told she had asthma. Since then, Pauline has experienced periodic episodes of dyspnea and wheezing that were managed with nonprescription antihistamines. The etiology of her asthma had never been identified.

A chest radiograph shows hyperlucent lungs, flattened hemidiaphragms, and increased space between the sternum and heart, all of which are consistent with the trapping of air frequently seen in those with asthma. A complete blood count (CBC) with differential was performed and revealed a white blood cell count of 6700/mm^3 (normal is 5000 to 10,000/mm^3) with 27% lymphocytes (normal is 20% to 40%), 62% neutrophils (normal is 40% to 60%), 8% eosinophils (normal is 1% to 3%), and 3% monocytes (normal is 4% to 8%).

QUESTIONS

3. *What is currently thought to be the pathophysiology of asthma?*
4. *What is the cause of Pauline's eosinophilia?*
5. *What is the role of corticosteroids in asthma?*

DISCUSSION

Asthma is the condition of an overly sensitive trachea and bronchi, which narrow in response to various stimuli. Its pathophysiology is poorly understood. Currently, the principal component of an asthma attack is thought to be an inflammatory process. Multiple complex mechanisms are involved, including blood basophils, tissue mast cells, neutrophils, eosinophils, platelets, histamine, leukotrienes, prostaglandins, bradykinin, neutrophil and eosinophil chemotactic factors, and platelet-activating factor.

Eosinophilia is frequently associated with asthma and allergic diseases. Eosinophil chemotactic factor of anaphylaxis is stored in the mast cell granules. Eosinophilia may also be seen in various parasitic diseases. Several pulmonary diseases also cause an elevation in eosinophils, as do many connective tissue diseases and drug reactions.

Corticosteroids are effective because they suppress both acute and chronic airway inflammation. They block breakdown of membrane phospholipids and interfere with the diapedesis of blood cells such as basophils through the vascular endothelium. Because their onset of action may take several hours, they are never used alone as primary treatment of an acute asthma attack. Corticosteroids are useful in controlling the late phase of asthma attacks.

The decision is made to admit Pauline at least overnight for further care and observation. The admitting physician wanted to test Pauline for possible allergies that may be triggering her asthma. He considered the radioallergosorbent test (RAST) and the scratch test, and decided to use the scratch test. Pauline did very well in the hospital and was discharged the following day with orders to complete a 7-day steroid treatment. Results of the scratch test indicated that she was allergic to goose dander. A call to the motel confirmed that the pillows contained goose feathers. Pauline's father purchased a hypoallergenic pillow, and the family proceeded on their vacation without further incident.

QUESTIONS

6. *Why did the admitting physician decide to perform the scratch test?*
7. *Is desensitization recommended for this patient?*
8. *Are there any medications that asthmatics should routinely avoid?*

DISCUSSION

The radioallergosorbent test (RAST) is only available for a limited number of allergens (e.g., ragweed) and is used only in patients with the appropriate allergy. The scratch test is extremely rapid (within minutes) and permits the use of the largest sample of potential allergens.

Desensitization is not recommended for this patient because environmental control and avoidance of goose feathers will suffice. A thorough allergy work-up should be started at the earliest convenience.

As stated, the pathogenesis of asthma remains unknown. The most popular hypothesis is airway inflammation. Stimuli cause mast cells, basophils, and macrophages to release chemical mediators that exert their effects on airway smooth muscle and increase capillary permeability. Drugs that are commonly associated with triggering asthmatic episodes include aspirin, β-adrenergic antagonists, and sulfating agents.

The aspirin-sensitive respiratory syndrome begins with vasomotor rhinitis, which progresses to hyperplastic rhinosinusitis and may give rise to nasal polyps. This is followed by progressive asthma. Even very small quantities of aspirin may trigger an attack, resulting in ocular and nasal congestion with severe episodes of airway obstruction. Nonsteroidal anti-inflammatory drugs (NSAIDs) share a significant cross-reactivity with aspirin in the triggering of asthma attacks. Acetaminophen is well tolerated and may be used by these individuals.

β-Adrenergic antagonists cause bronchoconstriction via the β_2 receptors in the tracheobronchial tree. Because even selective β_1 agents tend to produce airway obstruction in asthmatics and those individuals with increased airway reactivity, their use should be avoided in these patients.

Case 8

A 27-year-old woman is brought to the emergency department by ambulance 15 minutes after suffering a generalized tonic-clonic seizure, which lasted approximately 5 minutes and resolved spontaneously. The paramedics started an intravenous line en route to the hospital but gave no medication.

According to family members, the woman has never had a seizure before, and there is no history of recent head trauma. The patient's sister states that the patient has been ill for the past 4 years, when her symptoms began as arthralgias and erythema of her fingers, wrists, and elbows. Since then, the patient has been treated by a general practitioner, but the sister does not know the diagnosis or what medications the patient may be taking.

A physical examination reveals a pale, semiconscious woman. Her breathing is not labored, and she began moving her arms and legs during the examination. The examination is unremarkable except for a butterfly rash over her cheeks and several ulcers on her buccal mucosa.

QUESTION

1. *What is the significance of the presence of a rash, particularly a "butterfly" distribution on the malar aspect of the face?*

DISCUSSION

A malar rash is highly suggestive of systemic lupus erythematosus (SLE). The 4-year history of arthritis is consistent with this diagnosis.

The emergency department physician placed the patient on supplemental oxygen and ordered: a complete set of serum level tests, a complete blood count, a urinalysis, a urine drug screen (UDS), a pregnancy test, a Venereal Disease Research Laboratory (VDRL) screen for syphilis, a fluorescent treponemal antibody absorption test (FTA-ABS), a computed tomography (CT) scan, and a lumbar puncture.

   The patient became alert enough that she could give a history. She stated that she had been diagnosed with SLE, three years ago. She developed painful episodes in her fingers whenever they were exposed to cold temperatures. She was told at the time that she had Raynaud's phenomenon. She has experienced moderate fatigue during her illness, and 2 years ago she developed hematuria. Her physician explained to her that the SLE was affecting her kidneys. Corticosteroid therapy was recommended but refused. One year ago she developed the malar rash that is characteristic of SLE followed by an episode of acute anterior chest pain, which was diagnosed as lupus pericarditis. At that time, she accepted treatment with prednisone and had marked improvement in her symptoms. However, because of the cushingoid side effects of the steroids, she discontinued them 6 months ago. Since that time, she has had a return of her fatigue, arthralgias, and malar rash.

QUESTIONS

2. *Based on this new information, what is the most likely cause of the patient's seizure?*
3. *Knowing that the patient has SLE, what additional tests should be ordered?*

DISCUSSION

Given that the patient has SLE, the most likely cause for her new-onset seizure is lupus cerebritis. Damage is brought on by the deposition of immune complexes in the central nervous system, an event that occurs in approximately 5% of patients with SLE. Although lupus cerebritis is probably the cause for her seizures, other potentially treatable causes still must be ruled out. Additional studies that may be ordered based on the fact that the patient has SLE include an anti-double-stranded DNA (anti-dsDNA) study, Coombs' test, and measurement of C3 levels.

The laboratory results revealed that serum glucose and electrolytes were within normal limits; white blood cell count, hemoglobin, and hematocrit were within normal limits; UDS and pregnancy test results were both negative; VDRL was positive; FTA-ABS was negative; CT scan was negative for gross structural abnormalities; and analysis of cerebrospinal fluid was within normal limits. The patient's blood urea nitrogen (BUN) and creatinine levels were 35 mg/dl (normal is 8–20 mg/dl) and 3.0 mg/dl (normal is 0.7–1.4 mg/dl), respectively. The urinalysis showed proteinuria (3+), 20–30 red blood cells per high-power field, and a trace of glucose. The direct Coombs' test and the anti-dsDNA tests were positive, and the C3 level was 65 mg/dl (normal is 80–175 mg/dl).

QUESTIONS

4. What is the cause of the urinary abnormalities?
5. What is the Coombs' test, and why is it positive in this patient?
6. What is the significance of the VDRL and FTA-ABS results?
7. Why is the patient's C3 level depressed?

DISCUSSION

The patient's renal glomeruli are being destroyed by the deposition of immune complexes. These complexes activate the complement cascade with resultant deposition of the C3b opsonin on the glomerular membrane and the release of the potent chemotaxin C5a. Polymorphonuclear leukocytes accumulate in the glomeruli and undergo exocytosis when they attempt to engulf the basement membrane. The released enzymes damage the glomeruli, leading to an elevated BUN, increased creatinine, proteinuria, and glucosuria.

The Coombs' test detects anti-red blood cell antibodies. The direct test examines erythrocytes for the presence of antibodies on the cell surface. If present, these antibodies will cause the cells to agglutinate when an anti-human gamma globulin antiserum (Coombs' serum) is added. An indirect Coombs' test starts with an unknown serum that might contain antibodies reactive with erythrocytes. This serum is mixed with red blood cells, the cells are then washed with a saline solution to remove excess gamma globulin, and the Coombs' reagent is added. Agglutination indicates that the unknown serum contained antibodies reactive with the erythrocytes used in the assay (usually O-positive human red blood cells). The direct Coombs' test is positive in this patient because she is making autoantibodies against her own erythrocytes. Approximately 25% of patients with SLE will make anti-red blood cell antibodies at some point during their disease.

The positive VDRL is due to an antibody in the serum that reacts with cardiolipin. It is detected in the nontreponemal screening test, which ruled out syphilis as a diagnostic possibility. The patient's C3 level is depressed because the circulating immune complexes in the blood have activated the complement cascade and consumed the C3 component faster than the liver can produce it. Anti-dsDNA titers may increase during acute SLE exacerbations. Anti-Sm, anti-Ro, and anti-La autoantibodies may also be found in some patients with SLE.

Case 9

Approximately 1 year ago, a 38-year-old unemployed man was a new patient seeking evaluation of fatigue that progressively worsened for 3 months and was occasionally associated with a low-grade fever. The patient had a medical history of syphilis and gonorrhea 14 years ago, for which he was treated with penicillin. He also had hepatitis 11 years ago but did not know which strain of the virus he had or how he contracted it. He denied using drugs and has never required hospitalization, surgery, or a transfusion.

On further questioning, the patient admitted that he is strictly, but covertly, homosexual, and that he has had "dozens of one-night stands" and two long-term relationships. He had been unwilling in the past to be tested for human immunodeficiency virus (HIV). He rationalized that because he felt healthy, the test was unnecessary, and that if he had contracted it, nothing could be done to keep him from dying from acquired immune deficiency syndrome (AIDS).

The patient refused an HIV test, despite the physician's insistence, and he left before the physician could examine him. He was lost to follow-up until 1 year later. He had done well until 2 months earlier, when he began to become exhausted performing even the most minor physical task. He has had a persistent, nonproductive cough.

During the physical examination, the patient's vital signs were blood pressure = 112/65 mm Hg; pulse = 98 beats/min; respirations = 28 breaths/min. He has diffuse rales throughout all of his lung fields, and there are several prominent cervical, axillary, and inguinal lymph nodes.

After a lengthy discussion, the patient agreed to submit to several baseline tests and follow-up in 1 week.

QUESTIONS

1. *What are the risk factors for HIV infection?*
2. *How should this patient be counseled regarding HIV serologic testing?*

DISCUSSION

The risk factors for HIV infection include sexual contact with an infected person, perinatal exposure, and parenteral exposure to infected blood via transfusion or needle sharing. The patient should be informed that there are several potential benefits to obtaining HIV testing. Testing should be done so that the patient can notify past partners of their potential exposure, modify his behavior so as to put no further contacts at risk of infection, and establish plans for medical care and follow-up. Although all HIV-infected individuals will eventually develop AIDS, the time course of progression is highly variable. Therapy directed at both the primary HIV infection and at the secondary opportunistic infections and malignancies that define AIDS can significantly prolong life.

The physician obtains an HIV antibody assay and a CD lymphocyte profile. The results are HIV antibody positive; The Western blot detects antibodies to p24, gp41, p55, and gp120. CD4 lymphocytes are 180/ml (normal is >500/ml). When the physician informs the patient of his laboratory results at the follow-up visit, the patient is initially stunned but then becomes tearful. The patient asks the physician if he will die of AIDS and whether anything can be done to help him.

QUESTIONS

3. *What is the significance of the laboratory results?*
4. *How should this patient be counseled regarding his long-term medical prognosis, lifestyle, psychosocial challenges, and potential risks of therapy?*

DISCUSSION

The HIV-ELISA is a screening test with a greater than 95% sensitivity. When used in conjunction with the Western blot, sensitivity approaches 99.9%. At least two HIV antigens must be positive for the test to be conclusive.

CD4 lymphocytes are significantly low. Antibiotic prophylaxis against opportunistic infections is typically started when the CD4 count decreases to below 200/ml.

Patients should be informed that HIV is a chronic disease, the outcome of which is likely to be AIDS. However, the prognosis for any particular person cannot be predicted. Therapy that is specific for HIV and is directed at opportunistic infections is available and effective in prolonging the quality of life.

The patient should be encouraged to try to improve his general well-being through discontinuation of cigarettes, alcohol, and recreational drugs. He should be given information on improving his nutrition and obtaining adequate rest and exercise.

The importance of a strong support system composed of family and friends should be stressed, and access to mental health professionals should be made available.

Although antiretroviral therapy has been shown to prolong life, it is not without side effects, including nausea, emesis, anorexia, headache, hypersensitivity rash, myositis, and bone marrow suppression, especially of erythropoiesis.

A chest radiograph reveals diffuse, "fluffy" pulmonary infiltrates. Immunofluorescence assay of sputum reveals pulmonary macrophages and clusters of yeast-like cells. The results of acid-fast

stain are negative, and Gram stain of sputum reveals few squamous cells, many white blood cells, and no bacteria.

QUESTIONS

5. *What pulmonary process may be taking place in this patient?*
6. *What is the diagnosis based on the sputum studies, and what is the drug of choice for treatment?*

DISCUSSION

The radiograph suggests an active pneumonitis, most likely caused by an infective process. Based on the low CD4 count and the presence of yeast cells, the patient has *Pneumocystis carinii,* the opportunistic pathogen that frequently infects immunosuppressed patients. Treatment consists of oxygen supplementation as needed and trimethoprim–sulfamethoxazole. *P. carinii* prophylaxis with trimethoprim—sulfamethoxazole is instituted when the CD4 count decreases to below 200/ml. Patients who are sensitive to trimethoprim—sulfamethoxazole may be treated with either pentamidine or dapsone.

The patient visits the physician 2 weeks later and reports that he is feeling better. He says he is willing to try the AZT that was prescribed because he met several people through an AIDS support group who were able to tolerate it.

Case 10

A26-year-old white woman has just given birth to a healthy infant boy at full term. Her pregnancy was uneventful, she received good prenatal care, and there were no complications during labor and delivery. As part of her pre-delivery screening tests, her physician discovered that her rapid plasma reagin (RPR) test result was reactive at 1:8. The RPR on the fetal cord blood was nonreactive. The mother admits that she had syphilis as a teenager. She received "two shots" at that time and was told to follow-up in 1 year but failed to do so. She denies ever having painless ulcers in her genital area or oropharynx, and she has no recollection of any enlarged, painless lymph nodes. She gives a history of progressive malaise, joint pain, and a tendency for her cheeks to sunburn easily, but attributes these symptoms to normal aging and her pregnancy. She has taken no medication other than her prenatal vitamins.

Realizing that several conditions may predispose her to false-positive RPR test results, her physician ordered a fluorescent treponemal antibody absorption (FTA-ABS) test, which was negative. The remainder of her screening test values were within normal limits.

QUESTIONS

1. *What is the difference between the RPR and FTA-ABS tests?*
2. *What causes false-positive results in the nontreponemal antigen tests?*
3. *If the patient's FTA-ABS test had come back positive, what would have been the next step in treatment?*
4. *What is the differential diagnosis for a false-positive RPR?*

DISCUSSION

The rapid plasma reagin (RPR) and Venereal Disease Research Laboratory (VDRL) tests are nontreponemal antigen tests. They use a component of normal tissue—beef heart cardiolipin—as an antigen to measure nonspecific antibodies formed in the blood of patients with syphilis. These tests are easy, rapid, and inexpensive to perform and are, therefore, used as screening tests. The fluorescent treponemal antibody absorption (FTA-ABS) test employs killed *Treponema pallidum* as antigen to detect antibodies specific for treponemes. It is used primarily in determining whether a positive nontreponemal test result is false-positive or is diagnostic of syphilis.

Some patients with certain connective tissue diseases may record a false-positive nontreponemal antigen test caused by anti-DNA antibodies cross-reacting with cardiolipin. Lyme disease may cause a false-positive result in a FTA-ABS test but rarely a false-positive RPR test result.

If the FTA-ABS test had confirmed a syphilis infection, treatment for both the mother and infant would have been started immediately. The drug of choice for all forms of syphilis is penicillin. For patients who are allergic to penicillin, oral tetracyclines are effective treatment.

Causes of false-positive RPR test results include systemic lupus erythematosus (SLE), malaria, infectious mononucleosis, infectious hepatitis, leprosy, brucellosis, atypical pneumonia, typhus, other treponemal infections, and pregnancy.

As part of the diagnostic work-up, the patient's physician ordered a complete blood count with differential, peripheral blood smears, liver function tests, a chest radiograph, and various antinuclear antibody tests. Over the next few days, all of the results appear normal except for positive reactions to antinuclear antibodies (ANA); anti–double-stranded DNA antibodies; anti-Sm, anti-Ro, and anti-La antibodies. The physician explained the test results to the patient and arranged for follow-up care with a rheumatologist.

QUESTIONS

5. *Based on the history and laboratory results, what is the diagnosis?*
6. *What drugs can cause false-positive results in serologic tests for connective tissue diseases?*
7. *What are some of the complications that this woman may encounter?*

DISCUSSION

This patient almost certainly has SLE, an inflammatory autoimmune disorder. Symptomatology is thought to be secondary to the trapping of antigen–antibody complexes within the capillary beds of multiple organ systems. Patients are typically women between the ages of 20 and 40 years. The most common complaint is joint pain. Positive antinuclear antibodies (ANA) and double-stranded DNA (dsDNA) values are found in 95% and 60%, respectively, of patients with SLE. Anti-Sm, Anti-Ro, and anti-La antibodies are very specific but poorly sensitive serologic markers of SLE.

It is important to realize that several drugs are known to cause a lupus-like syndrome, and the possibility of their use must be excluded before making a final diagnosis of SLE. The most common of these drugs include procainamide, hydralazine, and isoniazid. Also, chlorpromazine, methyldopa, and quinidine have been well documented to cause signs and symptoms as well as false-positive antibody test results similar to SLE.

Clinical features of SLE include fever, malaise, anorexia, and weight loss. The classic "butterfly" rash affects less than 50% of patients. Patients may complain of photo-sensitivity, oral ulcers, and joint pain. Further diagnostic testing may reveal serositis, renal disease, neurological findings, hematologic disorders, and immunologic abnormalities.

COMPREHENSIVE EXAMINATION

QUESTIONS

1. For the second time in 6 months, a 7-year-old girl presents with a lacerated wound from stepping on a broken bottle. As an infant, she received the standard tetanus immunizations, and 6 months ago she received a tetanus booster. What treatment should she receive today?

(A) The wound should be cleaned.
(B) Human toxin should be administered.
(C) Tetanus toxoid should be administered.
(D) Her infant diphtheria-pertussis-tetanus (DPT) injections should be repeated.
(E) Tetanus toxoid plus human antitoxin should be administered.

2. While eating at a seafood restaurant, a 47-year-old man develops urticaria, nausea, abdominal pain, chest tightness, and dyspnea. His blood pressure is 88/60 mm Hg. Which of the following is the mechanism most likely to be involved in this illness?

(A) Activation of the alternative complement pathway by proteins contained in the ingested seafood
(B) IgA-mediated activation of an intestinal inflammatory response.
(C) IgE-mediated release of histamine from mast cells
(D) IgG-mediated activation of the classic complement pathway
(E) IgM-mediated activation of the classic complement pathway

3. A 49-year-old man who had the "flu" last month is currently experiencing tingling in his fingers and toes and has marked muscular weakness in his extremities. Deep tendon reflexes are absent. A diagnosis of peripheral neuritis is made. Which of the following disorders most likely affects this man?

(A) Sjögren's syndrome
(B) Goodpasture's syndrome
(C) Systemic lupus erythematosus (SLE)
(D) Guillain-Barré syndrome
(E) Amyotrophic lateral sclerosis

4. After a bone marrow transplant from his human leukocyte antigen (HLA)-matched sister, a boy develops a syndrome characterized by pancytopenia, aplastic anemia, skin rash, diarrhea, jaundice, and weight loss. What is the correct term for this condition?

(A) Allograft rejection
(B) Graft-versus-host disease
(C) Failure of bone marrow engraftment
(D) Secondary infection
(E) Second set reaction

5. The immunosuppressant that blocks expression of the interleukin-2 (IL-2) gene in Th1 cells is

(A) antithymocyte serum
(B) monoclonal antibody versus CD3
(C) cyclosporine
(D) Cytoxan
(E) monoclonal antibody versus CD4

Questions 6–8

The data in the table below are the results of human leukocyte antigen (HLA)-A and HLA-B tissue typing using lymphocytotoxicity assay.

Antiserum	HLA Antigenic Specificities	Cytotoxicity*
A-1	A1, A11	10%
A-2	A2	8%
A-3	A2, A28	90%
A-4	A3	80%
A-5	A3, A10, A11	95%
A-6	A10, A11	5%
B-1	B7, B27	85%
B-2	B7, B45	95%
B-3	B8, B27	10%
B-4	B27, B44, B45	75%
B-5	B44	85%
B-6	B45	5%

*Percentage of dead cells observed.

6. The patient's HLA-A haplotype is

(A) A-1 and A-11
(B) A-2 and A-3
(C) A-2 and A-28
(D) A-3 and A-28
(E) A-10 and A-11

7. The patient's HLA-B haplotype is

(A) B-7 and B-27
(B) B-7 and B-44
(C) B-8 and B-45
(D) B-27 and B-44
(E) B-44 and B-45

8. The reaction with which one of the following serums shows that the patient's lymphocyte does NOT have an A-10 antigen on its membrane?

(A) A-1
(B) A-2
(C) A-3
(D) A-4
(E) A-5
(F) A-6

9. A patient has just been informed that his rapid plasma reagin (RPR) test to screen for possible infection with the syphilis spirochete has come back positive. His fiancé has asked that a more specific test be employed before their marriage. In the fluorescent treponemal antibody absorption (FTA-ABS) test used to diagnose syphilis, the patient's serum is added to a slide containing

(A) *Treponema pallidum* organisms
(B) fluorescein-tagged antibody to *T. pallidum*
(C) fluorescein-tagged antibody to human gamma globulin
(D) fluorescein isocyanate
(E) complement and sheep red blood cells (SRBCs)

10. The patient has a rash on his wrist immediately beneath his watch, the back of which is made of nickel. The most likely cause of this dermatitis is

(A) atopic dermatitis
(B) immune complex disease
(C) cytotoxic antibody-mediated disease
(D) contact dermatitis
(E) Arthus reaction

11. A patient has poor immunoglobulin A (IgA) response, an abnormal gait, and abnormal blood vessels, which are particularly noticeable in his eyes. Which one of the following disorders is the most likely diagnosis?

(A) Bruton's hypogammaglobulinemia
(B) DiGeorge syndrome
(C) Severe combined immune deficiency (SCID)
(D) Ataxia-telangiectasia
(E) Wiskott-Aldrich syndrome

12. A second-year medical student must be immunized before beginning to see patients at the Veterans Administration medical center. Which of the following would be the most appropriate treatment?

(A) Injection of killed virus vaccine and specific immune globulin
(B) Injection of live virus vaccine
(C) Injection of purified capsular carbohydrate vaccine
(D) Injection of specific immune globulin (horse)
(E) Injection of viral subunit vaccine prepared by recombinant DNA technology

13. In radioimmunoassay (RIA), it is essential that the substance to be detected have which one of the following characteristics? It

(A) can induce specific antibodies
(B) is protein in nature
(C) can be labeled with fluorescein isothiocyanate
(D) does not contain tritiated thymidine
(E) is an allergen

14. A 4-year-old patient has received the standard diphtheria-tetanus-pertussis (DTaP) immunization series starting at 3 months of age. He has been plagued by repeated pulmonary infections. A recent laboratory test revealed that he has no detectable antibody to diphtheria toxoid. The physician currently is faced with treating him for a deep puncture wound in his foot, which he obtained while playing in the street. Which of the following would be the best treatment to prevent tetanus?

(A) Tetanus spores plus toxoid
(B) Tetanus antitoxin (equine)
(C) Tetanus immune globulin (human)
(D) Tetanus antitoxin (human) plus tetanus toxoid
(E) Tetanus antitoxin plus antibodies

15. Patients with hypoplastic parathyroid glands may also suffer from recurrent fungal and viral infections. The functional capability of their T cells can be assayed by

(A) mixed lymphocyte culture
(B) fluorescent antibody assay with CD8 antiserum
(C) lipopolysaccharide mitogenic response
(D) erythrocyte (E)-rosette test
(E) fluorescent antibody assay with CD3 antiserum

16. Which of the antigens listed below has the highest correlation of occurrence in a patient with multiple myeloma?

(A) Prostate specific antigen (PSA)
(B) Alpha-fetoprotein (AFP)
(C) Carcinoembryonic antigen (CEA)
(D) Bence Jones protein
(E) Common acute lymphoblastic leukemia antigen (CALLA)

17. A new viral disease (Ebola) has recently emerged in Africa. It has a 60% mortality if untreated. Twenty-three newly diagnosed patients were treated with serum from patients who had recently recovered, and 22 of the 23 survived. Serum from United States blood donors had not been of help to previous patients with this disease. This observation proves that which one of the following is critical for recovery?

(A) Specific antibody
(B) Cytotoxic lymphocytes
(C) Natural killer (NK) cells
(D) Neutrophils
(E) Complement

18. Bacille Calmette-Guérin (BCG) is sometimes used for

(A) passive immunization for tuberculosis
(B) active immunization for tuberculosis is in the U.S.
(C) nonspecific suppression of the immune response
(D) potentiation of the humoral immune responses
(E) potentiation of the cell mediated immunities

19. A nine-month-old baby girl is brought to your office by her anxious mother. The child has lost most of her muscle control and can not even hold her head up. The child has been colicky for the past month; mother has used honey to control her hiccups. Injection of which of the following is the most appropriate treatment for this patient with neonatal botulism?

(A) Pooled human gamma globulin
(B) Specific human immune globulin
(C) Specific equine immune globulin
(D) Toxoid vaccine plus specific human immune globulin
(E) Toxoid vaccine

20. The cytoplasm of natural killer lymphocytes contains granules, the molecular contents of which are important in the cytotoxic activity of these cells. Which one of the following substances is found in these granules?

(A) Immunoglobulin G
(B) C3b
(C) Lysozyme
(D) Interleukin 1
(E) Perforin

21. Another name for an antigenic determinant is

(A) immunogen
(B) paratope
(C) carrier
(D) epitope
(E) antigen

22. What is the major protein component of the amyloid deposits seen in patients with primary amyloidosis?

(A) Complement protein fragments
(B) Intact IgM
(C) Immunoglobulin light (L)-chain fragments
(D) Aggregated IgG
(E) IgE heavy (H) chains

23. Which of the following is the most appropriate treatment for a patient with aplastic anemia?

(A) Bone marrow transplant
(B) Fetal thymus transplant
(C) Infusion of adenosine deaminase
(D) Thymectomy
(E) Splenectomy

24. Antibodies to beta cells of the pancreatic islets of Langerhans are a serologic clue for the presence of which of the following autoimmune diseases?

(A) Pernicious anemia
(B) Systemic lupus erythematosus (SLE)
(C) Myasthenia gravis (MG)
(D) Pemphigus
(E) Insulin-dependent diabetes mellitus

25. Which one of the following substances works to directly reverse bronchoconstriction and, therefore, is the treatment of choice in severe allergic respiratory distress?

(A) Cromolyn sodium
(B) Antihistamine
(C) Epinephrine
(D) Blocking antibody
(E) Methylxanthine drugs

26. A 37-year-old school nurse presents with arthritis, pleuritis, and low grade fever. She has anti-dsDNA antibodies in her serum. The symptoms began shortly after she began taking procainamide to control her cardiac arrhythmias. What disorder likely affects this woman?

(A) Amyotrophic lateral sclerosis (ALS)
(B) Systemic lupus erythematosus (SLE)
(C) Sjögren's syndrome
(D) Guillain-Barré syndrome
(E) Goodpasture's syndrome

27. Which of the following is a characteristic of innate immunity?

(A) Anamnesis
(B) B-cell mediation
(C) Complement participation
(D) Long induction time (days to weeks)
(E) Specificity

28. Which of the following statements about interferon-γ (IFN-γ) is true?

(A) It is released as a consequence of antigen- or mitogen-induced activation of B lymphocytes.
(B) It specifically binds to the antigen that induces its release.
(C) It activates macrophages to ingest and destroy bacteria and viruses.
(D) It is a potent immunosuppressant
(E) It activates T helper 2 cells.

29. A feverish 4-year-old African-American girl in excruciating pain who is jaundiced and has a tender spleen and hepatomegaly. A diagnosis of sickle cell disease is made after the laboratory data are obtained. The child requires immunization to protect her from bacterial septicemia. Which of the following would be the most therapeutic measure?

(A) Transfusion of erythrocytes
(B) Bone marrow transplant
(C) Injection of killed virus vaccine and specific immune globulin (horse)
(D) Injection of live virus vaccine
(E) Injection of purified capsular carbohydrate vaccine
(F) Thymectomy
(G) Injection of specific immune globulin (horse)

30. A 5-month-old patient has congenital hypoparathyroidism and an apparent absence of the thymus due to dysmorphogenesis of the third and fourth pharyngeal pouches. Facial and cardiac anomalies were noted at birth. The care of this child is complicated by episodes of hypocalcemic tetany. Which one of the following disorders is the most likely diagnosis?

(A) Bruton's hypogammaglobulinemia
(B) DiGeorge syndrome
(C) Severe combined immune deficiency (SCID)
(D) Ataxia-telangiectasia
(E) Wiskott-Aldrich syndrome

31. An immune response that mimics the response induced by natural infection is believed to be stimulated by administering agents via which route?

(A) subcutaneous
(B) percutaneous
(C) intradermal
(D) intravenous
(E) intranasal

32. The D region of the human major histocompatibility complex (MHC) contains loci that code for which of the following substances?

(A) Molecules found on the surface of macrophages and B cells
(B) Antigen-specific receptors on T cells
(C) Gene products that control the production of IgD
(D) β_2-microglobulin
(E) Cellular differentiation antigens (CD)

33. Antibodies to thyroid microsomal antigens are a serologic clue for the presence of which of the following immune diseases in a patient with a hypothyroid condition?

(A) Hashimoto's thyroiditis
(B) Multiple sclerosis (MS)
(C) Myasthenia gravis (MG)
(D) Goodpasture's disease
(E) Graves' disease

34. Rebecca, a 19-month-old child, was hospitalized for a yeast infection that would not respond to therapy. The patient had a history of acute pyogenic infections. Physical examination revealed that the spleen and lymph nodes were not palpable. A differential white count showed 95% neutrophils, 1% lymphocytes and 4% monocytes. From the list below, select the disease that Rebecca has?

(A) Severe combined immunodeficiency disease (SCID)
(B) AIDS
(C) Chronic granulomatous disease
(D) Neutropenia
(E) DiGeorge syndrome

35. If the emergence of forbidden clones is not continuously suppressed throughout life, a person may develop

(A) hypergammaglobulinemia
(B) allergic conditions
(C) autotolerance
(D) autoimmune disease
(E) serum sickness

36. Patients with Bruton's X-linked hypogammaglobulinemia may fail to produce immunoglobulin G in response to immunization with diphtheria toxoid because they

(A) have a decreased number of B cells
(B) have an increased number of T-suppressor cells
(C) lack CD4+ T-helper cells
(D) have a faulty antigen processing macrophage
(E) have a faulty class switching mechanism

37. A patient who is allergic to ragweed develops IgE myeloma. The myeloma IgE does not react with the ragweed pollen. What would be the effect of the patient's myeloma on the severity of his allergic symptoms during hay fever season?

(A) No change
(B) Increase due to increased production of IgE
(C) Increase due to the blocking effect of the myeloma
(D) Decrease due to the displacement of IgE anti-ragweed on mast cells by myeloma IgE
(E) Decrease due to chemotherapy used to treat his malignancy

38. The anamnestic response is defined as

(A) a gradual rise in antibody titers
(B) true immunological paralysis
(C) the prompt production of antibodies after a second exposure to antigen
(D) species-specific antibodies
(E) the lag in antibody production after initial antigen exposure

39. An 8-year-old boy has been bothered nearly all his life by a fungal pathogen that causes large, scaly lesions on his back and arms. Nystatin has been used therapeutically with some success. He has not had problems with any other infectious agent. What immune deficiency does the boy have?

(A) Severe combined immune deficiency (SCID)
(B) DiGeorge syndrome
(C) Chronic mucocutaneous candidiasis
(D) Wiskott-Aldrich syndrome
(E) AIDS

40. Which one of the following white blood cells is a major source of the mediators of atopic allergies?

(A) Neutrophil
(B) Basophil
(C) Monocyte
(D) Lymphocyte
(E) Eosinophil

41. DNA recombination is important in the development of immunologic diversity. Which one of the following is involved in this process?

(A) Recombinase enzymes
(B) Pentameric recognition signals
(C) 7–11 spacer sequence
(D) Transduction
(E) Transformation

42. Which of the following disorders is characterized by overproduction of monoclonal IgG?

(A) Serum sickness
(B) Asthma
(C) Waldenström's macroglobulinemia
(D) Hypersensitivity pneumonitis
(E) Multiple myeloma

43. Immunosuppressive measures are most effective when administered

(A) immediately before antigen exposure
(B) 1 week before antigen exposure
(C) 1 week after antigen exposure
(D) 1 month before antigen exposure
(E) 1 month after antigen exposure

44. A 28-year-old woman has recently been placed on hydralazine therapy to control her high blood pressure. She is now experiencing some arthralgic pain, and her urine has a pink color. A butterfly rash is noted on physical examination. Which of the following is the most likely diagnosis?

(A) Amyotrophic lateral sclerosis
(B) Systemic lupus erythematosus (SLE)
(C) Sjögren's syndrome
(D) Guillain-Barré syndrome
(E) Goodpasture's syndrome

Grouped questions, 45 and 46:

A 36-year-old woman is stung on the neck by a wasp. Within minutes, she develops urticaria and tightness in the chest and is brought to the emergency department.

45. This reaction is caused by

(A) IgA antibody
(B) Tdth lymphocytes
(C) IgG antibody and complement
(D) IgM antibody and complement
(E) IgE antibody

46. The most appropriate next step is to administer which one of the following?

(A) Antihistamine
(B) Cardiopulmonary resuscitation (CPR)
(C) Corticosteroids
(D) Epinephrine
(E) Cromolyn sodium

47. The major immunoregulatory effect of interferon-γ (IFN-γ) seems to be

(A) differentiation of plasma cells
(B) enhancement of natural killer (NK) cells and macrophages
(C) suppression of cell-mediated immunity
(D) enhancement of antibody production
(E) provision of passive immunity

48. Which of the following statements about natural killer (NK) cells is true?

(A) They lack granules in their cytoplasm.
(B) They lack Fas protein in their membrane.
(C) They lack Fc receptors in their membrane.
(D) They secrete interleukin (IL)-1.
(E) They kill malignant cells by inducing pore formation in the target cell membrane.

49. The most likely combination for producing erythroblastosis fetalis (a hemolytic disease of the newborn) is

(A) Rh+ mother, Rh− father, Rh− child
(B) Rh− mother, Rh+ father, Rh+ child
(C) Rh− mother, Rh+ father, Rh− child
(D) Rh+ mother, Rh+ father, Rh+ child
(E) Rh+ mother, Rh+ father, Rh− child

50. Erythroblastosis fetalis can be prevented if the mother is injected with an antibody specific for the Rh antigen. The recommended schedule for this immunoprophylactic injection is

(A) a single injection given before conception
(B) a single injection given immediately after the birth of the first Rh-positive offspring
(C) single injections given at parturition for each pregnancy
(D) injections given at 26 weeks of gestation and again at parturition for each pregnancy and at the termination of any abortion
(E) injections given at 26 weeks of gestation in each pregnancy

51. A diminutive 5-year-old boy who has had repeated pulmonary infections with agents such as *Staphylococcus epidermidis* and *Klebsiella pneumoniae* and had a normal recovery from chickenpox at 16 months. Which of the following would be the most appropriate therapeutic measure?

(A) Injection of pooled gamma globulin (human)
(B) Fetal thymus transplant
(C) Injection of purified capsular carbohydrate vaccine
(D) Injection of specific immune globulin (human)
(E) Bone marrow transplant

52. Which of the antigens listed below has the highest correlation of occurrence in a patient with primary carcinoma of the liver?

(A) Carcinoembryonic antigen (CEA)
(B) α-Fetoprotein (AFP)
(C) Common acute lymphoblastic leukemia antigen (CALLA)
(D) Prostate specific antigen (PSA)
(E) Hepatitis B surface antigen (HBsAg)

53. Macrophages are the phagocytic cells that predominate in a chronic inflammatory lesion such as seen in the lungs of a patient with tuberculosis. They are derived from blood monocytes. Which of the following is a product of macrophages that induces an antiviral state in neighboring cells?

(A) Complement
(B) Properdin
(C) Lysozyme
(D) Interferon (IFN)-α
(E) Interferon (IFN)-γ

54. Which one of the following is true about the T-cell receptor (TcR)?

(A) It has a hinge region that gives it flexibility.
(B) It is bivalent.
(C) It is associated with the CD3 protein complex in the membrane.
(D) It is present in low numbers on T-helper lymphocytes.
(E) It is readily secreted from the cell.

55. An Rh-negative 23-year-old mother who has recently become engaged to her high school sweetheart (not the father of her child) is concerned about the possibility of Rh disease in subsequent children. She received $Rh_o(D)$ immune globulin after delivery of her first child. The most important step to be taken at this time is to determine the

(A) ABO blood group of her fiancée
(B) Rh antigen profile of her fiancée
(C) Rh antibody level in her serum
(D) Rh antigen profile of her first child
(E) Rh antibody level in her first child

56. Which one of the following substances secreted by tumor cells can favor tumor growth?

(A) Antibodies
(B) Interleukin-1 (IL-1)
(C) Muramyl dipeptide
(D) Tumor-specific transplantation antigens (TSTAs)
(E) Tumor necrosis factor (TNF)

57. Which of the following infectious agents can infect and activate B cells?

(A) Epstein-Barr virus
(B) Herpes zoster
(C) Measles virus
(D) *Bordetella pertussis*
(E) Bacille Calmette Guérin (BCG)

58. Most antibody is synthesized within which of the following structures?

(A) Central lymphoid organs
(B) Peripheral lymphoid organs
(C) Thymus
(D) Macrophages
(E) Golgi apparatus

59. An 18-month-old infant who has had thrush almost constantly since birth, although he seems to have no problem fighting other infectious agents. Which of the following would be the most appropriate therapeutic measure?

(A) Injection of pooled gamma globulin (human)
(B) Injection of specific immune globulin (human)
(C) Transfusion of erythrocytes
(D) Bone marrow transplant
(E) Fetal thymus transplant

60. An 8-year-old boy had a sore throat for 1 week. Three weeks later he developed fever and had pain in his right knee. His mother gave him aspirin, and he improved. Three days later, his urine turned pink. Urinalysis reveals 3+ protein and numerous red blood cells (RBCs). Of the following diseases, which one is the proper diagnosis for this boy?

(A) Goodpasture's disease
(B) Poststreptococcal glomerulonephritis
(C) Systemic lupus erythematosus (SLE)
(D) Wegener's granulomatosus
(E) Reye's syndrome

61. Molecules involved in opsonization of bacteria include which of the following?

(A) Immunoglobulin E (IgE)
(B) C3a
(C) C5a
(D) C3a receptor
(E) C3b receptor

62. The patient has been on dialysis for 3 years waiting for an organ match. One is finally found and the surgery is performed. Which of the following drugs could be used to inhibit the transcription of the interleukin-2 (IL-2) gene?

(A) Azathioprine
(B) Cyclophosphamide
(C) Cyclosporine
(D) Corticosteroid
(E) Antilymphocyte globulin

63. The process of phagocytosis is extremely important in protection from, and recover after, microbial infections. Opsonins sensitize particles for engulfment and hence are an integral part of this process. Which of the following is a glycoprotein that reacts nonspecifically with bacteria to enhance phagocytosis?

(A) Immunoglobulin G1 (IgG1)
(B) Fibronectin
(C) C3a
(D) Lysozyme
(E) Leukotriene B_4

Grouped question, 64 and 65:

A married couple requests blood typing of their 2-year-old son. His pregnant mother is type A negative. Results of hemagglutination assays of the child's blood are as follows: (+ = hemagglutination; − = no hemagglutination)
Anti-A plus child's RBC: +
Anti-B plus child's RBC: −
Anti-D plus child's RBC: +

64. Which one of the following is the child's blood type?

(A) A +
(B) B +
(C) C +
(D) AB +
(E) O −

65. What blood group antigen (inherited from the father) would most likely cause serious hemolytic disease in future children?

(A) A
(B) B
(C) Either A or B
(D) D
(E) Neither A or B

66. A 23-year-old pregnant woman is exposed to German measles (rubella) while student teaching at a local elementary school. She should be injected with what vaccines/immunogens?

(A) Recombivax (HBsAg)
(B) Measles–mumps–rubella (MMR)
(C) Bacille Calmette Guérin (BCG)
(D) Immune globulin (IG)
(E) Specific immune globulin

67. A 36-year-old man has recently developed hemoptosis, hematuria, and signs of severe glomerulonephritis. Examination of his serum reveals the presence of an antibody specific for an antigen shared by the kidney and lung. Which of the following is the most likely diagnosis?

(A) Amyotrophic lateral sclerosis
(B) Systemic lupus erythematosus
(C) Sjögren's syndrome
(D) Guillain-Barré syndrome
(E) Goodpasture's syndrome

68. Which of the following is a component of acquired immunity?

(A) Turbulence in the upper airway
(B) Natural killer (NK) lymphocytes
(C) Lysozyme
(D) T lymphocytes
(E) Complement

69. A 72-year-old man presents with shingles; biopsy and radiographic evidence support a diagnosis of multiple myeloma. From the list below, select the antigen whose occurrence is most highly correlated with the disease.

(A) α-Fetoprotein (AFP)
(B) Bence Jones protein
(C) Carcinoembryonic antigen (CEA)
(D) Oncofetal antigen
(E) Hepatitis B core antigen (HBcAg)

70. The delicate balance between effective chemotherapy and iatrogenic (physician-induced) disease is well exemplified in the treatment of human malignancies. Many of the therapeutic agents used to arrest the growth of the cancer cells also will cause which one of the following conditions?

(A) Hepatotoxic manifestations
(B) Aplastic anemia
(C) Immunosuppression
(D) Drug allergies
(E) Autoimmune diseases

71. A kidney transplant from a cadaver donor is most likely a(n)

(A) autograft
(B) isograft
(C) allograft
(D) xenograft
(E) lifesaving event in a patient with systemic lupus erythematosus

72. Autoimmune diseases due to antibody may be prevented by the emergence of which of the following?

(A) Formation of antigen–antibody complexes
(B) Antibody blocking a cell receptor
(C) Antibody-induced phagocytosis
(D) Antibody-induced complement-mediated lysis
(E) Antigen-induced deletion of T helper cell clones

73. A healthy 24-year-old woman requires immunization prior to beginning a job as a dental hygienist. She has had no immunizations since 15 years of age. Which of the following vaccines should she receive?

(A) Pneumovax
(B) *Haemophilus influenzae* type B vaccine
(C) Cholera vaccine
(D) Hepatitis B subunit vaccine
(E) Oral polio vaccine

74. A 4-year-old patient has a history of repeated infections. History reveals congenital absence of the parathyroid glands, accompanied by rudimentary development of the thymus. Which of the following is the most appropriate treatment for this patient?

(A) Transfusion of neutrophils
(B) Bone marrow transplant
(C) Fetal thymus transplant
(D) Infusion of adenosine deaminase
(E) Thymectomy

75. A 29-year-old pregnant woman is exposed to rubella virus when her son who is in kindergarten contracts a case of German measles. Realizing the potential for in utero damage to her fetus, the physician elects to immunize her. Which of the following immunizations should she receive?

(A) Injection of pooled gamma globulin (human)
(B) Injection of specific immune globulin (human)
(C) Measles–mumps–rubella (MMR) vaccine
(D) Live attenuated varicella virus vaccine
(E) Killed rubella virus vaccine

76. This 18-year-old drug abuser brings her 15-month-old son into the emergency room. The child has a sore throat, pulmonary rales and a severe yeast infection of 2 months duration. Cervical lymph nodes and spleen are somewhat enlarged. Laboratory report reveals normal immunoglobulin (Ig) levels, and a complete blood cell count (CBC) that is unremarkable except for a moderate lymphopenia. Which of the following is the most appropriate laboratory procedure used in serodiagnosis of AIDS?

(A) Enzyme-linked immunosorbent assay (ELISA)
(B) Immunofluorescence
(C) Hemagglutination inhibition
(D) Virus neutralization
(E) Latex agglutination

77. The patient is a 24-year-old woman with arthralgia, joint inflammation, and IgM antibodies specific for her own IgG molecules. Immune complex deposition and complement activation are causing localized inflammation. Which of the following is the most appropriate laboratory procedure used in serodiagnosis of this disease?

(A) Enzyme-linked immunosorbent assay (ELISA)
(B) Immunofluorescence
(C) Hemagglutination inhibition
(D) Virus neutralization
(E) Latex agglutination
(F) Radioimmunoassay
(G) Radial immunodiffusion
(H) Coombs' test

78. During inflammatory responses and the immune response, the body recruits progenitor cells from the bone marrow. Which of the following interleukins causes stem cell proliferation?

(A) Interleukin (IL)-2
(B) IL-3
(C) IL-4
(D) IL-8
(E) IL-12

79. Which of the antigens listed below has the highest correlation of occurrence in a patient with cancer of the prostate?

(A) α-Fetoprotein (AFP)
(B) Common acute lymphoblastic leukemia antigen (CALLA)
(C) Prostate specific antigen (PSA)
(D) urinary Bence-Jones protein
(E) Carcinoembryonic antigen

80. The patient has a significant weight loss in spite of robust eating habits. Serum analysis detects anti-thyroid-stimulating hormone (TSH) antibodies. Which of the following is the most appropriate treatment for this patient with Graves' disease?

(A) Infusion of adenosine deaminase
(B) Thymectomy
(C) Splenectomy
(D) Thyroidectomy
(E) Injection of specific equine immune globulin

81. Lysis of foreign cells is an important aspect of immunity. Which of the following describes a group of serum proteins that can lyse gram-negative bacteria that have antibody on their surface?

(A) Complement
(B) Lactoferrin
(C) Lysozyme
(D) Lactoperoxidase
(E) Interferon (IFN)-γ

82. A substance that can evoke either a humoral or a cell-mediated immune response is termed a(an)

(A) immunogen
(B) hapten
(C) epitope
(D) antigen
(E) adjuvant

83. Which of the antigens listed below has the highest correlation of occurrence in a patient with colorectal carcinoma?

(A) Carcinoembryonic antigen (CEA)
(B) α-Fetoprotein (AFP)
(C) Common acute lymphoblastic leukemia antigen (CALLA)
(D) Prostate specific antigen (PSA)
(E) Bence-Jones protein

84. During a normal immune response, an individual makes IgM antibodies first followed by IgG or another class of antibody. Which of the following interleukins plays an important role in this class switching?

(A) Interleukin 1 (IL-1)
(B) IL-2
(C) IL-3
(D) IL-4
(E) IL-10

85. Which of the following is prepared from human volunteers that have been immunized against a particular microbe?

(A) Immune globulin (IG)
(B) Specific immune globulin
(C) DNA vaccine
(D) RhoGAM
(E) Antivenin

86. Asthma is a serious allergy which kills approximately 5, 000 people (usually children) in the United States each year. IgE is the antibody that is primarily involved in this sensitivity. Which of the following interleukins promotes IgE production?

(A) Interleukin 12 (IL-12)
(B) IL-8
(C) IL-4
(D) IL-2
(E) IL-1

87. A 39-year-old pathologist with chronic active hepatitis, which he acquired in a work-related incident 8 years ago, has lost 15 pounds in 2 months; there is tenderness and a friction rub over his liver. Which of the proteins below is the one whose occurrence is most highly correlated with the disease?

(A) α-Fetoprotein (AFP)
(B) Anti- hepatitis B surface antigen (HbsAg) antibody
(C) Hepatitis B core antigen (HbcAg)
(D) Myeloma protein
(E) Carcinoembryonic antigen (CEA)

88. A jaundiced premature infant has a total serum bilirubin concentration of 15mg/dl, and 10% nucleated erythrocytes in a peripheral blood smear. Which of the following is the most appropriate laboratory procedure used in serodiagnosis of erythroblastosis fetalis?

(A) Hemagglutination inhibition
(B) Latex agglutination
(C) Radioimmunoassay
(D) Radial immunodiffusion
(E) Coombs' test

89. An 18-month-old boy presents with severe recurrent *Haemophilus influenzae* otitis media. Serum analysis reveals absence of all five immunoglobulin classes. The child has had two episodes of pneumonia has also had trouble with boils. From the list below, select the hereditary immune deficiency disease with defective maturation of pre-B cells.

(A) Bruton's X-linked agammaglobulinemia
(B) Severe combined immunodeficiency disease
(C) AIDS
(D) Chronic granulomatous disease
(E) Neutropenia

90. Which of the following substances blocks interleukin 2 (IL-2) gene expression?

(A) IL-2 receptor
(B) IL-1
(C) Interferon-γ (IFN-γ)
(D) Cyclosporine
(E) IL-10

91. Human plasma can kill and lyse gram-negative bacteria. This is the result of the presence of which of the following molecules?

(A) Immunoglobulin E (IgE) antibody against the organism
(B) Complement
(C) Lactoferrin
(D) Hydrogen peroxide
(E) Lactoperoxidase

Grouped questions—92 and 93.

A 9-year-old boy's mother received a frantic call from the teacher who was hosting a picnic as part of the class visit to the zoo. The boy's tongue, lips, and cheek were grossly swollen. He was having difficulty breathing.

92. This boy is experiencing a severe

(A) anaphylactic reaction
(B) bronchospasm brought on by exertion
(C) cardiovascular collapse
(D) delirium episode
(E) panic attack

93. The therapy for this boy should include

(A) cromolyn sodium
(B) epinephrine
(C) histamine
(D) antihistamine
(E) phosphodiesterase

94. A 6-year-old boy is hospitalized for lobar pneumonia. A culture of his sputum yielded many colonies of catalase-positive, gram-positive cocci. Past history indicated that the patient had numerous recurrent infections including boils and other staphylococcal infections. Complement and immunoglobulin levels were normal. There was a 17-mm area of induration at the site of a candidin injection (read at 48 hours). A nitroblue tetrazolium (NBT) test is negative (i.e., no dye reduction). Therapy for this patient should include antibiotics to control the infection and which one of the following actions?

(A) Injection of specific human immune globulin
(B) Infusion of neutrophils
(C) Bone marrow transplant
(D) Fetal thymus transplant
(E) Infusion of adenosine deaminase

95. A 9-year-old boy who is recovering from a serious viral infection of unknown etiology now has a petechial rash and blood in his urine and stools. His platelet count is severely depressed and serum studies reveal the presence of immunoglobulin G (IgG) antibodies on the patient's own platelets. Antinuclear antibodies and rheumatoid factor are absent. Which of the following is the most likely diagnosis?

(A) Rheumatoid arthritis
(B) Sjögren's syndrome
(C) Systemic lupus erythematosus (SLE)
(D) Idiopathic thrombocytopenic purpura (ITP)
(E) Atopic dermatitis

96. Which of the following is an accurate description of the complement component C1?

(A) It is composed of five polypeptide chains—one C1q, two C1r, and two C1s.
(B) It is part of both the classical and alternative pathways.
(C) The activated form is an opsonin.
(D) Deficiencies of this protein lead to hereditary angioedema.
(E) Its natural substrate is C3.

97. Immunity in the respiratory tract depends on which of the following?

(A) Lactoferrin
(B) Macrophages
(C) Lysozyme
(D) Flushing action of saliva
(E) Locally produced IgD

98. The patient has just experienced a complicated pregnancy and delivery. She had fatty liver of pregnancy which had destroyed all hepatic function. She has received a cadaver transplant. Which of the following drugs would most likely be used to reduce the number of circulating lymphocytes and interfere with the production of lymphokines?

(A) Azathioprine
(B) Cyclosporine
(C) Corticosteroid
(D) Antilymphocyte globulin
(E) Actinomycin D

99. Features of major histocompatibility complex (MHC) control of the immune response include which of the following?

(A) CD molecule recognition
(B) thymus independence
(C) regulation through the action of B cells
(D) class III molecule participation
(E) B7–CD28 interactions in B cell activation

100. A primary immune response differs from secondary immune response in that the former has (a)

(A) shorter latent period
(B) more antibody produced
(C) longer duration of antibody production
(D) different class of immunoglobulin produced
(E) different specificity of antibody produced

101. A 5-year-old boy has had repeated pyogenic infections. An immune status evaluation indicates that he has normal immunoglobulins in his serum. Recently, he had chickenpox with no unexpected clinical problems. While playing in an abandoned barn, the boy's foot was punctured by a nail. He received the standard diphtheria-tetanus-pertussis (DTP) immunization series beginning at 2 months of age. What should he receive now to protect him from tetanus?

(A) Tetanus toxoid
(B) Tetanus antitoxin (human)
(C) Both toxoid and antitoxin at the site of injury
(D) Toxoid in one arm and antitoxin in the gluteus maximus
(E) No treatment

102. Anti-tumor products of macrophages include which one of the following?

(A) Perforin molecules
(B) INF-γ
(C) Fas protein
(D) Granzymes
(E) Toxic oxygen metabolites

103. A 28-year-old woman has the recent on-set of joint stiffness, ankle edema, and facial swelling. Urinalysis shows 3+ protein with a sediment containing 5 erythrocytes per high-power field (hpf) and 4 leukocytes/hpf. A tentative diagnosis of systemic lupus erythematous (SLE) has been made. What diagnostic tests might confirm this diagnosis?

(A) Rheumatoid factor
(B) Salivary duct antibody
(C) Anti-centromere antibody
(D) Anti-ds DNA antibody
(E) Depressed C3 levels

104. A 5-year-old child has been injured in a motor vehicle crash. To protect him from tetanus, a single booster injection of toxoid is given. Which of the following characteristics best describes the anamnestic response to the toxoid in comparison with the primary immune response?

(A) Lag period is longer after antigenic stimulus.
(B) More antibody is produced.
(C) IgM production predominates.
(D) More immunogen is required.
(E) It characterizes the immune response to carbohydrate antigens.

105. Which of the following DNA segments contribute to the constant portion of the IgM heavy (H) chain?

(A) V_H genes
(B) J_H genes
(C) D_H genes
(D) C_μ genes
(E) N-region additions

106. Endotoxins of gram-negative bacteria cause fever by direct action on the hypothalamus. They also cause a second fever response. Which of the following is the endogenous pyrogen produced by macrophages?

(A) Interleukin 1 (IL-1)
(B) IL-2
(C) IL-3
(D) IL-8
(E) IL-12

107. A 72-year-old woman presents with shingles; biopsy and radiographic evidence to support a diagnosis of multiple myeloma. She should be injected with what vaccine?

(A) Immunoglobulins intramuscular (IGIM)
(B) Varicella-zoster immune globulin (VZIG)
(C) Recombivax hepatitis B surface antigen (HBsAg)
(D) Varicella live attenuated viral vaccine
(E) Bacille Calmette Guérin (BCG)

108. Tetanus neonatorum kills hundreds of thousands of children in third world countries each year. Which one of the following ways would best provide immunologic protection for these children?

(A) Inject the infant with human tetanus anti-toxin.
(B) Inject the newborn with tetanus toxoid.
(C) Inject the mother with antitoxin 72 hours before the birth of her child.
(D) Immunize the mother with tetanus toxoid in early pregnancy.
(E) Give the child antitoxin and toxoid for both passive and active immunization.

109. A 56-year-old man who presents with constipation and abdominal cramping that has persisted for 2 months has a guaiac-positive stool; digital examination detects a palpable rectal mass. Which of the antigens below is the one whose occurrence is most highly correlated with the disease?

(A) Bence Jones protein
(B) Carcinoembryonic antigen (CEA)
(C) Oncofetal antigen
(D) Hepatitis B core antigen (HbcAg)
(E) Hepatitis C antigen (HCAg)

110. A 32-year-old woman has a 10-year history of arthralgia, a rash that waxes and wanes in intensity, and symptoms of glomerulonephritis. She has recently developed dry mucus membranes. Which of the following is the most likely diagnosis?

(A) Amyotrophic lateral sclerosis (ALS)
(B) Systemic lupus erythematosus (SLE)
(C) Sjögren's syndrome
(D) Guillain-Barré syndrome
(E) Goodpasture's syndrome

111. Which of the following can interfere with development of anti Rho antibodies in mothers, thus protecting infants from erythroblastosis fetalis?

(A) Cytotoxic T cells
(B) $Rh_o(D)$ immunoglobulin (RhoGAM)
(C) Interferon-γ (IFN-γ)
(D) Coombs serum
(E) Interleukin 10 (IL-10)

112. A 4-year-old child suffering from repeated infections with staphylococci and streptococci was found to have normal phagocytic function and delayed hypersensitivity responses. Lymph node biopsy probably would reveal

(A) depletion of thymus-dependent regions
(B) intact germinal centers
(C) hyperplastic juxtamedullary regions
(D) lack of plasma cells
(E) absence of dendritic cells

113. This 3-year-old has a history of repeated chronic pulmonary infections. No antibodies are detected in his serum: complement and phagocytic functions are normal. Which of the following laboratory procedures was used in serodiagnosis of this disease?

(A) Enzyme-linked immunosorbent assay (ELISA)
(B) Immunofluorescence
(C) Latex agglutination
(D) Radial immunodiffusion
(E) Coombs' test

114. An 8-year-old boy was brought to his family pediatrician suffering from repeated painful bouts of inflammation of mucosal surfaces, especially the lips. The mother reports that similar symptoms occurred in previous generations of her family. From the list below, select the disease that has hereditary deficiency of a complement control protein.

(A) Hereditary angioedema
(B) Meningococcal meningitis
(C) Severe combined immunodeficiency disease
(D) Hemolytic disease of the newborn
(E) Chronic granulomatous disease

115. Which of the following infectious agents enhances macrophage and natural killer (NK) cell activity?

(A) *Listeria monocytogenes*
(B) *Candida albicans*
(C) *Herpes zoster*
(D) *Bordetella pertussis*
(E) Bacille Calmette Guérin (BCG)

116. Compared with the other classes of immunoglobulins, IgG is predominant in which one of the following ways?

(A) Complement activation
(B) Major component of primary immune response to most antigens
(C) Enhanced phagocytosis
(D) Production by the fetus
(E) Response to thymus independent antigens

117. A 2-year-old girl with partial albinism is suffering from recurrent bacterial infections. Polymorphonuclear (PMN) leukocytes contain peroxidase-positive inclusions. A diagnosis of Chédiak-Higashi disease is made. Which of the following antimicrobial products would be ineffective in this patient?

(A) Lysozyme
(B) Hydrogen peroxide
(C) Superoxide anion
(D) Myeloperoxidase
(E) Singlet oxygen

118. Which of the following interleukins down regulates Th 1 cells and thus inhibits the cytokine synthesis?

(A) IL-4
(B) IL-6
(C) IL-8
(D) IL-9
(E) IL-10

119. Which of the following vaccines should a veterinarian receive to protect him from an occupational hazard?

(A) Rabies vaccine
(B) Tetanus toxoid vaccine
(C) Cholera vaccine
(D) Influenza vaccine
(E) Anthrax vaccine

120. An important characteristic of inflammatory responses is the influx of phagocytic cells into the area of damage. Which of the following interleukins is a chemotaxin?

(A) Interleukin 1 (IL-1)
(B) IL-8
(C) IL12
(D) IL-4
(E) IL-9

121. A previously healthy 18-year-old naval seaman is brought to the emergency department because he is comatose. His temperature is 41° C (106° F) and pulse is 200 beats per minute. His blood pressure is unobtainable. He has a dusky rash over the extremities. Laboratory studies show a platelet count of 30,000/mm3 and a prolonged prothrombin time. Which of the following vaccines would have protected this recruit?

(A) Adenoviral vaccine
(B) Pneumovax
(C) Cholera vaccine
(D) Meningococcal capsule vaccine
(E) Anthrax vaccine

122. A 4-year-old child suffering from repeated infections with staphylococci and streptococci was found to have normal antibody levels and delayed hypersensitivity responses. A diagnosis of chronic granulomatous disease is made on the basis of nitroblue tetrazolium dye reduction assay. Which of the following is the most appropriate treatment for this patient?

(A) Injection of specific human immune globulin
(B) Infusion of neutrophils
(C) Bone marrow transplant
(D) Fetal thymus transplant
(E) Injection of pooled gamma globulin

123. Which of the following vaccines should an individual with advanced sickle cell disease complicated by functional asplenia receive?

(A) Tetanus toxoid vaccine
(B) Pneumovax
(C) *Haemophilus influenzae* type B vaccine
(D) Hepatitis B subunit vaccine
(E) Meningococcal capsule vaccine

124. Transplantation of the thymus gland from an aborted fetus to an immunodeficient neonate has been beneficial in which of the following immunodeficiency disorders?

(A) Chédiak-Higashi syndrome
(B) DiGeorge syndrome
(C) Bruton's hypogammaglobulinemia
(D) Hereditary angioedema
(E) Wiskott-Aldrich syndrome

125. Which of the following cells is the most susceptible to tolerance induction?

(A) T helper cell
(B) B cell
(C) Macrophage
(D) Cytotoxic T cell
(E) Plasma cell

126. Eczema, low platelet numbers (thrombocytopenia), and low levels of immunoglobulin M (IgM) are clues for the presence of which of the following immune deficiency diseases?

(A) Bruton's disease
(B) Graves' disease
(C) Wiskott-Aldrich syndrome
(D) DiGeorge syndrome
(E) CREST syndrome (calcinosis, Raynaud's phenomenon, esophageal dysmotility, sclerodactyly, and telangiectasia)

127. Several types of immunologic rejection reactions can occur following organ transplantation. The rejection reaction caused by preformed antibodies in the recipient is referred to as

(A) acute
(B) hyperacute
(C) chronic
(D) immediate
(E) accelerated

128. A 3-year-old presents with a high fever and a stiff neck. Spinal fluid analysis reveals an elevated opening pressure, pleocytosis, a decrease in glucose content (20% of blood glucose levels), and increased levels of immunoglobulins. Patient has received no childhood vaccinations. What vaccine could have prevented this disease?

(A) Pneumovax
(B) *Haemophilus influenzae* type B conjugated vaccine
(C) Cholera vaccine
(D) Hepatitis B subunit vaccine
(E) Rabies vaccine

129. An outbreak of meningitis and septicemia is occurring at Ft. Leonard Wood. Twenty-five percent of the recruits are ill; a true medical epidemic. One soldier has already died; autopsy revealed bilateral adrenal cortical necrosis. What vaccine has been developed by the Department of Defense to prevent this type of epidemic?

(A) Pneumovax
(B) Meningococcal capsule vaccine
(C) Anthrax vaccine
(D) Adenoviral vaccine
(E) Cholera vaccine

130. Which of the following substances is a cytokine that enhances proliferation of B cells?

(A) Interleukin-1 (IL-1)
(B) Lipopolysaccharide
(C) Interferon-γ
(D) IL-4
(E) IL-2

131. A bone marrow transplant from mother to daughter can be characterized as which of the following types of transplants?

(A) Allogeneic
(B) Autologous
(C) Heterogenic
(D) Idiotypic
(E) Syngeneic

132. A bone marrow transfer between identical twins can be characterized as which of the following types of transplants?

(A) Allogeneic
(B) Autologous
(C) Heterogenic
(D) Idiotypic
(E) Syngeneic

ANSWERS AND EXPLANATIONS

1. The answer is A. [Chapter 5 VII A 1 b (1); Figure 5-8]. There is no need to give this child another tetanus toxoid booster shot. Her anamnestic response has already been activated, and she has plenty of antitoxin in her blood. The wound should be cleaned to prevent infection.

2. The answer is C. [Chapter 7 II C 2 a]. IgE has been produced in this man as a result of prior exposure to something he ate—most likely a shellfish, such as lobster or crab. These homocytotropic antibodies have coated basophils and mast cells. Cross-linking of this cell-bound antibody by allergen causes these cells to degranulate and release histamine, which is causing the symptoms seen in this individual.

3. The answer is D [Chapter 8 II E]. Guillain-Barré syndrome (acute idiopathic polyneuritis) manifests as progressive weakness, first of the lower extremities and then of the upper extremities and respiratory muscles. Peripheral nerve tissue shows perivascular mononuclear cell infiltrate and demyelination. It is a transient autoimmune disease triggered by viral infections or vaccines (e.g., influenza viral vaccine). Patients recover full function of affected nerves and muscles between 6 and 12 months after the onset of the disease. Sjögren's syndrome is a chronic inflammatory disease that primarily affects secretory glands such as the lacrimal and salivary glands, producing dry eyes (keratoconjunctivitis sicca) and dry mouth (xerostomia). Goodpasture's syndrome is a relatively rare disorder with symptoms referable to both the lungs (e.g., pulmonary hemorrhage) and kidneys (e.g., glomerulonephritis). The immunoglobulin G (IgG) deposited on alveolar and glomerular basement membranes appears to be specific for type IV collagen shared by the kidneys and lungs. Systemic lupus erythematosus (SLE) is a chronic, inflammatory systemic (multiorgan) disease that primarily affects women. A characteristic feature is the erythematous butterfly rash that occurs on the face of some patients. Death usually results from renal failure or infection. Amyotrophic lateral sclerosis (ALS; Lou Gehrig's disease) causes progressive degeneration of motor neurons of the spinal cord. ALS typically affects males older than 40 years of age. Some patients have a monoclonal IgM with specificity for ganglioside components of neural membranes. Other autoantibodies have been demonstrated, but immunosuppressive drugs have not proven to be effective.

4. The answer is B [Chapter 10 I C 7 c]. Graft-versus-host disease occurs when immunocompetent T cells are transferred into an immunologically immature or incompetent recipient. A critical step in preparation for bone marrow transplantation is severe immunosuppression, which makes the recipient particularly susceptible to graft-versus-host disease. Cytopenia, rash, diarrhea, and weight loss are characteristic symptoms of this condition.

5. The answer is C [Chapter 5 IX B 2 b (2) (c)]. Cyclosporine (cyclosporin A) is a fungal antibiotic that binds to the membrane phospholipids of lymphocytes and is internalized by pinocytosis. In the cytoplasm, it binds to an enzyme called cytophilin. By interfering with proper protein-chain folding, cyclosporine blocks transmission of cytosolic messages from the antigen receptor to the nucleus. Thus, interleukin-2 (IL-2) gene expression is blocked, and the Th cells are unable to synthesize this lymphokine. Cyclosporine also inhibits the production of interferon-γ (IFN-γ) by activated T cells.

6–8. The answers are: 6-D, 7-B, 8-F [Chapter 10 I C 3b,-c]. Human tissue typing is accomplished by exposing donor or recipient lymphocytes to a battery of antisera of known human leukocyte antigen (HLA) specificity. Peripheral blood lymphocytes are used because they are a convenient source of cells that have a high concentration of HLA antigens on their surface. The typing sera are obtained from multiparous women who have been exposed to HLA antigens of the male partner, from graft recipients who have rejected a graft, from individuals who have had multiple transfusions, or from sensitized donors. Complement (usually rabbit serum) is added to the mixture as the lytic agent. When the cells are killed by the antiserum and complement, the cell is presumed to have the same HLA antigen as the specificity of the antiserum. To visualize the dead and living cells microscopically, a vital dye such as eosin Y is added; dead cells take up the dye, and live cells exclude it. The antigen profile of the cells in the assay can be determined by examining the HLA specificities of the antisera that gave the highest cytotoxicity. Thus, antisera A-3, A-4, and A-5 were the most active. Because A-4 reacted only with A3 HLA specificity, it is known that one of the antigens must be A-3. That A-28 is the other HLA-A specificity is inferred from the observation that antiserum A-3 (specificity versus A-2 only) was only minimally toxic to the cells.

The HLA-B profile is deduced in a similar manner. B-7 is identified because antiserum B-1 was highly cytotoxic (suggesting either specificity B-7 or B-27). This is corroborated by the fact that antiserum B-2 (active versus B-7 and B-45) was cytotoxic but antiserum B-6 (single specificity versus B-45) was not. Antiserum B-5 (single specificity versus B-44) was highly cytotoxic.

The absence of cytotoxicity when the cells were incubated with antiserum A-6 shows that the patient's lymphocyte does not have the A-10 nor A-11 antigens on its membrane.

9. The answer is A [Chapter 6 III B 2]. In the fluorescent treponemal antibody absorption (FTA-ABS) test, *Treponema pallidum,* the etiologic agent of syphilis, is fixed to a slide that is then flooded with the patient's serum. If the patient's serum contains antibodies to *T. pallidum,* the antibodies will react with the spirochetes on the slide. The reaction can be visualized under a fluorescence microscope if fluorescein-labeled anti–human gamma globulin is added to the slide. The FTA-ABS test is an indirect immunofluorescence technique. Direct and indirect immunofluorescence techniques conjugate fluorescent dyes, such as fluorescein isocyanate, to antibody molecules in order to identify antigens.

10. The answer is D [Chapter 7 V C 1 c (1)]. Contact dermatitis (cell-mediated; type IV) reactions are Tdth–cell-dependent reactions manifesting as inflammation at the site of antigen exposure. Tissue damage results from the interaction between sensitized (antigen-reactive) T cells and specific antigen; antibody and complement are not required for these reactions. Contact dermatitis is a form of delayed hypersensitivity, which occurs in response to antigen exposure on skin. In this patient the al-

lergen was nickel which was acting as a hapten that had complexed with carrier proteins in the skin. Delayed hypersensitivity reactions also occur in response to tumors as well as viral, bacterial, fungal, and parasitic infections.

11. The answer is D. [Chapter 9 V D]. Ataxia-telangiectasia is an inherited immunodeficiency disease in which the patient has lack of muscle coordination (ataxia), dilated small blood vessels (telangiectasia), and an increased incidence of sinopulmonary infections, which is probably related to the selective immunoglobulin A (IgA) deficiency. Other immunoglobulins and T-cell functions also may be deficient. Ataxia and telangiectasia are not seen in Bruton's hypogammaglobulinemia, DiGeorge syndrome, severe combined immunodeficiency syndrome (SCID) or Wiskott-Aldrich syndrome. Bruton's is an absence of all immunoglobulins, not just IgA. In SCID not only are immunoglobulins low, but the patient also has depressed cell mediated immunities. DiGeorge syndrome is characterized by hypoplasia of both the thymus (with deficiency of T cell functions) and parathyroid (with calcium metabolism problems). Wiskott-Aldrich syndrome is a defect in IgM synthesis associated with eczema and thrombocytopenia.

12. The answer is E [Chapter 2 V B 6]. Medical students are at risk of exposure to blood contaminated with the hepatitis B virus. The same is true of many health care professionals, technicians, and students who handle human blood as part of their job or training. These people should be immunized with the recombinant vaccine before any exposure. Injection of killed virus vaccine plus passive immunization with specific immunoglobulins is used to immunize infants born to hepatitis B viremic mothers (although more commonly in the U.S. the recombinant vaccine is used instead of the killed virus). There is no live vaccine for hepatitis; however, female health care workers of childbearing age should have full rubella immunization. (Rubella is one of the 3 live, attenuated viruses in the measles-mumps-rubella vaccine [MMR]). Purified capsular vaccines are used in individuals at risk for pneumococcal disease, *Haemophilus influenzae* meningitis, meningococcal meningitis, and whooping cough. Specific immune globulin of equine origin is never given to humans if a human antiserum is available.

13. The answer is A [Chapter 6 III F]. In a radioimmunoassay (RIA), the material being assayed must be immunogenic, because an essential ingredient in the procedure is specific antibody. Further, the immunogen must be labeled with radioactive materials without undergoing any immunologic alterations that would interfere in its reactivity with its homologous antibody. Fluorescein is not used in RIA; it is used to label antibodies for visualizing pathogens or detecting antibodies, and it is used in the fluorescent cell sorter technique for enumeration of T-cell subsets. An antigen containing tritiated thymidine would not emit gamma rays and therefore would not be confused with the iodine-125 detected in the RIA.

14. The answer is D [Chapter 2 V A 1, VI A 3; Chapter 9 III B 1]. The child has not responded to toxin injections received as an infant, so he must be protected with tetanus antitoxin. It would also be advisable to give the young man a primary series of diphtheria-pertussis-tetanus (DPT). In the event that his original antibody deficiency disease was not Bruton's but was transient hypogammaglobulinemia of infancy, he will now be able to respond to the vaccine and develop an active immunity.

15. The answer is A [Chapter 6 IV C 2 c]. Of the tests listed in the question, only the mixed lymphocyte culture reflects the functional status of T cells. The mixed lymphocyte culture, fluorescent antibody assay with CD3 or CD8 antiserum, and erythrocyte (E)-rosette test all measure some T-cell characteristic. CD8 is the membrane marker seen on suppressor and cytotoxic T cells (Ts and Tc cells); CD3 is on all peripheral T cells. T cells form E rosettes when they are mixed with sheep red blood cells (SR-BCs); the E-rosette test is used to quantitate T cells regardless of their subtype. Lipopolysaccharide from the cell walls of gram-negative bacteria (endotoxin) is a potent B-cell mitogen and is used to assay the ability of B cells to proliferate.

16. The answer is D [Chapter 10; Chapter 3 V B 1 b]. Bence Jones protein is one of the myeloma proteins that is produced in the malignant plasma cell during the progression of the tumor. It is commonly excreted in the urine and is found almost exclusively in patients with multiple myeloma. It is composed of light-chain dimers of immunoglobulins and has the unique characteristic of precipitating at 56°C (a pyroglobulin). Prostate-specific antigen (PSA) is associated with prostate disease. Alpha-fetoprotein (AFP) is associated with liver disease. Carcinoembryonic antigen (CEA) is associated with cancer of the colon. Common acute lymphoblastic leukemia antigen (CALLA) is a de-differentiation antigenic marker of B cell leukemias.

17. The answer is A. [Chapter 1 I B 3]. The protective serum contained antibodies against the virus that had been developed in the recovered patients. The antibodies neutralized the virus and aborted its spread through the body. Because the disease had not been detected in the United States, there were no protective antibodies in those blood donors.

18. The answer is E [Chapter 5 XI B 3 b]. Bacille Calmette Guérin (BCG) is a live attenuated strain of *Mycobacterium bovis* that has been used with varying degrees of success for active immunization against tuberculosis. Administration of BCG can also nonspecifically stimulate the immune response. It appears to activate T cells and macrophages and to stimulate natural killer (NK) cells. Its primary effect is on cell-mediated immunity, not humoral antibody–mediated immunity.

19. The answer is B [Chapter 2 VI A 1; Table 2-3]. Botulism is a severe form of food poisoning in which the individual ingests botulinum toxin, which is a potent neurotoxin that interferes with the release of acetylcholine at synapses and myoneural junctions. Flaccid paralysis results. The intoxication can be treated by injection of a polyvalent antitoxin. (There are several different antigenic varieties of botulinum toxin.) The antitoxin is produced in horses and humans; the latter is the preferred therapeutic because its use diminishes the probability of serum sickness.

20. The answer is E. [Chapter 1 V A 3, Table 1-9]. Natural killer (NK) cells are large, granular lymphocytes that are present in the body before antigenic exposure. If they are incubated in the presence of interleukin-2 (IL-2), they are activated to heightened cytotoxicity and are called lymphokine-activated killer (LAK) cells. These cells kill by release of perforin molecules on contact with the target cell. Polyperforin channels form and protease and nuclease enzymes destroy the target, the Fas protein reacts with its ligand in the target membrane and initiates apoptosis. NK cells have receptors for the Fc region of IgG and can participate in antibody-dependent cellular cytotoxicity (ADCC). NK cells kill malignant cells and, as such, are sometimes referred to as the cells of immune surveillance (i.e., they patrol the body and eliminate premalignant conditions).

21. The answer is D [Chapter 2 II A]. The area of an antigen with which an antibody reacts is called an epitope, an antigenic determinant, or a determinant group. Epitopes are usually composed of 4–6 residues (amino acids or monosaccharides). These residues need not be linear within the molecule. They could be separated residues that come into proximity through folding of the molecular chain. The terms "antigen" and "immunogen" refer to the entire molecule. The paratope is the site on the antibody molecule that combines with an epitope. Carriers are molecules, usually proteins, that impart immunogenicity to haptens that are conjugated to them.

22. The answer is C [Chapter 3 V D]. Primary amyloidosis is a plasma cell dyscrasia characterized by the deposition of amyloid fibrils in the vascular endothelium. The amyloid fibrils (termed amyloid light chain, or AL, proteins) are primarily composed of immunoglobulin light (L)-chain fragments. Secondary amyloidosis is amyloidosis that is associated with chronic infection or inflammation; the amyloid fibrils in secondary amyloidosis (termed amyloid A, or AA, proteins) bear no structural resemblance to those seen in primary amyloidosis. All other choices are not related to the disease and should not have been in the differential.

23. The answer is A [Chapter 10 I A 3 b; Table 10-2]. Aplastic anemia is characterized by greatly decreased formation of erythrocytes with resultant low hematocrit and hemoglobin levels. It is usually associated with granulocytopenia and thrombocytopenia as a result of a hypoplastic or aplastic bone marrow. It is treated successfully by bone marrow transplantation, although the recipients have a serious threat of iatrogenic graft-versus-host disease. Recrudescence of latent viral infections (especially cytomegalovirus) is also a life-threatening consequence of the severe immunosuppression that the recipient must un-

dergo. Other diseases that are treated successfully by bone marrow transplantation include sickle cell disease, acute and chronic myelogenous leukemia, thalassemia major, and various immunodeficiency diseases, lymphomas, and solid tumors.

24. The answer is E [Chapter 8 II J 3]. Insulin-dependent diabetes mellitus (type 1) is an autoimmune disease characterized by production of antibodies and cytotoxic T cells reactive with beta cells in the islets of Langerhans. Destruction of these cells removes the source of insulin from the body, necessitating daily injections of the hormone to control glucose metabolism. Pernicious anemia is due to an antibody that blocks absorption of B_{12} from the diet. Systemic lupus erythematosus (SLE) is a multisystem disease with many different antibodies the primary target organs are the kidneys, cardiovascular and central nervous systems. The target in myasthenia gravis (MG) is acetylcholine receptors and skin keratinocyte membrane antigens are the target in pemphigus.

25. The answer is C [Chapter 7 Table 7-3]. The treatment of choice for severe asthma and anaphylaxis is epinephrine. This hormone has two levels of action that are of value in patients with asthma. Epinephrine increases the activity of adenyl cyclase intracytoplasmically in the mast cell, thus raising the level of cyclic adenosine monophosphate (cAMP), which inhibits degranulation. Epinephrine also reacts with a receptor on smooth muscle tissue and causes the muscle to relax, thus reversing the effects of histamine. In addition to these two actions, epinephrine is a potent vasopressor, increasing blood pressure and acting as a cardiac stimulant. Cromolyn sodium (sodium cromoglycate) prevents Ca^{++} influx and thus blocks phosphodiesterase activation. Methylxanthine drugs block the activity of this enzyme. Antihistamines will occupy the site of histamine reaction with host cells and thus interfere with an effect of histamine on smooth muscle; however, they cannot reverse the effect of this amine on tissues once it has reacted with its specific receptor. Blocking (IgG) antibodies react with the allergen and prevent it from reacting with IgE on mast cell and basophil membranes.

26. The answer is B [Chapter 8 II B 1]. Systemic lupus erythematosus (SLE) is a chronic, inflammatory systemic (multiorgan) disease that primarily affects women. A characteristic feature is the erythematous butterfly rash that occurs on the face of some patients. Death usually results from renal failure or infection. Amyotrophic lateral sclerosis (ALS; Lou Gehrig's disease) causes progressive degeneration of motor neurons of the spinal cord. ALS typically affects males older than 40 years of age. Some patients have a monoclonal IgM with specificity for ganglioside components of neural membranes. Other autoantibodies have been demonstrated, but immunosuppressive drugs have not proven to be effective. Sjögren's syndrome is a chronic inflammatory disease that primarily affects secretory glands such as the lacrimal and salivary glands, producing dry eyes (keratoconjunctivitis sicca) and dry mouth (xerostomia). Guillain-Barré syndrome (acute idiopathic polyneuritis) manifests as progressive weakness, first of the lower extremities and then of the upper extremities and respiratory muscles. Peripheral nerve tissue shows perivascular mononuclear cell infiltrate and demyelination. It is a transient autoimmune disease triggered by viral infections or vaccines (e.g., influenza viral vaccine). Patients will recover full function of affected nerves and muscles between 6 and 12 months after the onset of the disease. Goodpasture's syndrome is a relatively rare disorder with symptoms referable to both the lungs (e.g., pulmonary hemorrhage) and kidneys (e.g., glomerulonephritis). The immunoglobulin G (IgG) deposited on alveolar and glomerular basement membranes appears to be specific for a collagen antigen shared by the kidneys and lungs.

27. The answer is C [Chapter 4 I A, D]. The complement proteins are naturally occurring molecules that function to protect the body from various infectious agents. The biologic roles of these proteins include chemotaxis, opsonization, increased capillary permeability, and cell lysis. Anamnesis, B-cell mediation, specificity, and long induction time are all characteristics of acquired or adaptive immune responses.

28. The answer is C [Chapter 1 IV B 3 c]. Interferon-γ (IFN-γ) is a potent immunoregulatory molecule that activates (i.e., up-regulates) all of the cells of the immune system—not only the natural killer (NK) and phagocytic cells of the innate immune system, but the B and T cells of the acquired immune system as well.

IFN-γ is released from T cells, not B cells, when they are stimulated by an antigen or a mitogen. The cytokine is released from the T cell when that cell specifically binds the appropriate homologous antigen. IFN-γ then reacts with receptors on its target cells to effect its regulatory functions.

29. The answer is E [Chapter 2 V A 4]. The 4-year-old has functional asplenia due to the necrotic damage to her spleen caused by sickle cell disease. She has an increased risk of developing septicemia caused by *Streptococcus pneumoniae* or other bacteria. The pneumococcus is a common cause of serious disease in individuals who have a compromised immune system. It is the most common cause of pneumonia and meningitis in the elderly, as well as the major cause of septicemia in asplenic patients. The heightened incidence of septicemia occurs because the organism, which is part of the normal flora of the upper respiratory tract and causes transient bacteremia in most individuals, cannot be effectively cleared from the blood without a fully functioning spleen. Immunization of the patient with the capsular polysaccharide of the organism induces production of opsonic antibodies that will help clear the blood in the liver and other organs of the reticuloendothelial system.

30. The answer is B. [Chapter 9 IV A]. DiGeorge syndrome results from failure of development of the thymus and parathyroid glands due to faulty maturation of the third and fourth pharyngeal pouches during embryogenesis. Those affected have hypocalcemic tetany during the neonatal period and have a marked deficiency in T-cell immunities that results in recurrent infections with viral, fungal, protozoan, and certain intracellular bacterial pathogens. Immunoglobulins may be normal or decreased. Affected children usually die by the age of 2 years unless they receive grafts of fetal thymic tissue or thymic hormone injections. The major clues signifying the presence of DiGeorge syndrome are hypoplasia of the thymus and parathyroids, neither of which are seen in any other disease listed. (Bruton's hypogammaglobulinemia, severe combined immunodeficiency (SCID), ataxia-telangiectasia, and Wiskott-Aldrich syndrome)

31. The answer is E [Chapter 2 IV B 4]. Administering an immunizing agent intranasally appears to stimulate an immune response that mimics the response induced by a natural infection, particularly in upper respiratory tract disease. That is, this route results in the production of specific antibodies both in serum and in secretions at the local site of infection. Evaluation of the intranasal route for administering influenza vaccine is currently under way.

32. The answer is A [Chapter 10 I B 3 d]. The D region of the human major histocompatibility complex (MHC) encodes the class II human leukocyte antigen (HLA) molecules found only on the cells of the immune response, i.e., on activated T cells and on antigen-presenting cells such as macrophages and B cells. This specific encoding is the basis of the MHC restriction that prevents promiscuous antigen presentation by other cells of the body, which is an event that could result in life-threatening autoimmune disease. T cell receptors are encoded by genes involved in generation of immunologic diversity as are genes involved in IgD synthesis. β_2-microglobulin is not encoded by MHC genes but is associated with Class I MHC molecules. Cellular differentiation (CD) antigens are markers of cell function and they have no relationship with MHC.

33. The answer is A [Chapter 8 II H 2]. Chronic thyroiditis (Hashimoto's thyroiditis) is a thyroid disease that mainly affects women between 30 and 50 years of age. The thyroid gland may be enlarged and firm or hard. Hypothyroidism may be seen, and antibody to thyroglobulin and microsomal antigens are also detected. Graves' disease is a hyperthyroid disease with antibodies to the cell receptor for thyroid-stimulating hormone. The target antigen in multiple sclerosis (MS) is basic protein of myelin. Myasthenia gravis (MG) is an autoimmune disease where the antibody interferes with acetylcholine signaling at myoneural junctions by reacting with the acetylcholine receptor. In Goodpasture's disease, the patient dies of pulmonary and kidney dysfunction caused by an autoantibody against type IV collagen found in alveolar and glomerular basement membranes.

34. The answer is A [Chapter 9 V A 1 a]. Severe combined immunodeficiency (SCID) is a rare syndrome of infants caused by a profound deficiency of T lymphocytes and a variable deficiency of B cells. Affected infants are extremely susceptible to opportunistic bacterial, viral, and fungal pathogens, and they usually

succumb to overwhelming infection in early childhood. SCID may be inherited as an X-linked recessive or an autosomal recessive trait. In autosomal recessive SCID, most of the infants have an adenosine deaminase (ADA) deficiency or a purine nucleotide phosphorylase deficiency. Bone marrow transplants have proved beneficial in infants with X-linked SCID. Gene therapy has been successful in children with ADA deficiency.

35. The answer is D [Chapter 5 X A 2 a]. One theory concerning the origin of autoimmune diseases hypothesizes that these diseases are caused by the emergence of clones of cells that are autoreactive. These "forbidden" clones are triggered to proliferate and mature into immunologically competent effector cells that attack self-antigen by contact with antigens or altered native molecules. Another theory suggests that B cells reactive with self-antigen are present naturally and their development into plasma cells secreting autoantibodies occurs because a helper T (Th) cell has been recruited by a second epitope on the immunogen.

36. The answer is A [Chapter 9 III A 2 b]. Bruton's X-linked hypogammaglobulinemia manifests as very low levels of immunoglobulins of all classes. The B cells have a defective tyrosine kinase and cannot mature past the pre-B cell level. Thus, they lack B cells and all subsequent developmental form, although they have cells in the bone marrow with cytoplasmic (mu) μ chains (the pre-B cell).

37. The answer is D [Chapter 7 II B 3 a]. The basophil and mast cell receptor for the FC portion of epsilon (ε) chains cannot distinguish between a functional IgE molecule and the product of an IgE myeloma; therefore, the FC receptors will be saturated with this abnormal immunoglobulin. The cells will lose reactivity to allergens as a result of this displacement, and the severity of allergic symptoms should decrease.

38. The answer is C [Chapter 5 VII A 1 b(i)]. The anamnestic response, anamnesis, is also called the booster response, memory response, or secondary immune response. It is characterized by the prompt production of high levels of antibody (i.e., a rapid rise in antibody titers) following secondary exposure to antigen. Anamnesis is due to the presence of B and T memory cells that were induced during the primary immune response. Immune paralysis is the inability to mount a response to a normally immunogenic substance.

39. The answer is C [Chapter 9 IV B 1]. Chronic mucocutaneous candidiasis affects both males and females. It is inherited as an autosomal recessive trait. The disorder is associated with a selective defect in T-cell immunity, which results in an increased susceptibility to chronic candidal infections. B-cell immunity is intact, and the patients have a normal antibody response to *Candida* antigens. Studies of T-cell immunity reveal a specific defect. Patients usually have a normal total lymphocyte count, and these cells respond normally to T cell mitogens, allogeneic cells, and fungal antigens other than those of *Candida albicans*.

40. The answer is B [Chapter 7 II B 4 a (1)]. The granules in basophils and mast cells are very rich in histamine combined with the acidic polysaccharide heparin. During atopic reactions, these granules release their contents, and the symptoms of edema and smooth muscle contraction become evident. As the reaction continues, phospholipids of the cell are broken down to arachidonic acid, which is further degraded by lipoxygenase enzymes into the leukotrienes, which also have vasoactive potential.

41. The answer is A [Chapter 3 IV A 6; Figure 3-7]. The V-J and V-J-D DNA rearrangements are accomplished by endonuclease and ligase enzymes collectively called "recombinases." There are two recognition signals: a heptameric and a monomeric sequence. The spacer is 12–23 bases in length. The recognition signals are heptameric and nonameric, not pentameric. The spacer sequence is 12–23 bases, not 7–11. Transduction and transformation are genetic exchange mechanisms seen in bacteria.

42. The answer is E [Chapter 3 V B]. Multiple myeloma is one of several plasma cell dyscrasias (i.e., one of the diseases in which a single clone of plasma cells overproduces an immunoglobulin or an immunoglobulin fragment). Most cases of multiple myeloma involve plasma cell tumors of bone marrow that over-produce IgG. Serum sickness, asthma, and hypersensitivity pneumonitis are allergic

reactions to exogenous antigens (allergens). Obviously, Waldenström's disease is an over production of macroglobulins.

43. The answer is A [Chapter 5 IX B 1]. Immunosuppressive therapy is usually directed at cells in the process of proliferation and hence is most effective if given just before, or at the time of, antigen administration. It is far more difficult to block ongoing responses and booster responses because the need for cell proliferation is not as marked. If the suppression occurs too far in advance of the immunization, the drug effect will have worn off.

44. The answer is B [Chapter 8 II B 1].]. Systemic lupus erythematosus (SLE) is a chronic, inflammatory systemic (multiorgan) disease that primarily affects women. A characteristic feature is the erythematous butterfly rash that occurs on the face of some patients. Death usually results from renal failure or infection. Amyotrophic lateral sclerosis (ALS; Lou Gehrig's disease) causes progressive degeneration of motor neurons of the spinal cord. Sjögren's syndrome is a chronic inflammatory disease that primarily affects secretory glands such as the lacrimal and salivary glands, producing dry eyes (keratoconjunctivitis sicca) and dry mouth (xerostomia). Guillain-Barré syndrome (acute idiopathic polyneuritis) manifests as progressive weakness, first of the lower extremities and then of the upper extremities and respiratory muscles. Goodpasture's syndrome is a relatively rare disorder with symptoms referable to both the lungs (e.g., pulmonary hemorrhage) and kidneys (e.g., glomerulonephritis).

45. The answer is E [Chapter 7 II C 2 a]. Immunoglobulin (Ig)E has been produced in this woman as a result of prior exposure to wasp venom. These homocytotropic antibodies have coated basophils and mast cells. Cross-linking of this cell-bound antibody by allergen causes these cells to degranulate and release histamine, which is causing the symptoms seen in this individual.

46. The answer is D [Chapter 7 II D 4 c (2)]. Epinephrine is the drug of choice for anaphylactic reactions. It relaxes smooth muscle, thus reversing some of the effects of histamine and is also a cardiac stimulant. Beta-adrenergic drugs, such as epinephrine, also activate adenyl cyclase, thus elevating the level of cyclic adenosine monophosphate (cAMP) within the basophil and mast cells and inhibiting degranulation. Antihistamine cannot *reverse* the effects of histamine so they aren't much good once symptoms present. Steroids are useful to stop synthesis of slow-reacting substance of anaphylaxis (SRS-A) (leukotriene) compounds. Cromolyn sodium blocks calcium ion influx with resultant activation of phosphodiesterase and decrease in cAMP levels.

47. The answer is B [Chapter 10 II E 2 b (2)]. Interferon-γ, while it was originally associated with antiviral effects, is now recognized as having important immunoregulatory properties, mainly enhancement of natural killer (NK) cells and macrophages. Interferon can thus be expected to enhance cell-mediated immunity but to have little effect on antibody–mediated immunity. Plasma cell differentiation is influenced by IL-4, -5 and -6. INF-γ does downregulate $T_H 2$ cells and thus favors delayed hypersensitivity, but this is a minor role for this potent immunoregulatory molecule.

48. The answer is E [Chapter 1 V A]. Natural killer (NK) cells kill malignant cells and, as such, are sometimes referred to as the cells of immune surveillance (i.e., they patrol the body and eliminate premalignant conditions). Interleukin 1 (IL-1) is produced by macrophages, particularly if they are activated by endotoxin, interferon-γ (IFN-γ), and a wide variety of other stimulants. The contact between helper T cells and macrophages is also an effective signal for the secretion of IL-1. NK cells are large, granular lymphocytes that are present in the body before antigenic exposure. These cells kill by release of perforin molecules on contact with the target cell. Polyperforin channels form and protease and nuclease enzymes destroy the target, the Fas protein reacts with its ligand in the target membrane and initiates apoptosis. NK cells have receptors for the Fc region of IgG and can participate in antibody-dependent cellular cytotoxicity (ADCC).

49. The answer is B. [Chapter 7 III C 1 b (1) (b)]. Erythroblastosis fetalis is a cytotoxic antibody disease that occurs in Rh-positive children born of Rh-negative mothers. Prior to the current pregnancy, the mother becomes sensitized to the $Rh_o(D)$ antigen due to a previous pregnancy (Rh-positive infant), a transfusion of Rh-positive blood, or, rarely, a transplant. The immunoglobulin G antibody crosses the placenta and sensitizes the infant's red blood cells to lysis or phagocytic destruction.

50. The answer is D [Chapter 7 III C 1 b (4)]. Current obstetric practice recommends that an injection of RhoGAM be given during the pregnancy as well as immediately upon parturition. This inclusion of the injection at 26 weeks has decreased the incidence of Rh sensitization from 10% to 1%. Because RhoGAM is a human IgG antibody, it may be expected to cross the placenta and affect the infant. However, this does not occur because the antibody is greatly diluted in the mother's circulation and the injection is given when the IgG transport system functions poorly.

51. The answer is A [Chapter 9 III A 4]. The 5-year-old child probably has Bruton's hypogammaglobulinemia, although a phagocytic defect could not be ruled out on the basis of the history. Treatment for Bruton's hypogammaglobulinemia is maintenance therapy with pooled human gamma globulin. The patient must be monitored closely to ensure early detection of bacterial infections. Pneumonia is the most serious and life-threatening condition.

52. The answer is B [Chapter 10 II B 3 a]. α-Fetoprotein (AFP) is an oncofetal antigen seen in fetal liver and again when the organ is damaged later in life. It is used prognostically to predict success of therapy in patients with hepatocellular carcinoma. AFP levels will also be elevated in alcoholics, people with hepatitis, and a variety of other conditions—hence, it is not diagnostic. Carcinoembryonic antigen (CEA) levels are elevated in many conditions, including pregnancy and cancer of the colon, and in individuals who smoke. The other tumor markers are associated with specific malignancies. Hepatitis B surface antigen (HbsAg) is associated with hepatocellular carcinoma, but so is hepatitis C viral antigen, and this agent has a much higher concordance with liver cancer.

53. The answer is D [Chapter 1 IV B 3 a (1)]. Macrophages secrete interferon (INF) α during an inflammatory response. Interferon (IFN) γ, also known as immune interferon, is secreted by specifically sensitized T lymphocytes when they come into contact with their homologous antigen. The interferons induces an antiviral state in other nearby cells by inducing the production of proteins that interfere with viral messenger RNA activity. Complement is a group of more than a dozen serum proteins that react with antibody in a cascading manner and are able to disrupt the cell membrane of gram-negative bacteria. Properdin is a serum protein that stabilizes C3 convertase [C3bBb] generated by the alternative pathway of complement activation. Lysozyme is a mucopeptidase that hydrolyzes the bacterial cell wall, rendering the cell susceptible to osmotic lysis.

54. The answer is C [Chapter 5 IV A 1 a (1) (b), b (1) (c)]. The T-cell receptor (TcR) is the T-cell analogue of surface immunoglobulin on B cells. It is a monovalent molecule that has great functional and structural similarity with the Fab portion of an antibody molecule. In the membrane of the T cell, this receptor is closely linked to the CD3 heterodimer, and they both play a role in cell activation once the antigen has been presented to the T cell.

55. The answer is D. [Chapter 7 III C 1 b (1) (b)]. The Rh type of the first child will determine if she could have been sensitized. If the first child is Rh negative, then a subsequent pregnancy should not pose a risk. If the first child is Rh positive, then the mother's serum should be studied for Rh antibodies to determine if the $Rh_o(D)$ immune globulin had successfully aborted sensitization. The Rh antigen profile of her fiancée is also important because if he is Rh negative, the offspring would all be Rh negative, and Rh disease would not be a concern.

56. The answer is D [Chapter 10 II D 2]. Soluble tumor-specific transplantation antigens (TSTAs) can favor tumor growth by reacting with and neutralizing host anti-tumor defenses such as antibodies and cytotoxic T cells. Antibodies, interleukin-1, muramyl dipeptide, and tumor necrosis factor work to control the growth and spread of malignant cells.

57. The answer is A [Chapter 5 IV E 2 d (3) (a)]. Epstein-Barr virus has a tropism for B lymphocytes. It binds to CD 21 in the B cell membrane as the initial interaction with this target [this is analogous to the gp 120 spike on HIV virus reacting with the CD4 molecule in the membrane of the T cell.] The effect on the B cell of this interaction is activation and, in some cases, proliferation. *Bordetella pertussis* has the intrinsic ability to favor immunoglobu-

lin class switching to the production of immunoglobulin E (IgE) class antibodies. This is probably the result of ill-defined bacterial effects on lymphokine secretion, especially interleukin-4 (IL-4). IL-4 has been shown to favor the synthesis of IgE by plasma cells. This adjuvant effect of the whooping cough bacillus may play a role in the pathogenesis of this infection, because the patients exhibit an exaggerated hypersensitivity of the respiratory apparatus that lasts far beyond the acute phase of the disease. Up to 1 year after recovery, during the convalescence phase of the disease, affected children experience recurrences of their paroxysmal coughing episodes brought on by other respiratory insults, such as viral infections.

58. The answer is B [Chapter 5 III C 2]. Antibody synthesis occurs in peripheral (secondary) lymphoid organs such as the tonsils, Peyer's patches, lymph nodes, and spleen. The central (primary) lymphoid organs are the thymus and the bursa of Fabricius or its mammalian counterpart, the bone marrow. These are the sites where lymphocytes receive their immunologic education and become committed to life as T or B cells.

59. The answer is E [Chapter 9 IV B 2]. The 18-month-old child has chronic mucocutaneous candidiasis, which is a unique immunodeficiency disease in which the only failure of the immune system is in the cell-mediated response to the yeast *Candida albicans.* This organism is among the normal flora, and it usually does not cause much disease except in infants and in adults when the normal flora becomes imbalanced due to dietary or hormonal changes or in immunodeficiency diseases such as AIDS. The transplantation of fetal thymus tissue has been reported to be of some benefit in these patients. The other therapies listed (injection of pooled gamma-globulin or specific immune globulin, transfusion of erythrocytes, or bone marrow transplant) would not be beneficial in this patient.

60. The answer is B [Chapter 7 IV C 3]. The child has poststreptococcal glomerulonephritis, which is an immune complex disease. The streptococcal pharyngitis was not treated appropriately (no antibiotics), and immune complexes of streptococcal antigens and the patient's antibodies have formed and deposited on the glomerular basement membrane. Complement chemotaxin (i.e., C5a) has been released, and neutrophils are accumulating in the kidney. They are attempting to engulf the complexes and, being unable to do so, are releasing oxygen metabolites and enzymes that damage the basement membrane. Goodpasture's is an autoimmune disease where the patient makes antibodies to type IV collagen and destroys alveolar and glomerular basement membranes. Systemic lupus erythematosus (SLE) is another autoimmune disease where the kidney is the target, but, in this instance, the damage is due to immune complex deposition on the basement membrane. Wegener's granulomatosus involves the kidney and has serious consequences. Its etiology is unknown. Reye's disease is associated with some viral infections (e.g., chickenpox), especially if the children were given aspirin. It is characterized as an encephalopathy with associated hepatic dysfunction.

61. The answer is E [Chapter 1 III H; Table 1-7; Chapter 4 IV B 2 b]. C3b is the most potent opsonin in the body and is deposited on surfaces that are coated with IgG and IgM antibody molecules. The IgG molecule is also opsonic in its own right. Complement can also be activated by the alternative pathway (no antibody is needed), and C3b is found on membranes in this case as well. Phagocytic cells have membrane receptors (C3bR) for these potent opsonizing molecules. The interaction of these ligands creates a firm union between the cell and the microbe. C5a is not bound to phagocytic cell membranes; however, it does find a receptor in the mast cell membrane, which, when bound, induces mediator release. IgE is the antibody associated with atopic disease. C3a is an anaphylotoxin that causes degranulation and histamine release when it reacts with the C3a receptor in the mast cell membrane.

62. The answer is C [Chapter 10 I C 6 (3)]. Cyclosporine is one of a group of peptide antibiotics produced by various fungi; another is FK-506. These drugs interfere with the transcription of genes that encode interleukin peptides and interferon γ; thus, they downregulate the T-cell arm of the antigraft response. Azathioprine is used as an anti-inflammatory and immunosuppressant drug in the control of autoimmune diseases. Cyclophosphamide is a cancer therapeutic agent that is also immunosuppressive. Corticosteroid drugs are immunosuppressants used in treatment of autoimmune diseases; they

are also used in management of asthma. Anti-lymphocyte globulin is used to suppress graft rejection in transplant patients.

63. The answer is B [Chapter 1 III H 2 c (1)]. Fibronectin is an adhesive glycoprotein that is important in connective tissues where it cross-links collagen. One form of fibronectin circulates in plasma and acts as an opsonin; another is a cell-surface component that mediates cellular adhesive interactions. IgG1 is an important opsonizing antibody that reacts *specifically* with bacteria. C3a is an anaphylatoxin that reacts with a specific receptor in the membrane of mast cells and basophils and causes them to degranulate and release their vasoactive contents. Lysozyme is a mucopeptidase that hydrolyzes the bacterial cell wall, rendering the cell susceptible to osmotic lysis. It is found in secretions and in the granules of phagocytic cells. Leukotriene B_4 is produced from arachidonic acid via the lipoxygenase pathway during inflammatory reactions. It is able to increase vascular permeability, and it attracts (i.e., is chemotactic for) and activates neutrophils and eosinophils.

64. The answer is D [Chapter 6 II A 1]. The child's red blood cells were agglutinated by antiserums specific for the A, B, and D antigens, which means these three antigens must be on the cells of the young boy.

65. The answer is D [Chapter 7 III C 1 b (1) (b)]. The child is Rh positive (his cells were agglutinated by an anti-D antiserum). The mother is Rh negative so the presence of the D antigen on fetal cells presents 2 problems: first, the D antigen could cause antibody production in the mother (of no consequence to her); and, second, this antibody could cross the placenta (if of the IgG isotype) and cause hemolysis of the infant's RBCs resulting in a particular type of hemolytic disease of the newborn, erythroblastosis fetalis.

66. The answer is D [Chapter 2 VI B]. Immune globulin (gamma globulin) is prepared from pooled normal adult human plasma or serum by cold ethanol fractionation. Immune globulin contains antibodies to many common infectious agents (e.g., rubella, measles, hepatitis A) and is used for passive immunization in people at risk of developing measles or rubella or for maintenance of passive immunity in immunodeficient people. Recombivax is used to induce active immunity against hepatitis B. Measles-mumps-rubella (MMR) is the trivalent vaccine that can induce active immunity to rubella; however, it would not be used in this patient. There would not be time to induce immunity and, in fact, the vaccine could possibly make the disease worse. Bacille Calmette Guérin (BCG) is a live, attenuated tubercle bacillus that has been used in the U.S. as an immunostimulant. Specific immune globulin is obtained from hyperimmunized donors and contains high levels of selected antibodies (e.g., human botulinum immune globulin).

67. The answer is E [Chapter 8 II K 2 a]. Goodpasture's syndrome is a relatively rare disorder with symptoms referable to both the lungs (e.g., pulmonary hemorrhage) and kidneys (e.g., glomerulonephritis). The immunoglobulin G (IgG) deposited on alveolar and glomerular basement membranes appears to be specific for type IV collagen shared by the kidneys and lungs. Amyotrophic lateral sclerosis (ALS; Lou Gehrig's disease) causes progressive degeneration of motor neurons of the spinal cord. Systemic lupus erythematosus (SLE) is a chronic, inflammatory systemic (multiorgan) disease that primarily affects women. Sjögren's syndrome is a chronic inflammatory disease that primarily affects secretory glands such as the lacrimal and salivary glands, producing dry eyes (keratoconjunctivitis sicca) and dry mouth (xerostomia). Guillain-Barré syndrome (acute idiopathic polyneuritis) manifests as progressive muscular weakness, first of the lower extremities and then of the upper extremities and respiratory muscles.

68. The answer is D [Chapter 1 I B]. Antibodies and specifically sensitized T cells are characteristic of the acquired, or adaptive, immunities. They are produced in response to an antigenic challenge. Natural killer (NK) cells are not induced by immunization and are the cells of immune surveillance. Turbulence in the upper airway, shedding of epithelial cells, lysozyme in tears, and complement are all factors in nonspecific, or innate, immunity. These factors occur naturally to protect animals from microbes in the environment.

69. The answer is B [Chapter 3 V B 1 b; Table 10-4]. The 72-year-old man has a B-cell malignancy. He is producing abnormal immunoglobulins (a monoclonal gammopathy) and is excreting light-chain dimers (Bence-Jones protein) in his urine. Lytic bone lesions occur in approximately 60% of these patients. Alpha-fetoprotein (AFP) is associated with hepatic dysfunction. Carcinoembryonic antigen (CEA) is found to be elevated in several diseases but is used as a prognostic assay in colon cancer. Both AFP and CEA are oncofetal antigens. Hepatitis B core antigen is found in the serum of patients in the early stages of hepatitis caused by this virus.

70. The answer is C [Chapter 5 IX B 2 b]. Immunosuppression is an unwanted side effect of cancer chemotherapy. The agents that are toxic to dividing cells (DNA base analogues for example) will not discriminate between malignant and lymphoid tissues. The neutrophil has a very short half-life, and severe neutropenia is another consequence of cancer therapy. The end result is that opportunistic infections are a major cause of complications and death in cancer patients. None of the other conditions listed are associated with cancer chemotherapy.

71. The answer is C [Chapter 10 I A 1 c]. Allografts, or homografts, are tissue or organ exchanges between individuals of the same species (i.e., from one human to another). These transplants are routinely recognized as foreign by the recipient and are rejected unless immunosuppression is employed. Autografts are within the same individual; isografts are between genetically identical individuals. Xenografts are across species barriers (e.g., baboon to human heart transplant). A kidney graft would not be done in a patient with systemic lupus erythematosus, as the disease would destroy the new kidney as well.

72. The answer is E [Chapter 5 X B 1 b] Most autoimmune diseases are due to an antibody response to an autoantigen. Elimination of autoreactive T helper cells by clonal deletion induced by contact with autoantigen is the major controlling process. Some tissue damage in autoimmune diseases is caused by immune complexes being deposited on basement membranes (e.g., glomerular basement membrane). This certainly is not a method of prevention. Antibodies blocking a cell receptor are a cause of autoimmune phenomena, not a mechanism of control. The same can be said of antibody-induced phagocytosis and complement–mediated lysis.

73. The answer is D [Chapter 2 V B 6]. Veterinary students are routinely immunized against rabies, because it is a serious occupational threat. For similar reasons, dental hygienists should receive hepatitis B vaccine. Cholera vaccine is for people traveling to endemic areas. Pneumovax is for the elderly. *Haemophilus influenza* type B and polio are childhood vaccines.

74. The answer is C [Chapter 9 IV 4]. DiGeorge syndrome results from failure of development of the thymus and parathyroid glands due to faulty maturation of the third and fourth pharyngeal pouches during embryogenesis. Those affected have hypocalcemic tetany during the neonatal period and have a marked deficiency in T-cell immunities that results in recurrent infections with viral, fungal, protozoan, and certain intracellular bacterial pathogens. Immunoglobulins may be normal or decreased. Affected children usually die by the age of 2 years unless they receive grafts of fetal thymic tissue or thymic hormone injections.

75. The answer is A [Chapter 2 V B 1; Table 2-3]. Rubella (German measles) virus is highly teratogenic, particularly during the first trimester of gestation, when the majority of organ development occurs. Because this woman is pregnant, it is advisable to protect her from developing an active case of rubella. If she has a history of immunization, a blood sample could be taken and checked for IgG anti-rubella antibodies. If these are absent, she could be given a pooled human immunoglobulin preparation to passively protect her from the virus. Even if she had been immunized before, there would not be any harm in giving her the gamma globulin injection. The desirability of actively immunizing her with the attenuated vaccine is somewhat controversial, although more than 200 women have been inadvertently immunized during the first few months of their pregnancy and no harm was done to the developing embryos. However, as she has already been exposed, she would not have time to develop protective antibodies if we immunized her with measles-mumps-rubella (MMR) or a killed rubella virus vaccine. There is no hyperimmune anti-rubella serum available. Varicella vaccine is used for chickenpox.

76. The answer is A [Chapter 6 III G]. The enzyme-linked immunosorbent assay (ELISA) is used as the initial test to screen serum samples for the presence of antibodies to the human immunodeficiency virus (HIV). If the test is positive, the serum is analyzed further by Western blot assay, in which the viral antigens are first separated in a gel by electrophoresis and are then allowed to react with the patient's serum. Anti-HIV antibodies bind to the individual proteins in the gel. Their presence is then detected by an antihuman gamma globulin, which is usually labeled with a radionuclide or an enzyme that can be detected by the production of a specific color when the substrate is added to the mixture. The other procedures listed (immunofluorescence, hemagglutination inhibition, virus neutralization, and latex agglutination) are not used in serodiagnosis of HIV infection.

77. The answer is E [Chapter 6 III D]. Latex agglutination is a form of passive agglutination in which one reactant, either antigen or antibody, is adsorbed onto the latex bead, and the other component of the reaction (i.e., antibody or antigen, respectively), is added to the suspension of coated latex beads. A lattice is formed when the second reactant bridges the latex beads. This aggregate can usually be visualized directly. In people with rheumatoid arthritis, the latex particles are coated with human IgG and mixed with the patient's serum. If the rheumatoid factor, which is an antibody (usually IgM against human IgG), is present, it agglutinates the latex beads. Other assays could be utilized but they are not because they are too expensive, too cumbersome, or not of the appropriate specificity.

78. The answer is B [Chapter 5 IV B 6 a; Table 5-2]. Interleukin 3 (IL-3) is the interleukin that causes stem cell proliferation and works in synergy with other colony stimulating factors to increase the rate of hematopoiesis and the production of eosinophils, neutrophils and monocytes.

79. The answer is C [Chapter 10 Table 10-4]. Prostate specific antigen (PSA) is useful as a screening test for cancer of the prostate. Elevation of this protein in the serum is highly suggestive of prostatic cancer. Another antigen with similar clinical significance is prostatic alkaline phosphatase. Presence of elevated levels of PSA will indicate the need for further evaluation. Alpha-fetoprotein (AFP) is associated with primary hepatocellular carcinoma, another oncofetal antigen. Carcinoembryonic antigen (CEA) is elevated in patients with colon cancer. Common acute lymphoblastic leukemia antigen (CALLA) is a membrane marker of pre-β cells; it will increase in concentration if the patient has lymphoblastic leukemia. Bence-Jones protein is a light chain dimer seen in the urine of patients with multiple myeloma.

80. The answer is D [Chapter 8 II I a]. Graves' disease is an autoimmune form of hyperthyroidism in which the patient makes an antibody to the thyroid-stimulating hormone (TSH) receptor in the membrane of thyroid cells. When this antibody reacts with the TSH receptor, an intracellular signal is transmitted that is identical to one that would have been sent had TSH reacted at the cell membrane. The result is that the cell is activated, and the thyroid gland becomes hyperplastic due to this continuous stimulatory signal. Therapy for this disease consists of removal of the thyroid gland and maintenance of the patient on levothyroxine.

81. The answer is A [Chapter 1 IV A 1] . Complement is a group of 20 or more serum proteins that react with antibody in a cascading manner and are able to disrupt the cell membrane of gram-negative bacteria. Interferon (IFN) γ, also known as immune interferon, is secreted by specifically sensitized T lymphocytes when they come into contact with their homologous antigen. Lactoferrin and lactoperoxidase are antimicrobial molecules found in human milk; lactoferrin competes for iron, an essential metabolite for microbial growth, and lactoperoxidase is an enzyme that oxidizes essential proteins in microbial cell membranes. Lysozyme is a mucopeptidase that hydrolyzes the bacterial cell wall, rendering the cell susceptible to osmotic lysis.

82. The answer is A [Chapter 2 I]. Immunogens are substances that are able to induce an immune response. The response may be humoral (resulting in the production of circulating antibodies) or cell-mediated (resulting in the production of specifically sensitized T lymphocytes). An antigen can react specifically with its homologous antibody or lymphocyte, but it may not be able to induce an immune response. A hapten can react with antibody, but it is not immunogenic unless it is coupled

to a carrier molecule. The epitope is the site on the antigen molecule that reacts with specific antibody or lymphocyte. An adjuvant is a substance that intensifies an immune response when administered with an immunogen.

83. The answer is A [Chapter 10 II B 3 b]. Carcinoembryonic antigen (CEA) is found in high concentrations in the serum of patients with colorectal cancer and other epithelial tumors. CEA is a fetal protein that is expressed during the dedifferentiation that accompanies the transformation to malignancy. Its presence is not diagnostic of malignancy, because other conditions such as smoking, viral infections and other insults can cause the level of this protein to increase. It is used, however, as a prognostic indicator of the continued presence (or re-appearance) of the cancer in the patient following surgical and chemotherapeutic interventions. Plotting the concentration of serum CEA against time allows the oncologist to determine the success of surgical resection. A reappearance of the antigen, or an increase in the concentration of CEA, signals recurrence of the cancer. AFP is associated with primary hepatocellular carcinoma, another oncofetal antigen. CALLA is a membrane marker of pre-B cells; it will increase in concentration if the patient has lymphoblastic leukemia. Bence-Jones protein is a light chain dimer seen in the urine of patients with multiple myeloma. Prostate-specific antigen (PSA) is useful as a screening test for cancer of the prostate.

84. The answer is D [Chapter 5 IV B 2; Table 5-2]. Interleukin 4 (IL-4) plays a significant role in class switching and promotes the synthesis of IgG1 and IgE. IL-4 is produced by helper T (Th) cells of the Th2 subset. Acting synergistically with IL-5, IL-4 enhances the production of IgA; it also can stimulate mast cell proliferation and maturation in synergy with IL-3.

85. The answer is B [Chapter 2 VI C; Table 2-2]. Specific immune globulin is a gamma globulin obtained from people who have recently recovered from a specific infectious disease or from human volunteers who have been hyperimmunized against that disease. Examples include hepatitis B immune globulin and rabies immune globulin. Specific immune globulin is used to provide specific passive immunity. There are 2 preparations of pooled immune globulins, IGIM (for intramuscular route) and IGIV (for intravenous route). The latter, IGIV, has a higher antibody level and has been purified to remove aggregates of immunoglobulins which could activate complement and cause an anaphylactoid reaction. IGIV is also more expensive than IGIM. DNA vaccines are prepared from the genome of the infectious agent. RhoGAM is used to prevent erythroblastosis fetalis. Anti-venins are prepared in horses. Serum sickness is a common complication.

86. The answer is C [Chapter 5 IV B 2; Table 5-2]. Interleukin 4 (IL-4) plays a significant role in class switching and promotes the synthesis of IgG1 and IgE. IL-4 is produced by helper T (Th) cells of the Th2 subset. Interleukin 4 (IL-4) is the interleukin that enhances the production of IgE by plasma cells. It is produced by T helper 2 cells and acts to inhibit the activity of T helper 1 cells much like IL-10. Its major role is in the development of atopic allergies where it acts in the B cell (and plasma cells as well) to induce class switching to the epsilon heavy chain constant region genes. The antibody thus produced reacts with mast cells and basophils to sensitize them for degranulation in the event that the membrane-bound IgE molecules are cross-linked. IgE also is an important part of immunity to metazoan parasites.

87. The answer is A [Chapter 10 II B 3 a]. Approximately 10% of individuals who are infected with the hepatitis B virus become chronic carriers. Many of these patients develop cirrhosis of the liver or primary liver cancer, as this 39-year-old pathologist has done. α-Fetoprotein (AFP) is an oncofetal antigen produced by the embryonic liver. Its levels are also elevated in people with certain malignancies (e.g., primary hepatoma, prostatic and gastric carcinomas, and teratomas). AFP, like CEA, is not useful as a diagnostic test but is a valuable prognostic indicator of the presence of residual malignant cells. Hepatitis B and C are both associated with chronic hepatitis and cirrhosis, which this patient has. However, patients normally have antibodies to the following antigens: hepatitis B core antigen (HbcAg), hepatitis C antigen (HCAg), and hepatitis B surface antigen (HbsAg). Myeloma protein is the product of the B cell that has become malignant in myeloma (a monoclonal gammopathy).

88. The answer is E [Chapter 6 III E 1]. The Coombs' test uses an antiserum specific for human gamma globulin (Coombs' serum) to detect the presence of antibodies on human

erythrocytes. In the direct test, the Coombs' serum is added to red blood cells (RBCs) from a neonate. If the cells agglutinate, maternal antibodies are affixed to the cell surface. These antibodies usually cannot cause agglutination themselves; they are called incomplete, monovalent, or blocking antibodies because they can react with an antigen on the cell membrane but cannot induce the formation of a lattice. In the indirect Coombs' test, maternal serum is mixed with known Rh-positive cells but will not cause them to agglutinate. When the Coombs' serum is added to the antibody-coated cells, they form a lattice and agglutinate. The cells must be washed free of excess human serum components before the Coombs' reagent is added, because soluble gamma globulin could react with anti-human gamma globulin antiserum before a lattice of RBCs forms. Hemagglutination inhibition is used to identify certain viruses such as influenza A strains. Latex agglutination is used to detect capsular antigens in spinal fluid. Radioimmunoassays are extremely sensitive tests that are used to quantitate various materials such as hormones in body fluids. Radial immunodiffusion is used to quantitate immunoglobulin levels in human plasma.

89. The answer is A [Chapter 9 III A]. X-linked agammaglobulinemia was first observed in 1952 by Colonel Ogden Bruton, and his report is now acknowledged to be the first clinical description and precise diagnosis of an immunodeficiency disorder. Affected infants are unable to synthesize immunoglobulins of any isotype. They suffer from recurrent pyogenic infections beginning at the age of 6–8 months, when the maternal antibody levels decline. Their bone marrow contains normal numbers of pre-B cells, which contain μ chains in the cytoplasm. The defect is in a tyrosine kinase enzyme. The patients are unable to synthesize an intact IgM monomer and place it in the B cell membrane. Thus, they do not have surface immunoglobulin-bearing B cells in the peripheral blood and plasma cells will not be found in lymph nodes.

90. The answer is D [Chapter 5 IX B 2 b (2) (c)], Cyclosporine (cyclosporin A) is a fungal antibiotic composed of 11 amino acids arranged as a cyclic peptide. It binds to the membrane phospholipids of lymphocytes and is internalized by pinocytosis. In the cytoplasm, it binds to an enzyme called cytophilin, which is a member of the prolyl-isomerase (or conformase) family of catalytic proteins that can rotate the peptide bonds on either side of proline in a peptide chain and thus control the folding of the molecule. By interfering with proper protein-chain folding, cyclosporine blocks transmission of cytosolic messages from the antigen receptor to the nucleus. Thus, interleukin-2 (IL-2) gene expression is blocked, and the Th cells are unable to synthesize this lymphokine. Cyclosporine also inhibits the production of interferon-γ (IFN-γ) by activated T cells and so prevents lymphokine induction of class I major histocompatibility complex molecule expression in grafted tissues. This decreases graft rejection because it is the class I molecule that is the primary target in the rejection event.

91. The answer is B [Chapter 4 I D 3, Chapter 1 IV A]. Both antibody and complement are needed for immune lysis of gram-negative bacteria. However only immunoglobulin G (IgG) and IgM are able to activate complement for this lytic event; IgE is unable to react with C1q and initiate the hemolytic cascade. Complement can also be activated via the alternative (nonantibody) pathway when an activator surface, such as a bacterial cell wall, stabilizes C3b, and it reacts with factor B through the alternative pathway of complement activation to become a C3 convertase (C3bBb). Hydrogen peroxide is a bactericidal product of glucose metabolism generated during phagocytosis. Lactoperoxidase is an oxidizing enzyme found in milk that has antimicrobial properties. Lactoferrin is an iron chelating protein that competes with bacterial siderophores for iron and thus "starves" the microbe.

92. The answer is A [Chapter 7 II C 2 a]. Anaphylaxis is occurring in this young boy. He has probably eaten something to which he had an immunoglobulin E (IgE) allergy (symptoms in mouth, tongue, and cheeks). Attacks such as this to food allergens are frequent and may be life-threatening (he is having difficulty breathing).

93. The answer is B [Chapter 7 II D 4 c (2)]. Epinephrine is the drug of choice for anaphylactic reactions. It relaxes smooth muscle, thus reversing some of the effects of histamine and is also a cardiac stimulant. Beta-adrenergic drugs such as epinephrine also activate adenyl cyclase, thus elevating the level of cyclic adenosine monophosphate (cAMP) within the

basophil and mast cell and inhibiting degranulation. Cromolyn sodium is used before exercise to prevent histamine release triggered by exercise. Antihistamine drugs might be used as adjunct therapy to interfere with further histamine vasoactivity. Histamine is one of the major compounds contributing to the symptoms of anaphylaxis. It is released from mast cell and basophils following phosphodiesterase activation, which has reduced the intracellular level of cyclic adenosine monophosphate (cAMP), thus triggering degranulation.

94. The answer is B [Chapter 9 II B 1 c (2)]. The patient has chronic granulomatous disease which is caused by a nicotinamide-adenine dinucleotide phosphate (NADPH) oxidase deficiency. The defect results in a failure to recycle NADPH, which causes a failure to produce hydrogen peroxide during phagocytosis. As a result, the phagocytic cells are not efficient at microbial killing. Infusions of neutrophils will not correct the defect but will replace the defective cell, thus restoring intracellular killing activity. The phagocytic cells of this patient have intact oxygen independent killing capabilities (i.e., lysosomal granules are intact and fuse appropriately with phagosomes). Thus, gamma interferon may also be used therapeutically to activate phagocytic cells to heightened killing. Tissue transplantation has not been beneficial in these patients. Antibody synthesis is normal so gamma globulin injections would not help.

95. The answer is D [Chapter 8 II N 1, 2 a; Table 8-3]. In idiopathic thrombocytopenic purpura (ITP), immunoglobulin G (IgG) antibodies specific for platelets cause the platelets to be destroyed by macrophages of the spleen and liver. Although systemic lupus erythematosus (SLE) is primarily associated with antinuclear antibodies and rheumatoid arthritis with rheumatoid factor, both antibodies may be found in both diseases, as well as in other collagen-vascular diseases such as Sjögren's syndrome. This patient has thrombocytopenia which is not associated with atopic dermatitis.

96. The answer is A [Chapter 4 II A 5 a (1)]. The C1 complex is composed of five distinct polypeptide chains held together by calcium ions. C1q is the first to react, and it is bound by two adjacent Fc sections of immunoglobulin molecules. The rest of the cascade proceeds from this originating signal. C1r is activated by C1q. C1r activates (i.e., proteolytically cleaves) C1s. C1s has enzymatic activity (it is an esterase–peptidase whose substrate is C4). The alternative pathway of complement activation enters the cascade at C3, which is the fourth step in the classical pathway activated by antibody molecules' interaction with C1.

97. The answer is B [Chapter 1 III B 2]. The respiratory tract is protected from microbial assault by alveolar macrophages that engulf invaders, the mucociliary blanket that entraps microbes and sweeps them out of the lung, and by acquired immunities in the form of locally produced immunoglobulins and specifically-sensitized T lymphocytes. Antibodies and cytotoxic T cells are produced in the bronchus-associated lymphoid tissue (BALT). Lactoferrin is an iron-binding protein found in the lysosomal granules of neutrophils and in milk. It competes with the microbe for free iron in the environment and, thus, helps to control bacterial growth in vivo. Lysozyme is found in secretions such as tears and in lysosomal granules of phagocytic cells. The salivary flow to the back of the mouth provides a cleansing action for the oral cavity. IgD has no known antimicrobial action.

98. The answer is C [Chapter 10 I C 6 b (i)]. Corticosteroids are useful for controlling graft rejection because they are anti-inflammatory as well as immunosuppressive. They inhibit the release of inflammatory compounds from cells of the recipient and also alter the traffic pattern of lymphocytes to produce a functional lymphopenia. The other compounds are also immunosuppressive but would not be the first choice. Azathioprine has a great deal of extraneous toxicity, as does actinomycin D. Antilymphocyte globulin reduces the number of lymphocytes drastically, but does not do much to change cytokine synthesis. Cyclosporine is the opposite—it interferes with IL-2 and IFN-γ synthesis but does not alter lymphocyte numbers.

99. The answer is A [Chapter 10 I B 3 d]. Control of the immune response by the major histocompatibility complex (MHC) is thymus dependent. CD4 and CD8 molecules on T cells recognize class II and class I MHC molecules that are presenting foreign epitopes to the T-cell receptor. Class III MHC molecules are not involved in the immune response. B cells are only involved in control of the immune response when they act as antigen presenting cells. B7-CD28 interaction is involved in activation of B cells during the inductive phase of the immune response.

100. The answer is D [Chapter 5 VII A 2; Figure 5-8]. The secondary immune response differs from a primary immune response in that the interval between antigen exposure and antibody production is shorter in the secondary immune response and more antibody is produced for a longer period of time. Usually the immunoglobulin produced in the primary response is IgM, and during the secondary response IgG begins to appear due to immunoglobulin class switching. The antibody specificity does not change within a particular plasma cell line, although subtle mutations in B-cell immunoglobulin genes may produce a paratope with greater affinity for the epitope.

101. The answer is A [Chapter 5 VII A 1 b; Figure 5-8]. A single injection of tetanus toxoid induces an anamnestic response, and the child will be protected. It is possible to boost tetanus immunity up to 10 years after a full immunizing injection schedule. This patient has either a phagocytic defect or a C3 deficiency, because his immunoglobulin levels were normal and the T cell immunities also seemed intact as evidenced by normal recovery from chickenpox. The former could be treated with IFN-γ or neutrophil infusions. There is no treatment for complement deficiencies.

102. The answer is E [Chapter 1 III E 2 c]. Activated macrophages can kill tumor cells by secreting reactive oxygen metabolites such as superoxide anion, singlet oxygen, and nitric oxide. Phagocytic cells, under the influence of IFN-γ and tumor necrosis factor will have an increase in nitric oxide synthetase. The enzyme oxidatively cleaves arginine to yield the highly reactive nitric oxide, which is active against many infectious agents as well as malignant cells. Perforin and granzymes are found in Tc and natural killer (NK) cells. Perforin polymerizes in the target cell membrane and then the granzymes (enzymes of the granules = nucleases and proteases) destroy macromolecules in the tumor cell. The Fas protein of these same cells reacts with a Fas ligand in the target cell membrane and initiates apoptosis.

103. The answer is D [Chapter 8 II B 2 b (2)]. There are several different antibodies in the serum of patients with systemic lupus erythematosus (SLE). The most closely associated with disease occurrence and severity is anti-ds DNA. Rheumatoid factor will also be present, as will the syphilis reaginic antibody and a host of anti-nuclear and anti-ribosomal antibodies. Complement will also be depressed but that is true of many autoimmune diseases. Salivary duct antibodies indicate sicca complex.

104. The answer is B [Chapter 5 VII A b (1)]. A characteristic of the anamnestic (secondary) immune response is the greater amount of antibody produced during this response versus the primary immune response. In addition, there is a more rapid production of antibody during the anamnestic response. IgM is characteristic of a primary immune response; the antibody that predominates during the anamnestic response is IgG. It usually takes less immunogen to induce a secondary response than a primary response.

105. The answer is D [Chapter 3 IV A 4; Figures 3-1 and 3-6]. In IgM heavy (H) chain gene organization, three segments of DNA [the variable (V_H), diversity (D_H), and joining (J_H) gene regions] join together to generate the variable portion of the H chain. The D_H gene segment accounts for the third hypervariable (complementarity-determining) region of the H chain; this area included the N region. The C_μ segment of DNA codes for the constant region of the IgM H chain.

106. The answer is A [Table 5-2; Chapter 1 III F 4]. One of the actions of the monokine IL-1 is the production of fever; hence the name "endogenous pyrogen." IL-1 reduces the concentration of prostaglandins in the region of the hypothalamus and thus causes an increase in body temperature.

107. The answer is B [Chapter 2 VI C]. Specific immune globulin such as varicella-zoster immune globulin (VZIG) is a gamma globulin obtained from people who have recently recovered from a specific infectious disease or from human volunteers who have been hyperimmunized against that disease. Additional examples include hepatitis B immune globulin and rabies immune globulin. Specific immune globulin is used to provide *specific* passive immunity. IGIM would provide protection against the organisms experienced by the donors, which would probably include the childhood

infections and the vaccines the donors had received. So these antisera would have antibodies against varicella but at a much lower concentration. They would also have antibodies against hepatitis A, polioviruses, measles, mumps, and *Haemophilus influenzae*. Recombivax is the recombinant surface protein (antigen) from hepatitis B. We would not use the live attenuated varicella vaccine in this patient because the extra viral load could exacerbate the chickenpox infection. Also, there would not be time to induce immunity with an active immunizing agent. Bacille Calmette Guérin (BCG) is a live attenuated tuberculosis vaccine not used in the United States.

108. The answer is D. [Chapter 1 I A 3; 2 V A 1; Table 1-1]. Neonatal tetanus kills hundreds of thousands of infants every year in developing countries. Recently, the World Health Organization has instituted a program of tetanus toxoid immunization of prospective mothers as a part of routine prenatal care in these countries. Subsequently, there has been a dramatic decrease in the incidence of neonatal deaths because the passively acquired antitoxin protects the infants.

109. The answer is B [Chapter 10 II B 3 b]. The 56-year-old man has carcinoembryonic antigen (CEA), which is an oncofetal antigen produced during fetal development and in postnatal periods under certain conditions (e.g., smoking, cancer). CEA is found in high concentrations in the serum of individuals with colorectal cancer and cancer of the prostate and pancreas. The antigen is also elevated in nonmalignant conditions such as infectious mononucleosis and cirrhosis of the liver. Bence Jones protein is seen in the urine of patients with myeloma. Hepatitis B and C antigens will be found in the blood of patients with these hepatic diseases.

110. The answer is C [Chapter 8 II C 1]. Sjögren's syndrome is a chronic inflammatory disease that primarily affects secretory glands such as the lacrimal and salivary glands, producing dry eyes (keratoconjunctivitis sicca) and dry mouth (xerostomia). Guillain-Barré syndrome (acute idiopathic polyneuritis) manifests as progressive weakness, first of the lower extremities and then of the upper extremities and respiratory muscles. Peripheral nerve tissue shows perivascular mononuclear cell infiltrate and demyelination. Goodpasture's syndrome is a relatively rare disorder with symptoms referable to both the lungs (e.g., pulmonary hemorrhage) and kidneys (e.g., glomerulonephritis). The immunoglobulin G (IgG) deposited on alveolar and glomerular basement membranes appears to be specific for a collagen antigen shared by the kidneys and lungs. Systemic lupus erythematosus (SLE) is a chronic, inflammatory systemic (multiorgan) disease that primarily affects women. A characteristic feature is the erythematous butterfly rash that occurs on the face of some patients. Death usually results from renal failure or infection. Amyotrophic lateral sclerosis (ALS; Lou Gehrig's disease) causes progressive degeneration of motor neurons of the spinal cord. ALS typically affects males older than 40 years of age. Some patients have a monoclonal IgM with specificity for ganglioside components of neural membranes. Other autoantibodies have been demonstrated, but immunosuppressive drugs have not proven to be effective.

111. The answer is B [Chapter 5 IX B 2 c (2)]. $Rh_o(D)$ immunoglobulin (RhoGAM) is a commercial preparation of IgG antibodies specifically reactive with the $Rh_o(D)$ antigen of the human Rh blood type system. Although there are 6 antigens in the Rh system, D is the one that is the most common in erythroblastosis fetalis, a serious hemolytic disease of Rh-positive (i.e., D+) fetuses and neonates born of Rh-negative mothers. Indications for use of RhoGAM include abortion or termination of ectopic pregnancy at or beyond 13 weeks of gestation, in third-trimester amniocentesis, as antepartum prophylaxis at 26–28 weeks of gestation, and immediately postpartum. The amount of antibody administered is sufficient to abort an immune response to as much as 15 ml of Rh-positive red blood cells.

112. The answer is D [Chapter 9 III A 2 c]. The child described in the question probably has Bruton's X-linked hypogammaglobulinemia, which manifests as recurrent infections with such organisms as staphylococci and streptococci and is associated with a B-cell deficiency. Features of the disease include a lack of germinal centers and lack of plasma cells in lymph nodes, low serum levels of immunoglobulins, intact T-cell and phagocytic function, and hypoplastic tonsils and Peyer's patches. Normal delayed hypersensitivity would tell us that thymus-dependent regions of the node are normal. Juxtamedullary regions are thymus dependent

and would not be hyperplastic. Dendritic cells are antigen presenters and are not involved in immunodeficiencies.

113. The answer is D [Chapter 6 II C 2]. Radial immunodiffusion is the technique by which it is possible to quantitate levels of substances such as gamma globulin or complement components in serum or other body fluids. Antiserum is added to an agar solution before the agar is poured into a dish or onto a glass slide. Holes are then punched in the solidified agar, and serum or other body fluids are placed in the wells. The concentration of a particular antigen in the serum can be estimated by measuring the ring of precipitate that forms around each well. It is necessary to construct a standard curve with known reagents each time an assay is performed. The greater the diameter of the ring, the more reactant there was in the serum.

114. The answer is A [Chapter 9 VII A]. Hereditary angioedema is the result of a deficiency in C1 esterase inhibitor. It is sometimes called angioneurotic edema. The disease is characterized by recurrent episodes of swelling of subcutaneous tissues, the intestines, and the larynx. Swelling of the lips is a common physical sign of the disease. The defect in C1 esterase inhibitor leads to increased cleavage of C4 and C2 when C1s is activated. This leads to the production of a kinin-like peptide from C2, which increases vascular permeability. Hereditary angioedema is the only disease listed that would have the symptoms exhibited by this patient.

115. The answer is E [Chapter 5 XI B 3 b]. Bacille Calmette Guérin (BCG) is an attenuated bovine strain of *Mycobacterium tuberculosis* that is used as a vaccine against tuberculosis in many countries of the world; however, BCG is not used as a tuberculosis vaccine in the United States. In the United States, skin tests are used to detect exposure to *M. tuberculosis,* and the presence of BCG induces skin test reactivity identical to that seen in people who are infected with the tubercle bacillus. This vaccine is given to patients with certain types of malignancies in an effort to increase the antitumor activities of natural killer cells and macrophages.

116. The answer is C [Chapter 3 III A 1 b]. IgG is the most efficient antibody at opsonization due to the high number of Fcγ receptors on phagocytic cells. IgM is the most efficient immunoglobulin at activating complement. The major proportion of the primary immune response consists of IgM, whereas the secondary response consists almost entirely of IgG. IgM is synthesized before birth and represents the predominant antibody produced by the fetus. IgM is the only antibody made in response to thymus independent antigens.

117. The answer is A [Chapter 9 II B 4]. Chédiak-Higashi disease is due to a microtubular defect in which the lysosomes do not fuse with the phagosomes thus intracellular killing is compromised. Lysozyme is an antibacterial enzyme found in lysosomes that breaks down the carbohydrate backbone of peptidoglycan, thus rendering the microbe susceptible to osmotic damage. Antibody molecules and complement proteins enhance this antimicrobic action by enhancing phagocytosis (i.e., opsonizing the microbe). All other choices listed are part of the oxygen-dependent killing pathway and are intact in the patient with Chédiak-Higashi disease.

118. The answer is E [Chapter 5 IV B 5; Table 5-2]. Interleukin 10 (IL-10) is produced by T helper 2 cells. It down-regulates T helper 1 cells and inhibits cytokine release by macrophages. This cytokine also increases expression of class II major histocompatibility complex (MHC) molecules in B cell membranes and favors the expression of humoral immune (antibody) responses.

119. The answer is A [Chapter 2 V B 10]. Rabies is an occupational disease of all veterinarians and they are routinely immunized during their medical school training period. Boosters are administered periodically and the anti-rabies antibody levels are measured to be certain that all vaccine recipients have attained a protective level of immunity. Human anti-rabies specific immunoglobulins are commonly prepared from plasma donated by veterinary students.

120. The answer is B [Chapter 5 IV B 6 c; Table 5-2] Interleukin 8 (IL-8) is a cytokine produced by monocytes and macrophages. It is chemotactic for neutrophils and also activates these cells. It has been shown to play a role in angiogenesis as well.

121. The answer is D [Chapter 2 V A 3]. Because meningococcal disease may become epidemic among military recruits, the vaccine made from meningococcal polysaccharide capsular antigens is recommended. Adenoviral pharyngitis and conjunctivitis pose epidemic potential in the military and recruits also get vaccinated against these viruses. Currently the military are also giving hepatitis A and B injections to recruits. The administration of the anthrax vaccine has caused some concern, but is still used in the armed forces as of the date of this printing. Pneumovax is a vaccine composed of 23 serotypes of the pneumococcal capsule. It is given to the elderly and to people with compromised splenic function. Cholera vaccine is for individuals who are traveling into an endemic area.

122. The answer is B [Chapter 9 II B 1 c (2)]. Chronic granulomatous disease is caused by a reduced nicotinamide-adenine dinucleotide phosphate (NADPH) oxidase deficiency. NADPH oxidase is a multicomponent system for electron transport and energy generation. There are five mutational defects in NADPH oxidase that result in a failure to recycle NADPH, which causes a failure to produce hydrogen peroxide during phagocytosis. As a result, the phagocytic cells are not efficient at microbial killing. Infusions of neutrophils will not correct the defect but will replace the defective cell, thus restoring intracellular killing activity. Gamma interferon has also been used to activate phagocytic cells that still have an intact lysosomal killing pathway. Antibody levels are normal so injection of specific human immunoglobulin or pooled gamma globulin are not indicated. Transplantation of thymus of bone marrow has also not been of value.

123. The answer is B [Chapter 2 V A 4]. Individuals with sickle cell disease are uniquely susceptible to *Streptococcus pneumoniae* sepsis, as are patients who have undergone splenectomy. Immunization with the capsular carbohydrates of the organism confer an opsonic immunity and lessen the likelihood of septicemia developing as a consequence of a bacterial incursion into the bloodstream from the normal site of colonization, which is the throat.

124. The answer is B [Chapter 9 IV A 4 a]. Patients with DiGeorge syndrome (congenital thymic hypoplasia) are markedly deficient in thymic tissue owing to faulty development of the third and fourth pharyngeal pouches during embryogenesis. This results in profoundly impaired T-cell numbers. Treatment with fetal thymus transplantation can result in permanent reversal and the production of functioning T cells. Chédiak-Higashi is a phagocytic cell defect, Bruton's is a B cell defect, hereditary angioedema is due to a deficiency of the C1 esterase inhibitor, and Wiskott-Aldrich syndrome is a complex immune deficiency disease with patients having a low IgM response (associated with inability to respond to carbohydrate antigens with predictable problems with encapsulated microbes), eczema, and thrombocytopenia.

125. The answer is A [Chapter 5 X C 1]. The helper T (Th) cell is the most sensitive of the immunologically specific cells to the induction of immune tolerance. It is absent from an experimental animal 24 hours after the injection of a tolerogen; B-cell tolerance takes 5 days. Macrophages have no immunologic specificity and cannot be rendered tolerant. The autotolerance that protects humans from autoimmune diseases most likely is due to a lack of Th cells as well. In many experimental systems, it has been possible to detect autoreactive B lymphocytes in perfectly normal animals. Cytotoxic T cells and plasma cells are cells that are the end product of an immune response.

126. The answer is C [Chapter 9 V C]. Wiskott-Aldrich syndrome is a disease with a triad of symptoms—eczema, thrombocytopenia, and susceptibility to infections caused by encapsulated bacterial agents. The latter is due to faulty production of IgM. IgG will be normal, and IgA and IgE may be elevated. The specific deficit is an inability to respond to polysaccharide antigens. Bruton's disease is characterized by an inability to produce antibodies of any class. Graves' disease is an autoimmune disease in which the patient has a hyperthyroid condition. DiGeorge syndrome is congenital hypoplasia of the parathyroid and thymus glands coupled with facial and cardiac abnormalities.

127. The answer is B [Chapter 10 I C 5 b (1) (a)]. Hyperacute rejection occurs because the recipient had pre-formed antibodies against one or more antigens of the donor. These may have been induced by a previous graft, by a

transfusion, or by pregnancy. The antibodies cause a very rapid (less than 24 hours) rejection of the organ. Acute rejection is usually a T cell event. Chronic rejection can be due to either induced antibodies or T cells. The other terms are not normally used to describe graft rejection events.

128. The answer is B [Chapter 2 V A 2]. *Haemophilus influenza* type B conjugate vaccine is a highly recommended childhood vaccine. Veterinary students are routinely immunized against rabies, because it is a serious occupational threat. For similar reasons, dental hygienists should receive hepatitis B vaccine. Cholera vaccine is for people traveling to endemic areas. Pneumovax is for the elderly.

129. The answer is B [Chapter 2 V A 3]. Because meningococcal disease may become epidemic among military recruits, the vaccine made from meningococcal polysaccharide capsular antigens is recommended. Adenoviral pharyngitis and conjunctivitis pose epidemic potential in the military and recruits also get vaccinated against these viruses, although the availability of the vaccine is under question at the present. Currently the military are also giving hepatitis A and B injections to recruits. The administration of the anthrax vaccine has caused some concern, but is still used in the armed forces as of the date of this printing. Pneumovax is a vaccine composed of 23 serotypes of the pneumococcal capsule. It is given to the elderly and to people with compromised splenic function. Cholera vaccine is for individuals who are traveling into an endemic area.

130. The answer is E [Chapter 5 IV B 1, Table 5-2]. IL-2 is one of the lymphokines that enhances the proliferation and maturation of B cells during the induction of an immune response. It is actually a pluripotential lymphokine, and causes proliferation of T cells as well. It also is important in activation of macrophages and natural killer cells. IL-1 is a cytokine produced by antigen presenting cells that activates T helper 1 cells. It is also the endogenous pyrogen.

Lipopolysaccharide (LPS) is a B cell mitogen but it is not a cytokine, it is the endotoxin found in the cell walls of gram-negative bacteria. IFN-γ is a pluripotential cell activator. IL-4 is a cytokine, produced by T_H2 cells, that favors the induction of IgE synthesis by B cells.

131. The answer is A [Chapter 2 II B; Chapter 10 I A 1]. A bone marrow transplant from mother to daughter is allogeneic: the mother's bone marrow is antigenically different (al-loantigenic) and will be recognized by the daughter's immune system and rejected as for-eign. This is unfortunate and necessitates im-munosuppression of the bone marrow recipi-ent to prevent rejection of the graft. To accomplish this, the daughter would be treated with immunosuppressive drugs and, probably, with irradiation before the transplant was performed. Strict isolation procedures would have to be maintained because she would be very susceptible to nosocomial in-fections. A second threat to the recipient would be graft-versus-host (GVH) disease, in which mature lymphocytes in the grafted tis-sue (bone marrow) mount an immunologic at-tack on the recipient, with devastating results. Management after an allograft procedure in-cludes monitoring for GVH, and prompt and vigorous immunosuppression at the first sign of trouble. Because of the potential difficulties with allografts, bone marrow autografts have been used in the treatment of some malignan-cies, notably acute myelogenous leukemia, which has a mortality rate of over 90% in adults. In this instance, the patient's own bone marrow is removed during remission, treated with cyclophosphamide to kill residual leukemic cells, and frozen. The patient is then vigorously treated with antineoplastic drugs and reinfused with the stored marrow.

132. The answer is E [Chapter 2 II B; Chapter 10 I A 1]. Identical twins are syngeneic antigeni-cally. They behave immunologically, just like inbred animals, and do not reject grafted tissues. This is clinically fortunate, because it obviates the need for immunosuppression of the bone marrow recipient, as is done in homografts to prevent the host from rejecting the graft.

Appendix

Normal Laboratory and Physiologic Values

Physiologic Values

 Blood pressure: systolic, 115–190; diastolic, 70–110

 Pulse: 70 beats/min (resting)

 Respiration: 18–20/min (adults); increased in children

 Temperature: 98.6°F (37°C)

Blood Chemistry

 Acid phosphatase: 0–4.0 KA units

 Albumin (serum): 3.5–5.0 g/dl

 Alkaline phosphatase: 40–140 mU/m

 Bicarbonate (HCO_{3-}): 24–30 mEq/L

 Bilirubin: total, 0.2–1.2 mg/dl; direct, 0–0.3 mg/dl

 Blood gases:

  Po_2: 80–90 mmHg

  Pco_2: 35–45 mmHg

  pH: 7.35–7.45

  O_2 saturation: 95%–97%

 Blood urea nitrogen (BUN): 8–20 mg/dl

 Creatine: 0.2–0.6 mg/dl

 Creatinine: 0.7–1.4 mg/dl

 Electrolytes:

  sodium: 136–145 mEq/L

  potassium: 3.5–5.5 mEq/L

  chlorine: 95–106 mEq/L

  calcium: 8.5–10.5 mg/dl

  phosphorous: 2.5–4.5 mg/dl

 Glucose: 65–110 mg/dl

 Lactic dehydrogenase (LDH): 80–280 mU/ml

 Protein (total): 6–8 g/dl

 Serum glutamic oxaloacetic transaminase (SGOT): 7–40 mU/ml

 Serum glutamic pyruvic transaminase (SGPT): 5–36 mU/ml

 Uric acid: 2.4–8.0 mg/dl

Hematology

 Bleeding time (template): 2–7 min

 Fibrinogen (plasma): 200–400 mg/dl

 Hematocrit: men, 45%; women, 40%

 Hemoglobin: men, 14–18 g/dl; women, 12–16 g/dl; children, 12–14 g/dl; newborns, 14.5–24.5 g/dl

 White blood cells (WBC): 5000–10,000/mm^3

 Red blood cells (RBC): men, 5.0×10^6/mm^3; women, $4.5 \times 10_6$/mm^3

 Differential:

reticulocytes: 0%–1%
WBC, total: 100%
myelocytes: 0%
juvenile neutrophils: 0%–1%
band neutrophils: 0%–5%
polymorphonuclear neutrophils (PMN): 40%–60%
lymphocytes: 20%–40%
eosinophils: 1%–3%
basophils: 0%–1%
monocytes: 4%–8%

Platelets: 200,000–500,000/mm^3

Prothrombin time: 70%–110% of control value (10–12 sec)

Partial thromboplastin time (PTT): 26–40 sec

Immunoglobulins (serum)

IgA: 76–390 mg/dl

IgE: 0–380 mg/dl

IgG: 650–1500 mg/dl

IgM: 40–345 mg/dl

Urine

pH: 6

Creatinine clearance: men, 97–137 ml/min; women, 88–128 ml/min

Dipstix: blood, bilirubin, ketones, glucose, and proteins should all be negative in the urine. Trace amounts do not necessarily indicate abnormalities.

Index

Note: Page numbers in *italics* indicate illustrations; those followed by t indicate tables. Q and A denote questions and answers.